MATT RABIN AND ROBERT HICKS

THE PAIN-FREE CYCLIST

CONQUER INJURY & FIND YOUR CYCLING NIRVANA

BLOOMSBURY

LONDON · NEW DELHI · NEW YORK · SYDNEY

BLOOMSBURY SPORT
An imprint of Bloomsbury Publishing Plc

50 Bedford Square   1385 Broadway
London   New York
WC1B 3DP   NY 10018
UK   USA

www.bloomsbury.com

First published 2015

British Library Cataloguing-in-Publication Data
A catalogue record for this book is available from the British Library.

Library of Congress Cataloguing-in-Publication data has been applied for.

ISBN: PB: 978-1-4729-0659-5
         ePDF: 978-1-4729-2149-9
         ePub: 978-1-4729-2148-2

2 4 6 8 10 9 7 5 3 1

Designed by Austin Taylor   Typeset in DIN
Printed and bound in China by Toppan Leefung Printing

Bloomsbury Publishing Plc makes every effort to ensure that the papers
used in the manufacture of our books are natural, recyclable products made
from wood grown in well-managed forests. Our manufacturing processes
conform to the environmental regulations of the country of origin.

To find out more about our authors and books visit www.bloomsbury.com.
Here you will find extracts, author interviews, details of forthcoming events
and the option to sign up for our newsletters.

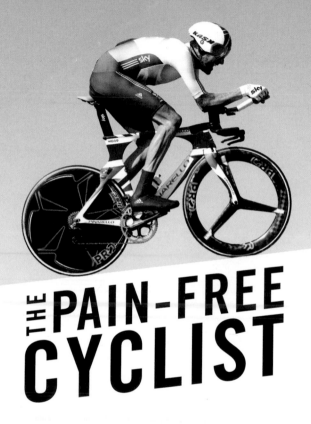

THE PAIN-FREE CYCLIST

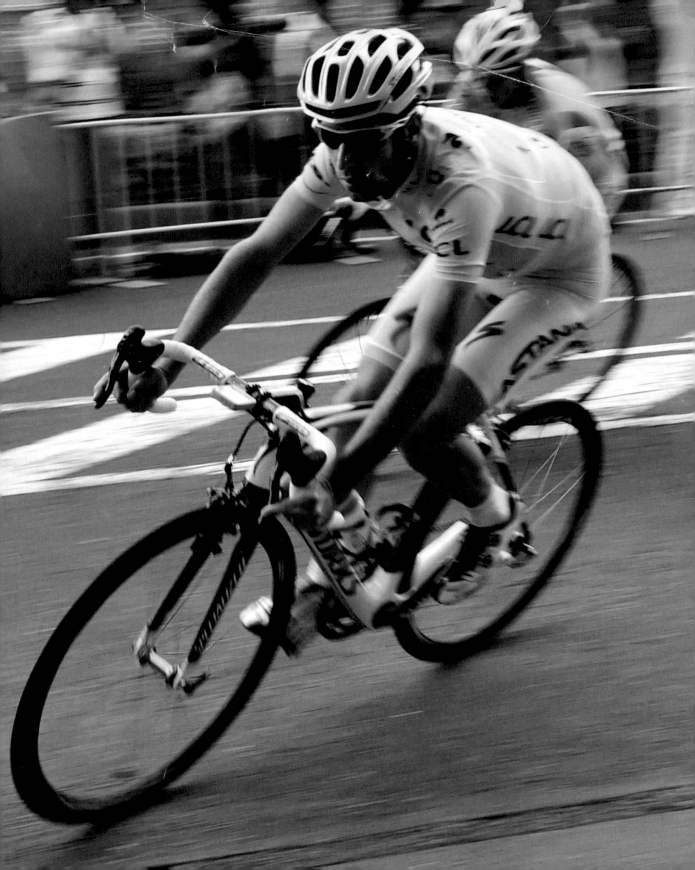

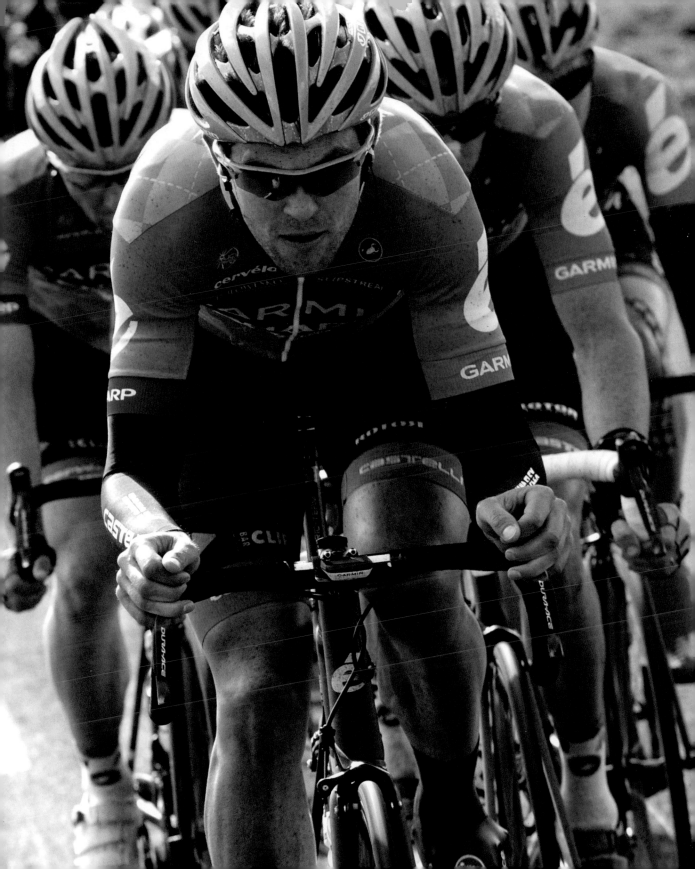

CONTENTS

PART 1
PREPARATION 12

PART 2
INJURIES 56

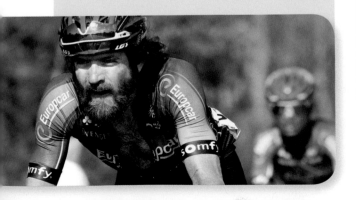

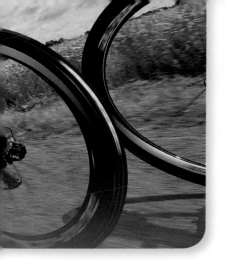

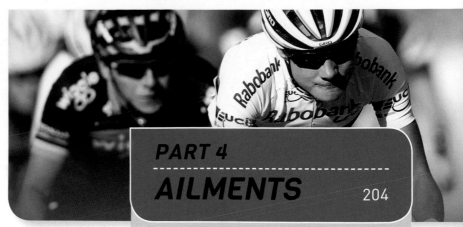

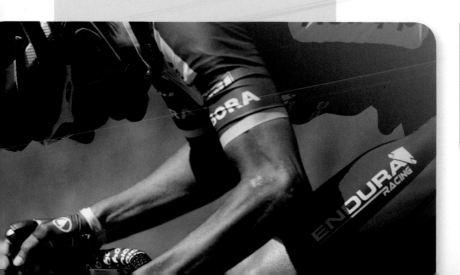

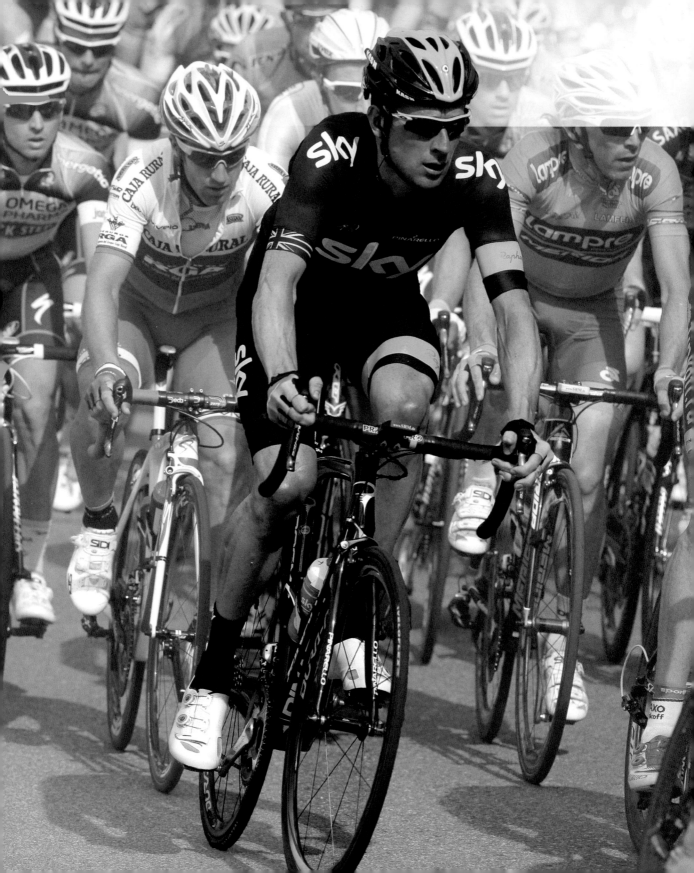

FOREWORD

There are good pains and bad pains. The good pains are the ones you get when you know they're there because you're pushing your body hard and digging deep – like the final time trial into Chartes at the 2012 Tour de France, or the closing laps of the Olympic team pursuit final in Beijing. You know your muscles are burning from the lactic acid build-up and your whole body hurts from exhaustion, but it's almost enjoyable as you're pushing your limits to get the most out of your performance.

For me, winning the Tour de France or an Olympic gold medal was the endgame at the time, the goal I set out to achieve, but I still remember training around Regent's Park and Paddington Rec in London as a 14-year-old kid dreaming of making it as a professional cyclist. The burning in my legs felt just the same then as it does now, only a lot less familiar.

Bad pain or injury on the other hand, for a pro-athlete, is our worst nightmare. It puts doubt in your mind, and often it seems there's no logic to it and many times you don't understand *why* it's happened. Injury can take you away from doing the things you enjoy – like riding your bike – and whichever way you look at it that's not fun at all. Injury forced me out of the 2013 Giro d'Italia when my knee pain got too much to continue. This frustratingly caused me to miss the chance to go into the 2013 Tour de France with race No. 1 on my back as the defending champion. Injury is no fun.

I've learnt over the years to listen to the signs my body is giving me. Learning what I can ignore and what I can push through versus when I should stop has been important to ensure small niggles don't become bigger injuries. Knowing when to rest, when and where to turn for advice, and who to see for certain treatment has also been invaluable to me. Over

the years, I have found out a lot more about my body, and having worked with Matt, I have learned that certain tightness, weakness and discomfort which I'd had at periods over my career in my lower back I shouldn't have had to put up with and that they could've been sorted. They are now. If you do need to seek help, for me it's about trusting that the person you are seeing can help you. Going with this approach has always worked for me.

I believe in this book, and you'll find out the best ways to deal with injury and the bad pain you can have on your bike. By reading this book you will be able to short cut some of the information it has taken me years and a career as a pro-cyclist to find out. Feeling strong on the bike and riding pain-free regardless of your level, from amateur to pro, is what we're all looking for. This book will help you to beat your injuries and prevent them returning, allowing you to slot back into riding your bike as the pain-free cyclist.

See you out on the road.

Sir Bradley Wiggins

FOUR-TIME OLYMPIC GOLD MEDALLIST, SEVEN-TIME WORLD CHAMPION AND TOUR DE FRANCE WINNER.

THE AUTHORS

Dr MATTHEW RABIN (BSc (Hons), MSc (Chiro), DC, ICSSD, PGDip, FRCC) graduated from the Anglo-European College of Chiropractic in 2002. He is team chiropractor for Cannondale-Garmin Pro Cycling team where he also consults on nutritional strategy. Matt has also worked with the American, Australian and Great Britain cycling teams at the World Championships and the Australian cycling team in the run up to the 2012 London Olympic Games. Matt has completed the International Chriopractic Sports Science Diploma (ICSSD) programme, the world recognised post-graduate qualification for sports chiropractors and has become the first chiropractor to complete the two-year post-graduate diploma (PGDip) in sports nutrition as awarded by the International Olympic Committee. When not on the road with Cannondale-Garmin, Matt works in clinic in London.

ROBERT HICKS is the Health and Fitness Deputy Editor across all the cycling titles at TimeInc, most notably, *Cycling Weekly*, the UK's biggest cycling magazine. He is also the author of two cycling books: *Fitter, Further, Faster: Get Fit For Sportives and Road Riding* and *Get on your Bike: Stay Safe, Get Fit and Be Happy Cycling*, both of which are published by Bloomsbury. Over the course of six years at TimeInc, the sport science graduate has written hundreds of fitness features and articles. Robert makes a habit of frequently meeting with readers, riders and coaches, to fully understand the real current health and fitness issues that cyclists face.

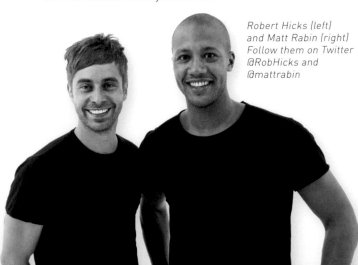

Robert Hicks (left) and Matt Rabin (right) Follow them on Twitter @RobHicks and @mattrabin

INTRODUCTION

Every cyclist can talk about the time when it all felt effortless. The time everything clicked and came together. It doesn't necessarily have anything to do with winning per se but has everything to do with a feeling, an emotion, a state of mind, a connection with cycling that is rare to come by, despite how many thousands of miles you have clocked up on the bike. Cycling Nirvana is winning inside your body, inside your head and the real sweet spot of the sport.

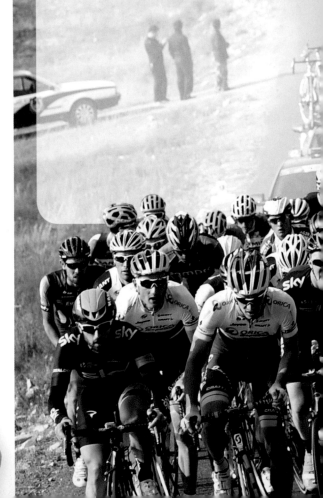

You've picked up this book because you know how to ride a bike. As a keen cyclist you're probably clued up on how important bike fit is and have, no doubt, done your homework on the right bike for you. Cycling injuries, however, are unlikely to have captured your attention in quite the same way. Yet, whether the result of a dramatic crash or just simply overworked muscles or overused joints, a cycling injury can dramatically hinder your performance, and cause significant pain and discomfort leading to unwanted time off the bike. Beating injuries before they take hold is the key to not only unlocking your potential as a cyclist but to enjoying every ride blissfully pain free.

When injuries or discomfort occur, a lot of cyclists simply don't know what to do. Very few find it easy to understand what their body is telling them, what the cause of their problem is, and most importantly how to address and treat it. Rest? Continue to ride? Struggle on through? It's these questions which go unanswered, leading to further complications and more harmful injuries, resulting in *substantial* time off the bike. Worse still, many cyclists see these feelings of discomfort as a natural by-product of bike riding. Not so. Cycling should and can be pain free.

There are more cyclists on Britain's roads than ever before, with over two million people cycling at least once a week. As enthusiasm for the sport grows, we want to see as many people as possible enjoying their bike rides pain free and heading towards their Cycling Nirvana. That's why we have written this book. We'll guide you through, explain what the injuries are, how to spot them and, most importantly, how to treat them in order to get you back on your bike as swiftly as possible.

But this isn't simply a book about injuries. It's also your number one tool for maximising your performance as a cyclist. By exploring every aspect of your life as a cyclist, from preparation such as warm-ups and fuelling to recovery, common ailments and more, we're giving you the ingredients to help you find your Cycling Nirvana – the sweet spot of the sport – and become a *pain-free* cyclist. But don't just take our word for it; we've called upon some of the biggest names in world cycling to tell you about the injuries they've battled and what they did to overcome them. There really isn't anyone better to help guide you through the world of cycling injuries than the pros themselves. Look out for their stories and what Cycling Nirvana means to them – it's a fascinating insight.

The Pain-Free Cyclist is the first and last book any cycling enthusiast will need on all things cycling-health related.

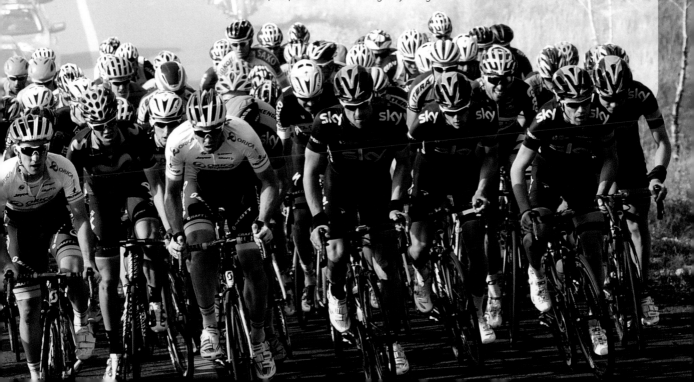

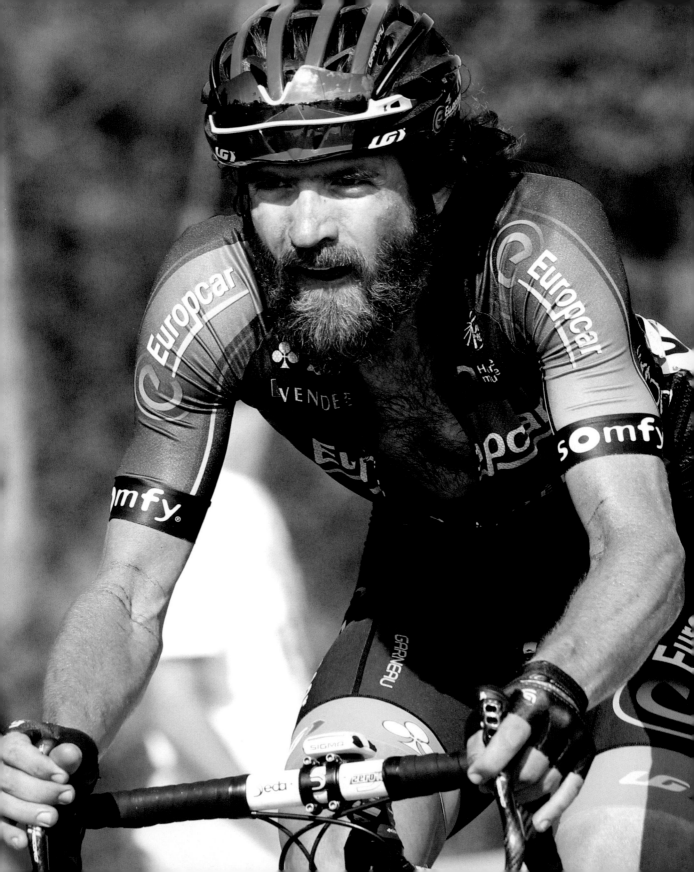

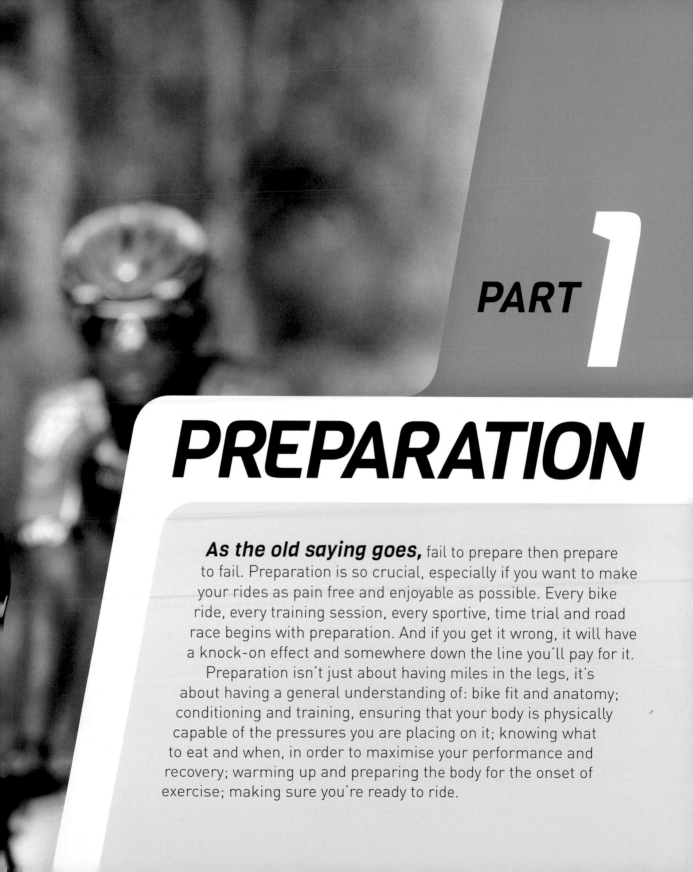

PART 1

PREPARATION

As the old saying goes, fail to prepare then prepare to fail. Preparation is so crucial, especially if you want to make your rides as pain free and enjoyable as possible. Every bike ride, every training session, every sportive, time trial and road race begins with preparation. And if you get it wrong, it will have a knock-on effect and somewhere down the line you'll pay for it. Preparation isn't just about having miles in the legs, it's about having a general understanding of: bike fit and anatomy; conditioning and training, ensuring that your body is physically capable of the pressures you are placing on it; knowing what to eat and when, in order to maximise your performance and recovery; warming up and preparing the body for the onset of exercise; making sure you're ready to ride.

1

SOMETIMES IT IS ABOUT THE BIKE

> *The right bike fit is not about being able to produce the most power; it's one you can ride 10,000 km on without getting injured.*

Nathan Haas AUSTRALIAN PRO CYCLIST AND TOUR OF BRITAIN WINNER

While this book is predominantly about the body, not about the bike, there's no denying that bike fit plays a significant role in the prevention of injuries. While it's naïve to believe that a proper bike fit instantly guarantees a pain-free ride, if you're not set up correctly on the bike, you *will* risk developing injuries, or exacerbating pre-existing aches and pains. It's not hard to see why – the riding position on the bike is completely unnatural.

It's not just the ungainly position, riding a bike for several hours requires both holding your position for an extended period of time and constant repetition of your pedalling motion. To put it into context, let's say you spin the pedals 90 times per minute – the average cadence of the majority of cyclists ranges between 80 and 90 rpm. If your Sunday morning ride lasts a couple of hours, that means you'll spin the pedals nearly 11,000 times. For a 4-hour sportive, your legs will go round over 20,000 times. It doesn't take a genius to work out that if you're not sitting comfortably, issues can arise quickly on the bike.

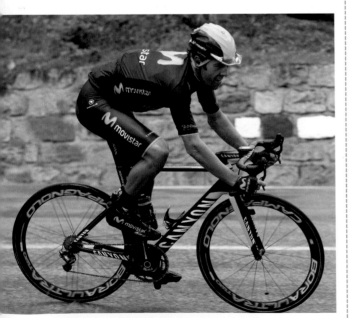

ABOVE A good fit will help you feel at one with the bike

So what can you do?

Well, the simple answer is to go and see a good bike-fitting specialist. True, the cost can seem a little steep (expect to pay around £150-£300, or 250-500 USD), but when you add up the money you've spent on a new bike, specialist clothes and the latest gadgets, a bike fit, which can significantly reduce your chances of injury, seems pretty reasonable. These trained professionals take into account not just your unique height, weight and reach ratios, but also your personal injury history, and tailor the bike just for you.

Do-it-yourself bike fit

If you're not willing to fork out a couple of hundred pounds for a bike fit, then there are some bike fit principles you can easily apply at home to get you started.

Step one: firstly, you need a bike – well a frame more specifically, that isn't too big or too small. When you're buying a bike, that's the priority. It sounds easy enough, but a lot of cyclists get distracted when choosing a frame size, worried more about brand names, gear ratios and the colour, and will end up buying the wrong-sized frame and then forever fight against their own position in a bid to *make the bike fit*.

Below is a table that gives some general guidelines for what size bike frame you should buy, based on your height.

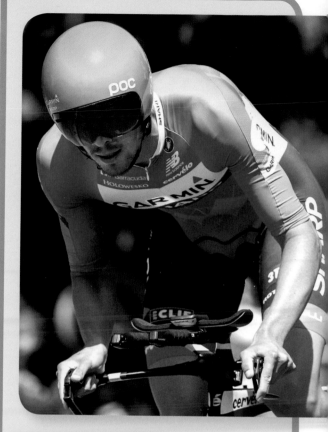

RIDER HEIGHT (MEN'S ROAD BIKE SIZING)		FRAME SIZE SUGGESTED	
Feet and Inches	Centimetres	Centimetres	Size
4' 10"–5' 0"	148–152	47–48	XXS
5' 0"–5' 3"	152–160	49–50	XS
5' 3"–5' 6"	160–168	51–52–53	S
5 6"–5' 9"	168–175	54–55	M
5' 9"–6' 0"	175–183	56–57–58	L
6' 0"–6' 3"	183–191	58–59–60	XL
6' 3"–6' 6"	191–198	61–62–63	XXL
RIDER HEIGHT (WOMEN'S ROAD BIKE SIZING)		FRAME SIZE SUGGESTED	
Feet and Inches	Centimetres	Centimetres	Size
4' 10"–5' 1"	147–155	44–45–46	XXS
5' 1"–5' 3"	155–160	47–48–49	XS
5' 3"–5' 5"	160–165	50–51–52	S
5' 5"–5' 8"	165–172	53–54–55	M
5' 8"–5' 10"	172–180	56–57	L

THE IMPORTANCE OF A BIKE FIT

Alex Howes AMERICAN PRO CYCLIST

■ *'Bike fit is very important because injuries can come out of nowhere if you don't know your fit or don't have a decent bike fit, it's as simple as that. You hear of pros sometimes that can't pee for a while after a stage or it's painful and stinging to pee, this is not good and bike fit can affect that. If injury doesn't persuade you to get a good bike fit, the thought of stinging pee or potential erectile dysfunction certainly should.'*

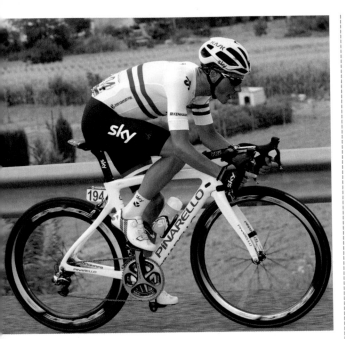

ABOVE Understand bike basics

Saddle height: At the bottom of your pedal stroke, your knee should be between 80 and 90 per cent fully extended. It should never be fully extended. Find what works for you, as it's largely dependent of the flexibility within your hamstrings.

Saddle position: When the cranks are horizontal with the ground – a three o'clock position – your knee should be vertically positioned over the pedal spindle. To start with, always set your saddle to horizontal – this is the standard. Avoid changing your saddle tilt, unless you know exactly what you are doing.

Handlebars (width, height and rotation): Handlebar width should be roughly equal to shoulder width and height is largely dictated by your preference and comfort. When you purchase your bike, enquire the width that is recommended for you. Generally, the upper arm should be between 80 and 90 degrees to the upper body, which will stabilise the shoulders, minimising hunching, and enable your body to withstand the load that is placed upon it. Provided that saddle height and stem length are correct, your hands

should fall naturally on to the hoods, in a neutral handshake position. Rotation of the levers is again down to preference, rotated slightly further forwards for improved aerodynamics, and more upright for improved comfort.

Torso angle: To maximise comfort and take load off the lower back, hamstrings and the neck, your torso should sit between 40 and 50 degrees while seated with hands on the hoods. This more relaxed comfortable position will compromise speed while a lower position (between 30 and 40 degrees) will improve aerodynamics and reduce comfort. The more aerodynamic, the more stress placed on the lower back and the more flexibility needed in your hamstrings.

Cleats: Place the cleat so that it sits under or slightly behind the ball of your foot. The ball of the foot should be positioned over the pedal spindle. The importance of the shoe/pedal interface and proper cleat alignment is so important, as a problem with the positioning of your cleats can have a knock-on effect causing problems further up the body – for example, on your knee or lower back.

■ *'You wouldn't drive a car with the seat right forwards if you are 6 ft tall, just as your wife wouldn't get in the car after you've driven it and leave the seat right back. Getting a good bike fit is key for comfort and avoiding problems.'*

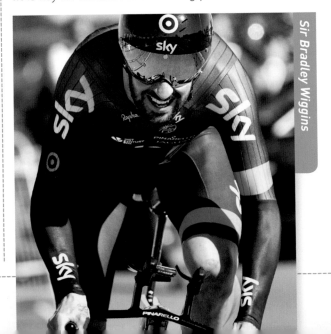

Sir Bradley Wiggins

Pedalling

The key parts of the body involved in the pedal stroke include all the muscles and joints of the legs and the lower back. It's important these have the appropriate range of motion, muscle length and freedom of movement in order to get optimal transfer of energy from the body into the pedals throughout the pedal stroke. An issue or injury with any of these muscles or joints could create a secondary problem elsewhere. For example, there is good evidence to demonstrate that a lower back issue can create a potential knee problem.

Aim to pedal between 80 and 100 rpm; pedal briskly and the mechanics of propelling the bike will naturally encourage the pedalling action to fall into place. You'll also start to optimise the use of the power phase from two o'clock to five o'clock (looking at the chain set from the right-hand side); remember, all you are doing from six o'clock to one o'clock is delivering the pedal deftly back to the power phase. Your ankle shouldn't flex too much and will mostly be flat or with toes slightly pointing downwards at the bottom of each stroke, but this will come naturally and doesn't need to be focused on as it will be determined by your body's mechanics and flexibility.

Clip-in pedals

These are a must for an efficient pedalling style. While the pedals will hold the shoe in place, many can be adjusted to allow some lateral float (movement) while pedalling. When buying cycling shoes, the degree of lateral foot movement can vary between 0–12 degrees depending on which brand you go for. Although the amount of lateral float is a personal choice, if you are new to cycling, opt for a shoe with some movement, as it can be altered until a comfortable position is found, or adjusted should an issue arise.

Fixated on the upstroke

Don't get fixated on the upstroke. Many cyclists work on pulling up, but there's little research to suggest it's beneficial to the pedalling stroke. There *is* some evidence suggesting that forcing the upstroke can actually lead to an *increased* chance of injury as you begin to use muscles in a slightly unnatural way. Remember, going with what feels natural to you is a good starting point.

SPECIFICS CAN MATTER

Andrew Talansky AMERICAN PRO CYCLIST

■ *'I notice if my saddle is off by 1–2mm; if it's too high, then, when I get off my bike, I am destroyed after the race or, if it's too low, I can't put the power out and wonder why I am not going so well. Above all the saddle height is the most important for me.'*

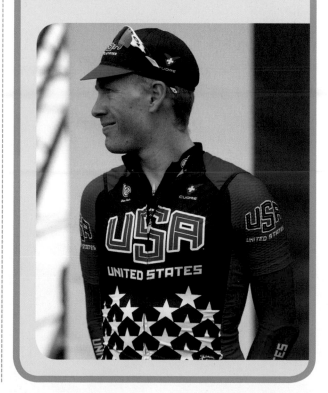

2

CORE STRENGTH:
A VITAL
COMPONENT

❝ *Five minutes a day is all I need to keep certain muscles activated and engaged. It's about knowing and finding out what works for you to keep your body strong on the bike.* ❞

Dan Martin IRISH PRO CYCLIST AND TOUR DE FRANCE STAGE WINNER

BELOW Core strength helps stability

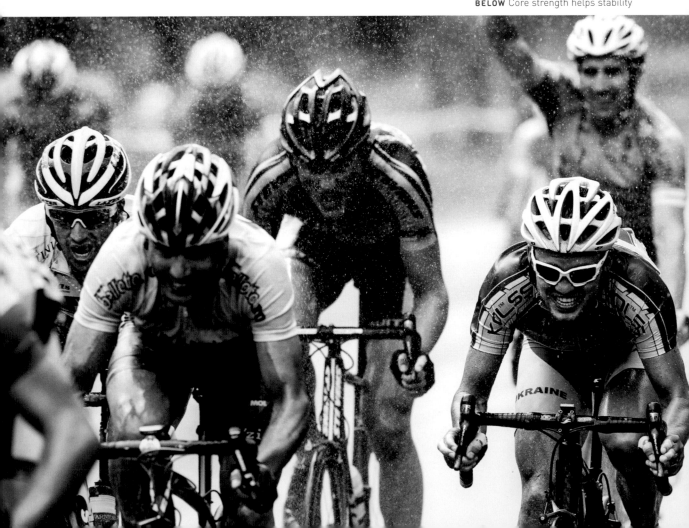

Once you have a bike that fits and understand some fundamentals of the pedalling action, it's now a case of building a body to ensure you are stable, strong and primed for action, which will undoubtedly see you on your way to Cycling Nirvana. Of course, aerobic training is a priority for any keen cyclist. But cycling involves the entire body; it's not just the legs that get the bike moving. A strong core that can withstand the pressures and stresses being placed on it is absolutely critical, not just for boosting your performance but also for preventing injury.

■ *'The older you get or the more you ride, the more you have to work on your core,'* says German pro cyclist, Fabian Wegmann. *'I focus on my posterior chain exercises to keep my glutes and lower back strong, which really helps me on the bike and has really reduced pain in my lower back after a hard stage. It makes no sense to have good strong legs when your upper body and core can't hold it and control it; it's a waste of power. Modern cycling means off-the-bike work like strengthening the core is critical for both comfort and stability.'*

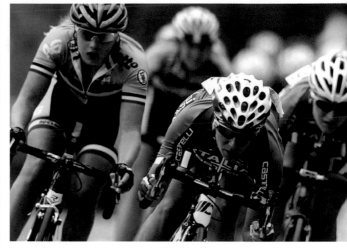

ABOVE Core strength improves cycling stability

Weak core = weak performance

When you're cycling, it's so important to keep still and steady, like a swan paddling on the water: the top half should be still and majestic while the legs are pedalling furiously underneath your stable body. A weak core will have a negative effect on your stability, and your lumbar/pelvic position (seated riding position) will significantly suffer. This can lead to excessive side-to-side movement, otherwise known as rocking. Although it might seem like a trivial issue, it's anything but, because you will lose power in your legs as you start to use your primary movers that power the bike and move you forwards – such as your gluteals (buttocks) and quadriceps (thigh) muscles – to compensate and keep you still. Put simply, the power you should be generating to propel the bike is now being wasted through your body. Rocking may even contribute to saddle sores due to excessive friction being generated, an additional concern you don't need.

In order to now sustain speed – without the use of the muscles you should predominantly use for pedalling – you may have to call upon other muscles such as your hamstrings to help. And if they aren't conditioned or prepared, this could

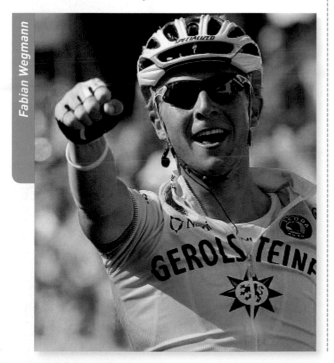

Fabian Wegmann

The Core –
Far from being the visible muscles

Whenever the core is mentioned, the superficial muscles of the torso such as the abdominal 'six-pack' muscles may spring to mind. However, it is often the deeper muscles that aren't necessarily in view that make up the 'real' core and its weakness and imbalance in these muscles that can lead to injury.

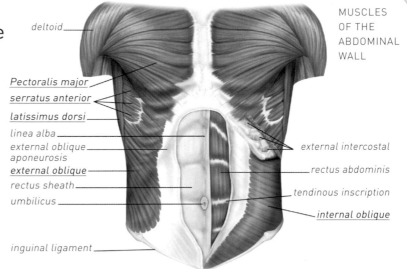

MUSCLES OF THE ABDOMINAL WALL

deltoid

Pectoralis major

serratus anterior

latissimus dorsi

linea alba

external oblique aponeurosis

external oblique

rectus sheath

umbilicus

inguinal ligament

external intercostal

rectus abdominis

tendinous inscription

internal oblique

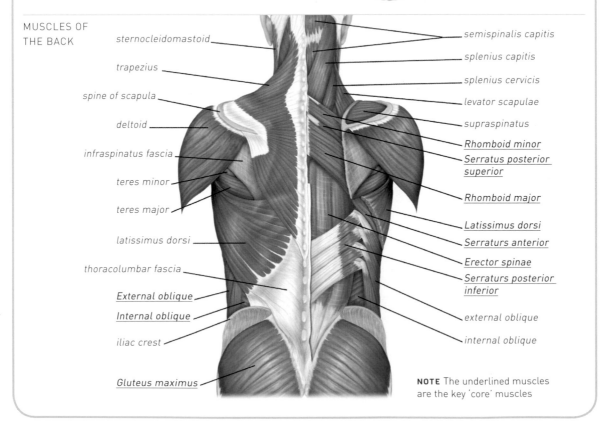

MUSCLES OF THE BACK

sternocleidomastoid

trapezius

spine of scapula

deltoid

infraspinatus fascia

teres minor

teres major

latissimus dorsi

thoracolumbar fascia

External oblique

Internal oblique

iliac crest

Gluteus maximus

semispinalis capitis

splenius capitis

splenius cervicis

levator scapulae

supraspinatus

Rhomboid minor

Serratus posterior superior

Rhomboid major

Latissimus dorsi

Serraturs anterior

Erector spinae

Serraturs posterior inferior

external oblique

internal oblique

NOTE The underlined muscles are the key 'core' muscles

➡ **The PFC core strengthening routine (see page 202) helps to both directly and indirectly strengthen these core muscles.**

result in pain elsewhere. For example, one cause of lower back pain could be insufficiently conditioned hamstring muscles.

The moment your body starts adjusting and compensating and as you move away from your ideal position, your set-up on the bike is being compromised. This can have a domino effect and lead to the development of pain and injuries elsewhere and notably hamper your performance. All the muscles are interconnected, they seldom work in isolation, and if there's any sort of muscular imbalance, other muscles will try and compensate to help and your body may naturally adjust itself. Once you can no longer compensate or adapt, pain and injury can creep in.

It requires just a little dedication and some aptitude and within a couple of weeks, you will improve your power to transfer through the pedals, your stability on the bike and reduce your chances of developing injuries.

➡ **See the rehab toolkit for a comprehensive core exercise programme.**

BELIEVE IN CORE WORK
Tyler Farrar AMERICAN PRO CYCLIST

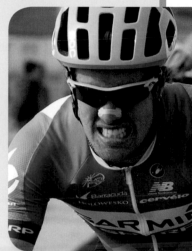

■ *'I'm a big believer in core work. It improves my energy transfer on the bike and helps prevent injuries. Cycling naturally strengthens some muscles but weakens others; that's why most pros slouch when they walk. I have specific gym days that involve core activities, where I'll spend an hour going through exercises, for example squats and dead lifting where you use the whole core to stabilise. I try to keep it cycling-specific, and finish every gym session with a difficult core workout where I'll do core exercises to fatigue.'*

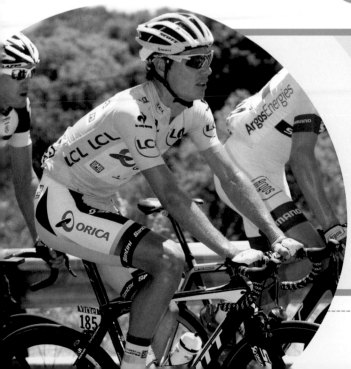

CYCLING NIRVANA
Daryl Impey SOUTH AFRICA | FIRST AFRICAN TO WEAR THE YELLOW JERSEY AT THE TOUR DE FRANCE

■ *'My Cycling Nirvana without question was the first day in the yellow jersey at the Tour de France in 2013. Just wearing the jersey took away any pain and made the whole day feel effortless. They say the yellow jersey gives you wings, I can attest to that. Maybe I was focusing on how awesome the moment was and how big it was that any pain I was experiencing, because of how hard the stage was, was worth it. What a special day.'*

3 WARMING UP TO THE IDEA OF WARM-UPS

❝The exercises I do give my body proper activation and my mind a few minutes to drift off before a hard workout or competition. An efficient warm-up is a true way to connect the mind and body.❞

Lucas Euser AMERICAN PRO CYCLIST AND UNIVEST GRAND PRIX WINNER

Warm-ups and stretching – it seems an unlikely topic to cause friction, but sport scientists can't quite agree on how beneficial they are. While various studies have shown that a decent warm-up can improve performance and reduce injury, others have shown it has little effect and some have even found them to be detrimental if the intensity of the workout isn't correctly tailored to the sport. So let's try and clear it up: *some* form of warm-up is necessary for cycling, and we'll explain why. The key is making sure it's the *right* type of warm-up for the intensity and length of ride you're doing that day.

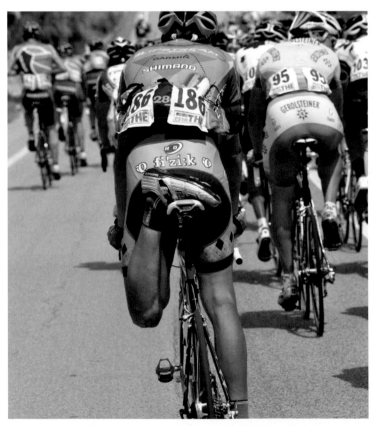

ABOVE An unconventional way to stretch, best left to the pros

Warm-Ups

The purpose of a warm-up

The purpose of a warm-up is to, quite literally, 'warm up' the body by increasing core body temperature. An increase of 1–2°C will create a number of physiological changes that will have a significant positive effect on performance, such as:

- Reduce sports-related musculoskeletal injuries by increasing the elasticity of muscles. Strains and tears are often a result of an abrupt, forceful muscle action where muscle fibres suddenly lengthen and a cold muscle will significantly increase the chances of muscle injury. A warm muscle is a looser, suppler, and more flexible muscle, which will be far more tolerant of forces and movement.
- An increased cardiac output means elevated blood flow so more blood is pumped around the body faster, carrying oxygen, nutrients and minerals to the working muscles.
- Muscles contract more forcefully and relax far quicker, enhancing both speed and strength.
- Increased speed of nerve impulses and heightened sensitivity of nerve receptors. During the initial onset of exercise, faster signalling within the body occurs.

What constitutes a warm-up?

Is a slow five-minute spin of the legs an adequate warm-up or should the body be pushed close to the point of fatigue in order to prepare the body for peak performance? If you're competing in a 10-mile time trial, should the warm-up replicate the event and is that same warm-up necessary for a 50- or 100-mile sportive? And what about stretches, should they be incorporated into a warm-up and if so, what type?

These are all valid questions, and the truth is, there isn't any one specific way to warm up. Warm-ups can be systemic on the bike, or they

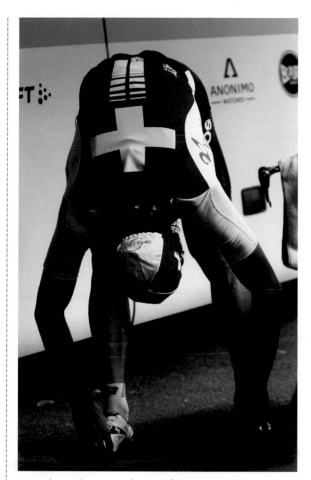

ABOVE Loosening up may be part of a warm up

can be exercises off the bike to get the muscles activated and ready for action. When you're watching TV coverage in the run-up to cycling events you'll see a whole range of warm-ups taking place, yet they all serve a similar purpose. For example, during Grand Tours before time trials, you'll see the pros spinning away on a home trainer, following structured plans, working to certain intensities, while concentrating on cadence and effort. It's a workout in itself, but they're preparing their body, so that they're ready to go from the starting gate. On other race days that start off more 'easily', you'll regularly find riders using the neutral zone – the 5–10 km as they roll out of town to the official start of the day's race – to loosen and warm up.

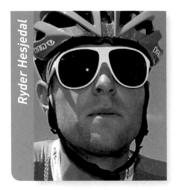

Ryder Hesjedal

■ _'If I'm doing a time trial when I know I need to go flat out 100 per cent from the line, then I'll do a specific, deliberate warm-up to get the body going and ready to race,'_ says Canadian pro cyclist and 2012 Giro d'Italia winner, Ryder Hesjedal. _'The majority of pro races have a 5 km or so neutral zone so you'll roll out easy and use this as the warm-up, but if you're trying to get in the day's breakaway or the stage starts up a mountain then I'll warm up as I don't want to get caught cold. If you see a whole team on the rollers before the start of a stage, buckle up as they're going to make the race hard, right from the start.'_

As Ryder points out, for short, specific sessions that require the body to be performing at its peak, it's imperative that your body is prepared and ready. Suddenly forcing cold muscles into all-out effort increases the chances of muscle tears and injury.

But what about rides that don't require such intense efforts straight away – is an intense warm-up necessary? The answer is no, and a slower, easier warm-up will suffice. For example, if you're heading out on a Sunday morning ride, then riding moderately, gradually increasing the intensity for the first 10–20 minutes, will be enough to raise body temperature by 1–2° – which is the important factor – and prepare the body. And yes, you guessed it, if it's cold outside to begin with, your warm-up may need to be longer by 10–15 minutes or so to have the same effect.

Remember, when performing warm-ups, it's not necessarily the duration of the warm-up

BELOW Stretching before the start of a race may help

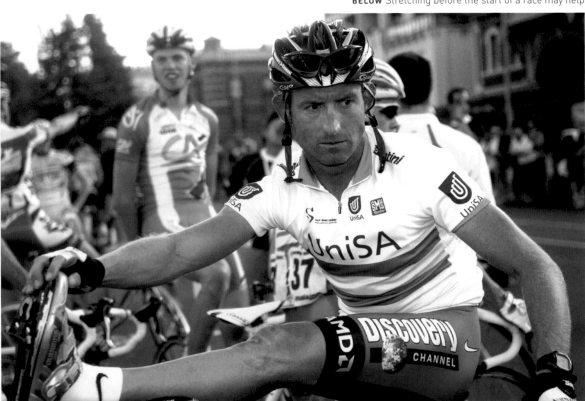

that counts, but rather what it consists of, how it activates parts of the body and that it raises body temperature.

So how do you know when the body is sufficiently warmed up? It's important to realise that there's a fine line between a warm-up that will signal the physiological changes you are looking for, and a warm-up that starts to eat away at precious energy levels. A reliable, quick barometer that will tell if you are suitably warm for exercise is when you can *almost* feel a bead of sweat about to drop down your forehead. Why? Well, in order to offload the extra heat that is being produced, the body's first mechanism is to sweat – simple. Otherwise, feel inside your jersey, if it's clammy, you've started sweating and you're warmed up.

To optimise performance and minimise injury, you must be sufficiently warmed up before riding hard. But there's another piece to the puzzle...

Stretching

■ *'When I'm heading out on a long ride, I'll take 20 to 30 minutes to begin with, to spin my legs easily,'* says American pro cyclist, Caleb Fairly. *'But before I get on my bike, I'll also do some glute and hamstring dynamic stretches and specific movement preparation to get the muscles firing and activated.'*

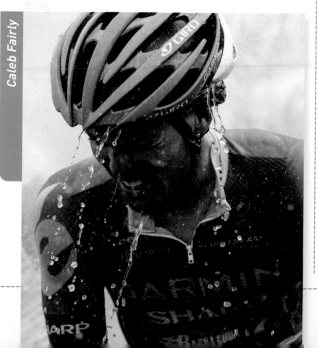

Caleb Fairly

Before Caleb even gets on the bike he will stretch specific parts of the body. A lot of other pros do, too.

■ *'I have a small core activation routine I do before heading out,'* says Tyler Farrar. *'Lower back, muscle activation, leg movements, superman track, some lying, some sitting and some standing exercises, some lunge work and shoulder mobility. It takes no more than five minutes, and it feels like I'm turning everything on, and straightens me out before I ride.'*

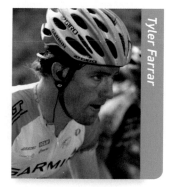

Tyler Farrar

And they're right to do so. Stretching, specifically dynamic stretching, is appropriate as part of an active warm-up. For many years, it was originally thought that static stretching – holding a position to its farthest point and maintaining it – was best to loosen muscles prior to training or competition. However, it's now advocated that the use of dynamic stretching is a more beneficial warm-up because according to research it improves the muscles' sustainable power and endurance.

Dynamic stretching is when muscles are stretched through their range of motion relatively swiftly, allowing the muscles to maintain their pliability. It involves moving parts of your body and gradually increasing reach and speed of movement. What's important to note is that dynamic stretches place emphasis on actively moving a joint through the range of motion that is specific for the sport.

For cyclists, it's beneficial to have a certain degree of movement in joints such as the ankles, knees and hips so that flexibility doesn't diminish your ability to hold good posture on the bike. Joints that can actively perform their full range of movement will also aid the pedalling action and performance. For example, if your ankle isn't able to move freely and is too tight, you may end up putting too much pressure on the knee and hips, affecting the kinematic chain, and if other structures of the chain aren't able to bear the load, injuries may occur.

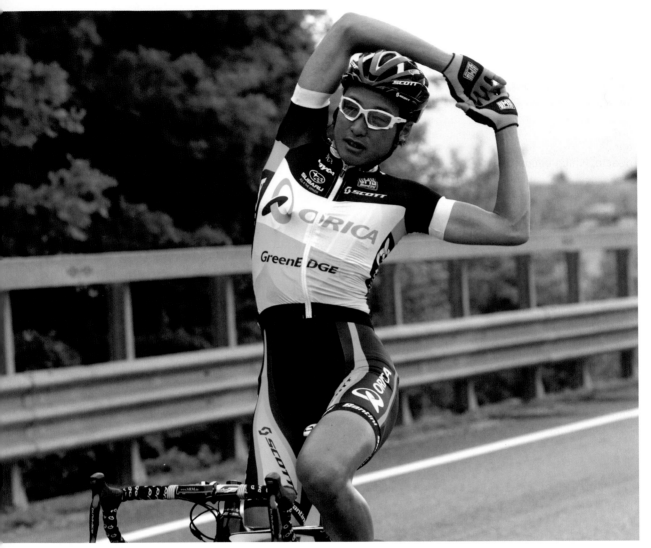

ABOVE Don't try this at home!

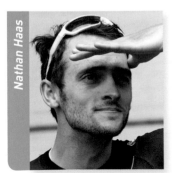
Nathan Haas

■ 'Every day before I ride I'll do 15 minutes of specific foam rolling,' says Nathan Haas. 'Then I'll do skipping – single and double legs – and kettlebell exercises (swinging upwards to horizontal, and kettlebell dead lifts), this way I benefit as I get improved movement, my proper range of motion working and it loosens up my muscles and fascia (connective tissue). I do this before every training ride, and if I don't for a while then I'll start to get ankle and knee soreness.

When I do the exercises I feel light, my coordination is better and I feel like I've switched on the body patterns I need to ride my bike properly and my body feels awake and alive as soon as I clip into the pedals.'

Dynamic stretching will also have a positive effect on muscle suppleness and allows muscles such as the hamstrings and gluteal muscles to extend and contract fully, and perform at their maximum. Increasing suppleness in muscles such as spinal erectors and quadratus lumborum (lower back muscles) will also support stability and minimise discomfort in the lower back. Dynamic stretching ultimately helps to increase muscle temperature, and a warmed muscle, which becomes more pliable, will be able to tolerate greater loads and won't tear as frequently when forces are placed on it.

Don't ignore dynamic stretches. They're an important part of a warm-up and movement preparation for cycling and may heighten performance, and reduce the risk of injuries.

➡ **Head over to the rehab toolkit where you'll find some exercises and stretches we recommend are a part of your warm-up *before* you get on the bike.**

CYCLING NIRVANA
Steve Cummings GREAT BRITAIN | VUELTA A ESPAÑA STAGE WINNER

■ *'Stage 13 of the 2012 Vuelta a España. I wouldn't say it was effortless, but I never felt I went full gas except for the last 1–2 km in the finale. I could sense the other riders in the breakaway group I was in were suffering and I felt like it was easy, so I decided to push on and make it harder to make them suffer more. I was gliding all day. I made several attacks before the break went, but just recovered quicker than normal after each attack. You don't get many days on a bike like that. I felt in total control and always felt I had another gear.*

I didn't think about winning until the last 5 km. I was feeling very strong, I was pushing the group along and we were moving fast. I knew it would be hard to chase behind and started to think the break might go to the line. I just tried to use my strength in the right place and not show my cards too early. I won the race alone with an attack from about 4 km to go and just went full gas and didn't look back.

I'd worked very hard for many years, often without a big reward, and I felt I finally got it on that day. Knowing I'd done everything right, and was able to execute a plan and feel amazing while I did it, was without question a Cycling Nirvana moment.'

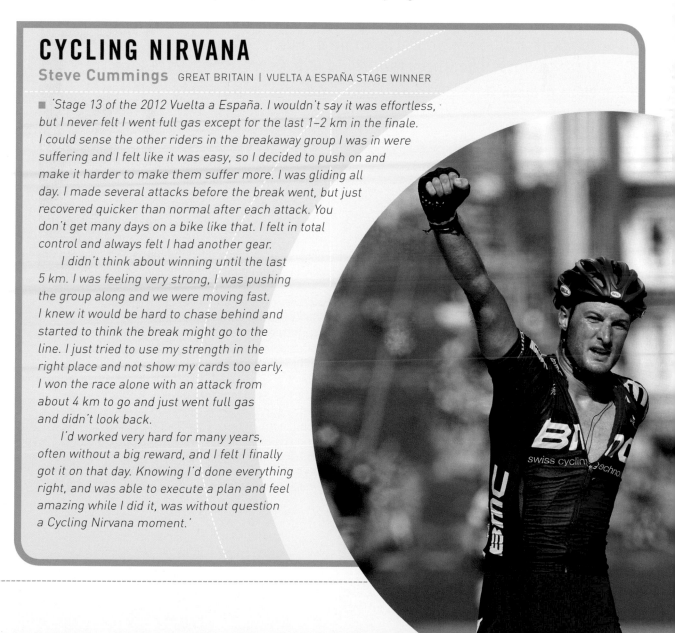

4

THE NEED TO FUEL

❝Nutrition plays such an important role in cycling and it has a massive influence on performance. Everyone gets it wrong from time to time. The important thing is to learn what works for you.❞

Philip Deignan IRISH PRO CYCLIST AND VUELTA A ESPAÑA STAGE WINNER

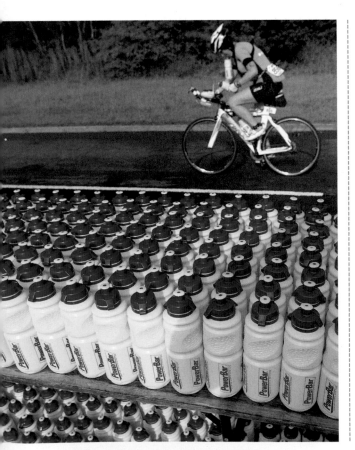

Every year as the Tour de France unfolds in front of our eyes, with the top names battling it out against one another, there's another race going on, one which is just as complex and strategic: the nutritional race. Everything is planned to the finest detail, right from what the riders are eating to the times they eat, and runs throughout the entire course of the day: from the moment they wake up, on the team bus before the start, during the stage itself, and even when they finish – the riders are forever fuelling and feeding their bodies.

While nutrition plans like these may be slightly excessive for amateur riders, the basic principles are just as important and it doesn't matter how fit you are or how many hours you've spent in the saddle, come the day of your ride, sportive or race, if you haven't fuelled the body efficiently, you won't get very far, and you'll be a million miles from your Cycling Nirvana.

The pain-free cyclist needs to know about nutrition, both before the bike and on it, paying particular attention to carbohydrates, the body's main source of fuel during cycling.

LEFT Maintaining hydration levels is important

All roads lead to glucose

Glucose is the carbohydrate used for energy, and is stored in the liver and skeletal muscle as glycogen. While it's true that during low to moderate cycling fats may provide the bulk of energy, they can't be broken down as quickly as carbohydrates and when the intensity of your ride ramps up – when the muscles require a faster supply of energy – it will have to start calling upon glucose and glycogen stores as the primary fuel.

The body has significant stores of fat, but unfortunately the same can't be said for our glycogen stores. In fact, the body can't store much – approximately 500g (2000 kcal) – and as the exercise intensity increases further, they will run out, fast.

It's so important you enhance your carbohydrate availability before you head off on your ride, which is achieved by eating the right foods at the right time. It's also vital they are kept topped up, so you are able to call on them when the going gets tough. Should you fail to do this, you will run into trouble...

Fill up before you go

Before you panic and head off stuffing your face full of carbohydrates, there are a few things you have to consider:

CYCLING UNDER 90 MINUTES (LOW TO MODERATE INTENSITY)

There's no point consuming large amounts of carbohydrates if you're only heading out for an hour's spin. In fact, if you're planning on a gentle ride for anything under 90 minutes then the need to optimise glycogen stores isn't paramount at all, as you should have enough stored already to fuel your ride comfortably.

A morning breakfast of porridge topped with bananas or a lunchtime snack of scrambled egg on toast will provide more than enough fuel for your ride.

CYCLING OVER 90 MINUTES (MODERATE TO HARD INTENSITY)

This is where things change slightly with regards to fuelling, and is where a lot of cyclists get caught short.

Let's use a simple analogy: if you were planning a road trip, you wouldn't fill the petrol tank up half way, would you? The same principle can be applied to cycling. When you're riding for many hours at a hard intensity, you want to maximise your energy systems, minimise the risk of breaking down and leave nothing to chance.

In order to fill the tank optimally and maximise your glycogen stores, you should consume a meal containing 1–4 g of carbohydrate per kg of body weight, 2–4 hours before your ride. This will allow your body to digest what you've eaten before you ride, reducing the risk of stomach upset.

It's also extremely important to eat foods that have a low glycaemic index (GI) rating. The GI is a table that records the rate at which blood glucose levels rise after eating certain foods. Foods that have a low GI will promote more stable blood glucose levels and minimise hunger pangs and sugar crashes throughout your ride.

A good rule of thumb to follow: low GI provides your base fuel over many hours; high GI provides a sudden injection of fuel, which lasts fleetingly.

In the hour or so leading up to your big ride, avoid eating anything too big, or things that could upset the stomach. Eating smaller snacks such as a piece of fruit or a bowl of muesli or even a sports drink or bar will help you keep on top of your glycogen stores, without filling you up.

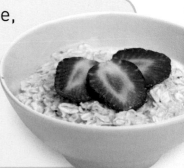

5 great pre-ride, low-GI foods:

- Porridge (traditional oats)
- Greek-style yoghurt
- Wholemeal pasta
- Banana
- Natural muesli

During your ride – nothing lasts forever

As we mentioned earlier, glycogen stores can last up to 90 minutes, providing the exercise intensity is moderate, but for higher-intensity exercise, glycogen stores will provide energy for only a limited period. In some extreme efforts, they may only provide energy for about 20 minutes. In other words, they are going to run out so they will need replacing.

Guidelines generally say that if you're cycling at a moderate intensity, and/or for over 90 minutes, you will need between 30–65 g of carbohydrates per hour to replace what's being lost and maintain performance.

It was always thought that a positive relationship between carbohydrate intake and performance was only observed up to 60g (1 g per minute) – anything more and the body would struggle to absorb and utilise it, which could be detrimental to performance. However, more recent research has revealed that the body can actually utilise more carbohydrates per hour without causing gastric distress, further enhancing performance.

In 2010, researchers discovered that, when glucose is consumed with fructose (fruit sugar) at a 2:1 ratio, carbohydrate consumption can exceed 1.5 g per minute, increasing the rate of delivery to the muscles to 90 g per hour, and in some cases even higher. This is due to the fact that fructose is transported and absorbed in the gut via different receptors than glucose, and these transporters

remain empty unless fructose is consumed. Imagine trying to empty a litre bottle of water from the bottom with a pierced hole. It takes time doesn't it? Now pierce the bottom of the bottle a number of times. The bottle will empty far more quickly and the rate of emptying increases, which is the same as the rate of carbohydrate absorption and utilisation when multiple carbohydrates – glucose and fructose – are ingested together.

While an elevation in carbohydrate consumption has been linked to an improvement in performance, such a high carbohydrate intake is only really necessary for extreme bouts of cycling, such as elite racing, where that extra intake could push the body further for longer. Lower down the cycling ranks, adhering to roughly 30–65g of carbohydrate per hour will suffice.

MATT SAYS

'It doesn't matter how you get your carbohydrates in during your ride. For example, foods such as jam sandwiches, cereal bars and bananas provide significant amounts of carbohydrates. However, the simplest way to get carbohydrates into your system is through energy drinks, gels and sport bars. An hourly intake of a 500–800 ml sports drink with a 6–8 per cent carbohydrate concentration will often meet your requirements.'

A failure to keep on top of your fuelling

When carbohydrate stores start to run low or are unable to be supplied quickly enough to the working muscles and you don't replace them, the body will have to rely on its fat and protein stores for energy, a process known as gluconeogenesis – synthesising glucose in the body from non-carbohydrate sources. These take longer to become available as the body needs to *first* break

down fat and the amino acids (broken-down protein) *before* transporting them to the working muscles so they can be used as energy.

This is why at a certain point in a ride you often instinctively have to slow down or run the risk of 'bonking', also known as the 'hunger knock', which occurs as energy availability becomes depleted – your muscles are almost running on empty.

Practise your nutrition

On your training rides, experiment with what works and what doesn't, devising your own fuelling strategy based on what you need. Eating such large quantities of food can be quite harsh on the stomach. It takes practice.

■ *'During races I usually eat bars because of the ease of their calorific intake, ease of opening and I know my digestion can cope with them,'* says Irish pro Dan Martin. *'Eating while riding is something that you need to practise otherwise indigestion can occur if you're not used to it as an amateur.'*

You may not think it, but eating, or even opening a packet, while riding is a skill; knowing when you need to refuel, what to eat and the effect it is having on performance and your body is important, and you don't want to be experimenting during competition. Practise your feeding during your training rides.

A cyclist who knows all too well about bonking is retired Swedish pro and winner of the 2004 Paris Roubaix, Magnus Bäckstedt.

BELOW Get your nutrition right during training rides

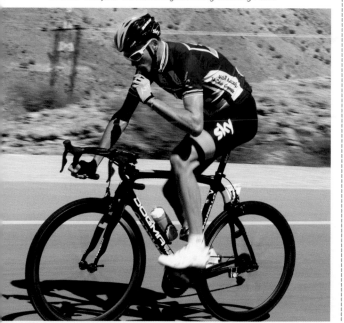

Supplement plan for riding

For longer rides over a few hours, sports drinks, gels and bars are very effective at getting carbohydrates and fluids into your body. All products display their carbohydrate content on their packaging so it's easy to work out how much you need an hour and prepare accordingly.

Sports drink 600–800 ml of 6–8 per cent carbohydrate drink: 50 g carbohydrate
Typical energy bar: 25 g of carbohydrate
Typical energy gel: 20 g of carbohydrate

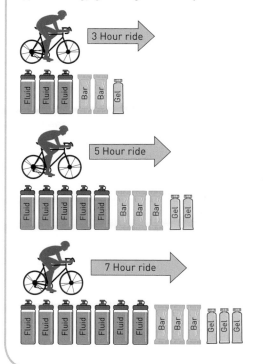

Refuelling

Examples of a 50 g serving of carbohydrates:
• 2 medium bananas
• 2 small cereal bars
• 1 small sandwich
• 475 ml coke

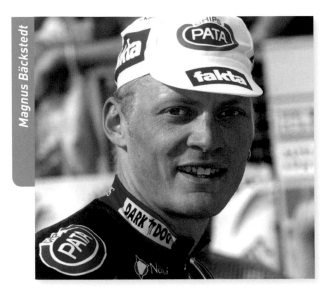

Magnus Bäckstedt

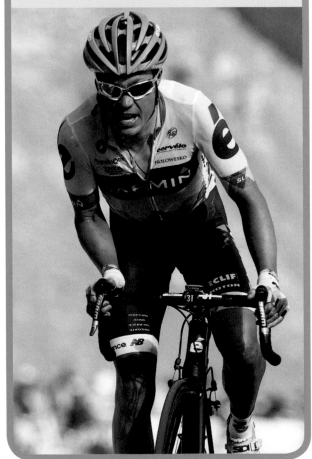

PERSONAL PREFERENCE

Tom Danielson AMERICAN PRO CYCLIST

■ 'I make my own rice cakes for training and have even started prepping my own for races. Using our team chef's recipe, I know exactly what's in them, they are real food, taste great and I know my body works well with them. Over the years as a pro I've recognised that some ingredients commonly found in energy bars, such as palm kernel oil, mess with my digestion and I can't afford to take the risk of this affecting my performance.'

■ 'It was stage seven of the 2008 Tour de France and I'd had some recent digestion issues before the race that meant I had to eat little and often to keep my fuel stores available.

The first 60 km of stage seven were really hard and undulating with never a minute's rest. From eating every 15–20 minutes the rest of the week, I suddenly had eaten nothing in the first hour as the intensity had been so hard I'd had no time. And boy did I pay for it. 60 km into the stage, I found myself running on empty, but it was too late; I was dropped from the peloton and riding solo. I immediately ate two gels to give me a quick pick-me-up and then whatever else I had in my back pocket. As soon as I'd eaten I started to feel better and ride better, but there was still 100 km to go. I rode as hard as I possibly could and kept feeding myself throughout as I had done all week.

With 15 km to go I was still inside the time cut and fancied my chances, then the road went uphill for the last 4–5 km and, being one of the bigger riders of the peloton, this did not suit me. The peloton ahead sped up, I ended up finishing just over 30 minutes down on the winner of the stage that day and I missed the time cut by about four minutes and was consequently eliminated from the Tour de France. While I didn't bonk properly, I had come close, and ultimately my poor fuelling in the first hour of racing meant I wouldn't be riding on to the Champs Élysées that year. I was devastated.'

Make your own rice cakes

Follow these instructions to make your very own rice cakes; perfect to be used before, during or after you ride. One cake provides approximately 85 kcals, 203 mg of sodium, 14 g of carbohydrates, 2 g fat, and 1.6 g of protein.

TIME: 30 minutes • SERVINGS: 16

STEPS:
- Combine 3 cups (approx 700 ml) of water and 2 cups (approx 360–400 g) of uncooked sticky (sushi) rice and cook on the hob or in a rice cooker.
- Mix in 2 tablespoons of soy sauce.
- Flatten half the rice mixture and spread with 3 tablespoons of almond butter.
- Roughly chop half a cup (90 g) of dates and spread over the almond butter.
- Cover the mixture with the remaining rice and press down into shape.
- Once pressed into shape, sprinkle with 1 tablespoon of brown sugar and ½ teaspoon of salt.
- Divide into 16 portions.

Ideally made the day before you ride, keep these refrigerated and consume within four days.

Are performance-enhancing supplements worth it?

The majority of cyclists, both amateur and elite, will at some point have used supplements in a bid to aid performance. It's nothing new. In fact, it's big business. There are many reasons for this boom; one of them being that if taken correctly, certain supplements will enable cyclists to train harder and for longer, and recover quicker, giving them a competitive edge.

Over the years the lines have been blurred as more and more supplements emerge – readily available in shops, supermarkets and online – capitalising on an ill-educated public and making spurious claims that they can help performance, weight loss and health. In truth, there are only a handful of legal supplements that can significantly help performance, and not all of these are relevant for cyclists. Let's be clear, doing the right training, getting the right amount of rest and eating a healthy balanced diet with good carbohydrate availability is far more important than any supplement you'll take. Supplements should be seen as the icing on the cake, not a short cut to success.

What works?

There's a commonly held belief in sports nutrition with regards to supplements. If it works, it's probably banned, and if it's not banned according to the World Anti-Doping Agency (WADA), then it probably doesn't work. There are some exceptions to this rule that are known to benefit performance when used in the correct way.

Creatine is not for cyclists. Though it does improve strength and power, it works over short bursts of time rather than for prolonged endurance exercise such as cycling. Creatine also encourages the body to retain water and put on weight – not ideal when you want to get up those hills and mountains quickly. Consequently, cyclists should steer clear of this supplement.

The next two are sodium bicarbonate and beta-alanine. Again, these work as they help buffer against excess lactic acid build-up in the muscles during exercise. But for long-endurance exercise, is it worth the potential stomach irritation of taking sodium bicarbonate, or remembering to take beta-alanine every day, sometimes twice a day, for four weeks in the lead-up to one event? We'd suggest not. It's not going to be *the* thing that helps you find Cycling Nirvana.

The fourth performance aid is good old fashioned caffeine. This is used by cyclists and is effective too; so much so that it was banned by WADA until 2004. Caffeine can provide the edge at a time you may feel you need it, it works on the same day, and will be cleared by your body by the end of the day so there are no real lasting effects. So let's take a closer look at caffeine and how it can benefit cyclists.

CAFFEINE

Caffeine is a stimulant (it's actually a drug) that can help improve concentration and sharpen reactions by speeding up messages to and from the brain. It has unanimously been shown to improve time to exhaustion in numerous studies from as far back as 1978 to the present day. It exerts its effects on the central nervous system by altering the perception of effort and fatigue, which is why it might be recommended for cyclists.

However, taking *too much* caffeine can cause nervousness, restlessness, nausea, stomach pain, vomiting and insomnia. Equally, some people are more sensitive to it than others.

Where can I get it?

Caffeine content of common foods and drink:

FOOD OR DRINK	SERVING	CAFFEINE CONTENT (MG)
Instant coffee	250 ml cup	60
Espresso	1 shot	100
Tea	250 ml cup	25
Coca Cola	330 ml can	32
Red bull	250 ml can	80
Sports gel	1 sachet	50–100
ProPlus	2 pills	100
No-Doz	1 pill	100

The dosage

1–3 mg/kg of body mass before you exercise. So if you weigh 70 kg, then 70–210 mg would be recommended. The range is determined by how sensitive you are, which you will become familiar with it as you use it. Its effects last in the body a few hours so one dose should be enough, but it's also used by many pros towards the end of races as a 'pick-me-up' before a hard finish.

Read the packaging to track how much caffeine you are consuming. From 2015, any product containing more than 150 mg of caffeine per litre (mg/l) must be labelled with the term 'high caffeine content'.

Some other supplements you may have read about

OMEGA-3

Unlike other fats, omega-3s (a group of long-chain fatty acids) can't be made by the body and so must come from the diet, for example, from oily fish. Essential for growth, development and the correct functioning of the brain and nervous system, evidence shows that omega-3s can protect against depression and heart disease. They also play a role in the regulation of body fat and may stimulate muscle protein synthesis. Plant-based omega-3 is also found in walnuts and flaxseeds, although these shorter-chain versions are less efficiently used in the body. Omega-3s are more frequently used as a cornerstone for health rather than for *performance* per se as there's little research linking supplementation with increased performance.

➡ **Instead of supplementing, eat two portions of oily fish, such as salmon and mackerel a week.**

ANTIOXIDANTS

Free radicals are a harmful by-product of the oxidative stress of exercise that can damage cells and attack the fats that provide structure to the walls of the cell membranes. Antioxidants help defend the body and mop up these free radicals by binding to them and nullifying their destructive effect. You can buy antioxidants in supplement form but save your money as they occur naturally within many fruits and vegetables. Provided that you eat a diet full of these foods, then you shouldn't need to take antioxidant supplements. In fact, it's recently been shown that artificially mopping up free radicals is potentially harmful, and can decrease positive adaptations that derive from training.

➡ **Instead of supplementing, eat 5–13 portions a day of fresh colourful fruit and vegetables (potatoes don't count!) depending on your required calorific intake (Harvard School of Public Health).**

NITRATES

Research is starting to show that nitric oxide (a conversion of nitrates) is beneficial to performance: increasing vasodilation, improving delivery of oxygen and nutrients, reducing oxygen uptake, making exercise less tiring and having a positive effect on the metabolism of the mitochondria – the cells' engines – within the muscles as well.

Nitrates are found in higher concentrations in certain foods such as beetroot and spinach, although concentrations can significantly vary, making it difficult to know how much to eat to gain a performance benefit. For cycling performance, the supplement may be a better choice. Many sports nutrition manufacturers now produce gels, drinks and bars that contain higher levels of concentrated nitrate, which the body can utilise far more easily. However, taking large quantities can cause gastric distress, so it's best avoided immediately before competition. In fact, because nitrates last in the body for a good few hours, you can take them in the morning for breakfast and still get the benefits in the afternoon when you ride.

Our advice on nitrates for now is to watch this space. Eat plenty of spinach and beetroot to naturally boost your nitrate availability through your diet, but remember, as with all supplements, it is more important to get the right amount of rest and eat a healthy balanced diet in addition to your training.

CYCLING NIRVANA
Tyler Farrar
UNITED STATES OF AMERICA | SECOND AMERICAN TO WIN STAGES IN ALL THREE GRAND TOURS

■ *'The Tour de France is something you dream about when you get into cycling and aspire to. I dreamed about it since I was 12 years old and finally got to ride it in 2009.*

The final stage into Paris has almost mythical status. You suffer through three weeks, especially in your first tour and you don't know if you will make it through or not. And then there's a moment on the stage into Paris when you make a left and right chicane through the Place de la Concorde on to a right turn, then the whole Champs Élysées is in front of you with the Arc de Triomphe at the end of the street.

That whole moment was the most amazing experience I've ever had. I'd lived the dream I'd had since I was 12 years old to be one of the best bike racers in the world and finish the tour. I've won my fair share of races, but that moment is my Cycling Nirvana.'

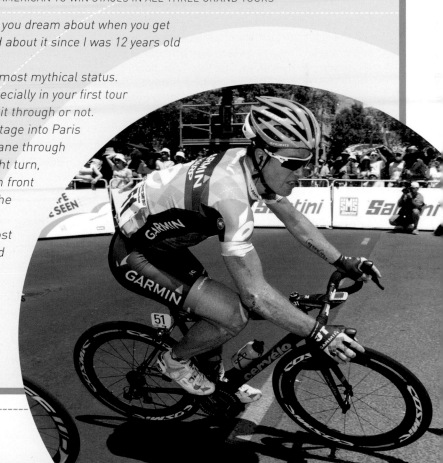

5

THE NEED FOR FLUIDS

> *Hydration is so important when out cycling for long periods of time. Get it wrong and it could severly hamper performance and in some cases, your health too. Understand the basics and it shouldn't ever become a problem.*

Alex Dowsett BRITISH PRO CYCLIST AND GIRO D'ITALIA STAGE WINNER

Current thoughts on dehydration suggest that 2 per cent body weight loss after exercise won't have as severe an effect on physiological functions (your performance) as was previously thought, which in turn has led to an amendment to guidelines on hydration. The International Olympic Committee (IOC) now advises that it's far better and easier to *minimise dehydration* rather than to *optimise hydration.*

It is now accepted that performance won't be significantly affected until a dehydrated state of above 3 per cent occurs. It is at this point the body has a more difficult time maintaining cooling capabilities to prevent an increase in core body temperature. Dehydration reduces the amount of sweat produced and thus the ability to dump heat from the body. This results in a rise in core temperature and it is *this* that causes problems.

■ *'I'm from Texas and it's super-hot,' says American pro cyclist, Caleb Fairly. 'When I was younger getting dehydrated happened a lot. I used to go out as a junior and ride for hours, forget to drink enough fluids and have to call my mum to pick me up. I've been out on training rides when people have got so dehydrated they've literally collapsed off their bike. It's not pretty or fun.'*

What happens?

For every 1 per cent of body weight lost through sweating during exercise, core temperature rises approximately 0.15–0.20°C. As core temperature increases and fluid loss reaches above 3 per cent of body weight you become dehydrated – this puts the cardiovascular system under huge strain, most notably:

- Blood thickness increases as the plasma volume reduces (so total blood volume reduces) as this fluid is lost in sweat. Thicker blood means the heart has to work harder to move it around the body.
- Increased heart and respiration rates. These rise to compensate for decreased blood volume, meaning what remains needs to be distributed around the body more quickly to maintain performance.

A rise in core temperature to 40°C leads to heat stroke, cramps and exhaustion, quickly putting the brakes on performance as well as placing your health in jeopardy.

So how do you stay relatively hydrated and minimise dehydration?

Start hydrated

Beginning training or competition with adequate hydration levels is paramount. Ensuring you have an optimised pre-hydration status will limit the risk of dehydration more efficiently than trying to hydrate while on the bike. What you've consumed over the last 24 hours will influence your hydration. Certain foods and fluids contain higher amounts of water than others, while some can promote fluid loss. Alcohol, for example, has diuretic properties that encourage the body to pass fluids.

RECOMMENDATIONS

- Drink 500 ml of water as soon as you wake up to replace the fluids your body lost overnight through respiration.
- Drink an additional 500 ml of water 2–3 hours before you get on the bike. Drinking several hours before riding gives your body sufficient time to excrete any excess fluid that hasn't been absorbed by the body.

Although it sounds simplistic, passing urine is a reliable indicator of hydration status. It's a good idea to check the colour of your urine. It should be a pale straw-like colour. Anything paler, and you may have taken on too much fluid; anything darker, and you haven't taken on enough.

■ *'I want my pee to be clear or light straw in colour,'* says American pro cyclist, Ben King. *'This lets me know I'm well hydrated. If it's bright yellow or dark like apple juice, you know you're dehydrated.'*

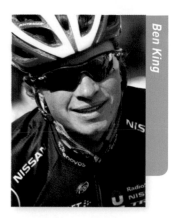

Ben King

Too much of a good thing?

It's easy to drink large quantities of water in a bid to avoid dehydration, but you may already be sufficiently hydrated, or not be riding hard enough, long enough or in hot enough conditions to warrant such an intake of fluids. At this point, hyponatremia becomes a risk. This occurs as a result of too much water consumption, which dilutes the body's sodium (electrolyte) levels. This is becoming more of a problem as the message has for a long time been *avoid dehydration at all costs*. Hyponatremia is also known as water intoxication and symptoms include: nausea and

ARE YOU DEHYDRATED?

1, 2, 3 – Well hydrated

4, 5 – Not well hydrated

6, 7, 8 – Dehydrated – you need to drink more

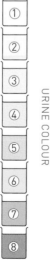

URINE COLOUR

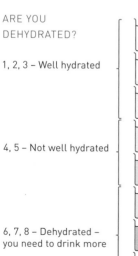

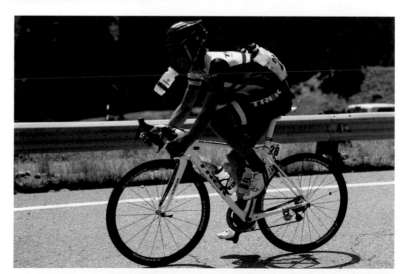

ABOVE It's important to stay hydrated

vomiting, headache, confusion, loss of energy and fatigue. It can lead to the more serious problems of seizures or falling into a coma – this needs to be avoided and our hydration recommendations should help you avoid this trap (see 'Applying the advice').

Aside from the more serious problem of hyponatremia, there are other less serious complications from drinking too much, such as feeling bloated or putting on short-term weight, which if you're riding up mountains isn't ideal as retired British pro cyclist Daniel Lloyd found out:

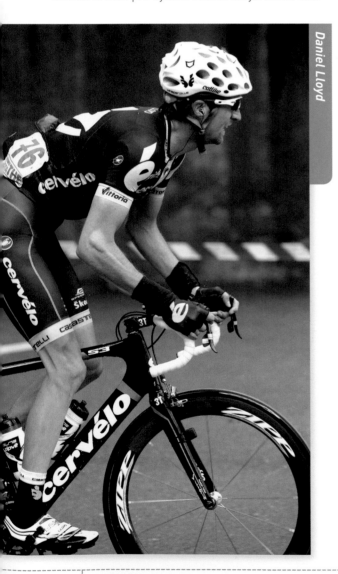

Daniel Lloyd

■ *'The 2009 Giro d'Italia was my first ever Grand Tour, and going into it I was nervous about staying hydrated enough and being able to recover properly after each stage to get me through the three weeks. The team doctor recommended I take some extra electrolytes because of the heat, which I did, and to ensure I had enough energy I ended up eating more than I actually needed to. I was weighing myself every morning and evening to ensure I was staying on top of my hydration after each stage. After two weeks, despite having ridden 14 stages of the hardest race I had ever done and burnt through thousands of calories, I had actually put on 4 kg. I realised firstly I didn't need to eat as much as I had been and secondly I didn't perhaps need as many electrolytes as I thought, as I figured some of the weight was from water retention. I didn't actually "feel" heavier but in the third week that extra weight as you go into the mountains only makes it harder.*

Through testing I did a few years later I consequently found out I don't actually lose that much salt through my sweat, which is why I probably didn't need to take so much on in the race. I now recommend to others to learn the signals your body gives you, and to start any event well hydrated and start drinking steadily as the event begins, and then you are not likely to find yourself dehydrated, which might make you start intuitively to drink heavily.'

Drinking on the go

To avoid dehydration and hyponatremia, the two ends of the scale, current trends advise drinking at a rate that replaces the majority of sweat losses. But how do you know how much you're sweating? Not an easy question to answer because there are so many factors that influence our sweat rates, from the outside temperature or your diet to the humidity in the air. Other factors such as your hydration status, fitness levels, body weight and clothing all play a role in how much you sweat.

Your hydration needs should be suited to you. Everyone is different and hydration is all about understanding how much you sweat and what is needed to cater to your specific needs. The content of sweat varies widely between people too. While all sweat contains salts, known as electrolytes, some cyclists naturally have more salty sweat than others.

Electrolytes are a combination of essential salts, which aid muscle contraction and relaxation. They also help to keep the nervous and cardiac system functioning and they need replacing when they're lost in sweat. There are four main electrolytes – sodium, chloride, potassium and magnesium – all with different jobs and roles to play, but it's sodium that has the most important role, helping maintain the fluid balance of the body. Sodium in sweat is measured in millimoles per litre (mmol/l), and concentrations can vary from anywhere between 15 to 93 mmol/l.

To find out how much you sweat and the content of your sweat, you'll need to undergo a laboratory test but the measures are a little extreme; a lot of pros don't adopt such an approach.

Applying the advice

Under 60 minutes: Hydration status is not a huge concern assuming you start in a hydrated state, unless you're riding at high intensity and it's hot outside.

Up to 90 minutes: Water is fine and effective at maintaining hydration levels, and drinking to thirst will be fine.

Over 90 minutes: It's advisable to consume a sports drink with a carbohydrate content of 4–8 per cent (4–8 g/100 ml). Known as 'isotonic' drinks they contain a similar concentration of salt and sugar as the human body, so are absorbed by the body as quickly as water. These drinks cover all bases, providing hydration, fuel and electrolytes, all key to performance when you're going hard on the bike.

In these longer rides, drinking to thirst isn't always reliable as riding hard or eating while riding may stop you feeling thirsty. So when you set out on longer training rides, adopt a strategy, and aim to drink 120–180 ml every 10–20 minutes – this will help replace most of your fluid losses while not overhydrating you. This roughly works

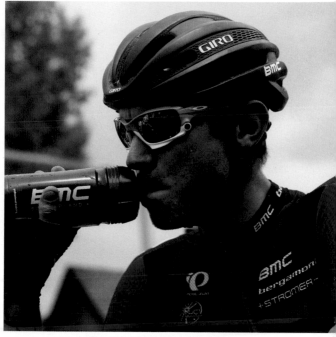

ABOVE Drink little and often to minimise dehydration

out at one regular sized bidon an hour. Remember, if it's hot outside (above 25°C) sweat rates can get as high as 2000 ml per hour, meaning you'll need to increase your fluid intake. Trying to drink 2 litres of fluid per hour to keep pace with fluid loss becomes difficult, uncomfortable and may be impractical, but you *will* need to increase your intake in hot conditions, so replacing 75 per cent of fluid losses – three bidons per hour should prevent you from going above 2 per cent dehydration. The more you become familiar with your weight before and after long rides, the more you can tailor your own individual fluid needs.

Make your own Isotonic drink

- 500 ml unsweetened fruit juice (orange, apple or pineapple work well)
- 500 ml water
- ¼ teaspoon of salt

■ 'I am a firm believer in the "drink your hydration, eat your nutrition" philosophy,' says American pro cyclist, Lucas Euser. 'Simple hydration drinks with sugar, electrolytes and few calories keep your body hydrated and able to absorb the food you consume. Getting behind on hydration can mean big performance decreases especially in severe temperatures, hot or cold. One trick I've found that is helpful: right before I leave for a workout or as I'm pedalling off in the neutral section of a race I will drink a 600 ml bottle of a light hydration mix as sometimes we forget to drink in the first hour of a workout/race. It's better to stick to light hydration mixes instead of just plain water as it helps with absorption. If you don't have any around, try adding a little honey, lemon and salt to water.'

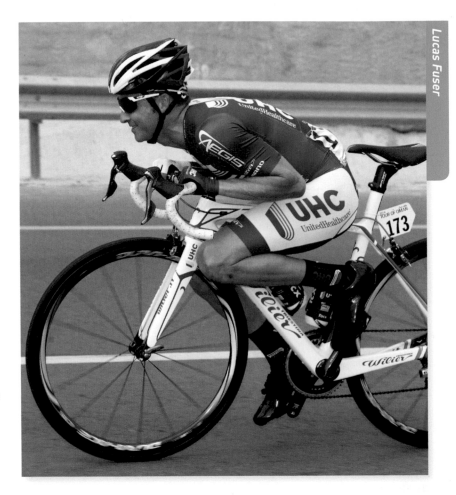

Lucas Fuser

Remember:

- Weigh yourself before and after each ride over 90 minutes to quickly assess your hydration status and replace 1.5 L of fluid for every 1 kg body mass for an optimal rehydration strategy – see page 52.
- Start your ride hydrated – drink 500 ml water 2–3 hours before you ride or on waking if you're riding in the morning (a good habit to adopt anyway).
- Check your urine: if it indicates dehydration before you ride, drink an isotonic sports drink before you head out.

- For rides under an hour, start hydrated and you won't need to take fluids with you (unless you're riding high intensity or it's hot outside).
- For rides up to 90 minutes, drinking cool water to thirst will keep you hydrated.
- Riding longer than 90 minutes, drink sports drinks as opposed to water to encourage good hydration status.1 bidon (700 ml) an hour will replace the majority of sweat loss at average rates of 800–1000 ml per hour; increase this if you're riding at high intensity or in hot weather.

CYCLING NIRVANA

Heinrich Haussler AUSTRALIA | TOUR DE FRANCE STAGE WINNER

■ 'It was the perfect situation, the perfect day, the only stage I had been given a free role in by the team during the race. It was stage 13 of the 2009 Tour de France. Months before the tour started I had that particular stage in the back of my mind as a potential target. I train in those areas a lot so I knew all the roads.

The stage started and it began raining straight away. Right from the gun there was an attack and I jumped on the wheel and followed. Another five guys bridged across and joined from behind and formed the day's breakaway. Then our group split, myself and two others broke away from the breakaway.

As we started to climb, it just got colder and colder, which I sensed was playing to my advantage. The day before had been 38 degrees heat so the change was a huge shock. We were 1400 m up and the other two riders didn't handle the cold as well as I did, I could just tell. I could feel they weren't as strong. Then one guy got dropped and my confidence soared.

With 50 km to go I attacked and rode the last 50 km solo. I was riding scared as I thought I was going to hunger flat and the peloton would catch me or that I'd crash on the descent, but at the same time I could sense the win. In the final kilometre, it all hit me that

I'd win. It was the best day of my career, of my life to that point, and I was crying like a baby. All my friends and family were there, they had come out as they knew it would be my only chance that tour. As I crossed the line I had all these flashbacks, all my childhood dreams of riding the Tour de France, riding when I started at six years old, waiting up late at night to watch the tour highlights. I knew my parents would be watching and going crazy; inside I was going crazy too and that was my Cycling Nirvana.'

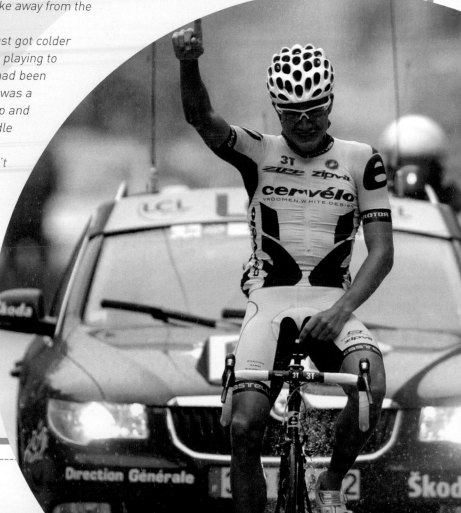

6 TRAIN THE MIND

> ❛Cycling is 95 per cent mental and 5 per cent physical. All the pro riders are very similar in physical abilities. So the big advantage is the mental side. That's the difference between the good riders and the best riders.❜

Carlos Sastre 2008 TOUR DE FRANCE WINNER

Cycling is physically challenging, pushing the body to its limits, but it's also a sport where you have to be mentally strong. Cyclists are forever faced with a number of mental challenges, such as willpower, focus and confidence. These are just some of the issues that are shaped through our psychological strength and that have a massive influence on performance. Without the mind, the body won't go as far. In fact without the mind, you'll never reach your Cycling Nirvana.

■ 'Mental approach is everything,' says Australia pro cyclist, Nathan Haas: 'If you've done all the training but you aren't prepared to suffer, you won't win even if you're the fittest guy there. Every race I've ever done well in, I've always put myself through it in training, visualised it and when I'm training and hurting I put it one gear harder and make myself suffer even more to simulate the mental suffering that comes with racing. The physical suffering is hard but the mental suffering is what I really have to train for to perform at my best.'

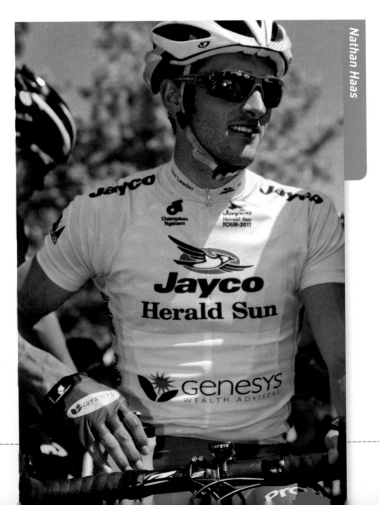

Nathan Haas

At the elite end of the cycling spectrum, the difference between the riders' physiological make up can be minimal. Very little may separate their strength, speed, skill and stamina. It's an individual's psyche that determines how well these function.

Look at the likes of Sir Bradley Wiggins, Mark Cavendish and Chris Froome: three completely different bike riders, all with their own riding style, goals, training techniques, attitudes and opinions. Yet they all share one thing in common: a strong set of psychological skills.

Sports psychology can be learned, just like any other skill, such as bunch riding or descending, and amateur cyclists can benefit from a set of strong psychological skills too. It might help you reach your full potential.

Concentration

Concentration is fundamental in cycling and can have a huge impact on performance. It doesn't matter whether you're a road racer, time triallist or sportive rider, you need to be able to concentrate and block out distractions.

■ *'Concentration is something you need to get on top of and learn to improve right at the start when you get into cycling,'* says retired Australian pro and 2011 Tour de France winner Cadel Evans. *'Training concentration is as important as training the legs. I see riders come into three-week stage races and their concentration can be a little off. You have to know when to focus and when to save yourself; if it doesn't come naturally, it can be a huge drain on energy.'*

In order to understand concentration, it's simplest to break it down into two areas: attention span (how long you focus on something) and selective attention (the ability to focus on certain things while paying less attention to others).

Selective attention is the most important ability for a successful cyclist. In a sport like cycling, an ability to identify and distinguish relevant information will aid early decision-making and allow more time to respond, for

example, descending at speed or reacting to an incident.

The direction of your attention can be internal or external. External is when attention is directed outwards on the events happening around you, such as other riders on the road or cars sharing the road with you. Internal is the need to analyse what is happening, reading the race as well as your own strategy.

Unsurprisingly, most of us have the same recurring problem when it comes to attention: distractions, either physical or emotional. A lot of amateur cyclists find it hard to maintain concentration for long periods of time but it can happen to the pros too. Remember the London 2012 Olympic men's road race? During the final few hundred metres, Colombia's Rigoberto Uran was distracted only momentarily, but it was enough for Kazakhstan's Alexandr Vinokurov to capitalise, attack and cross the finish line first and

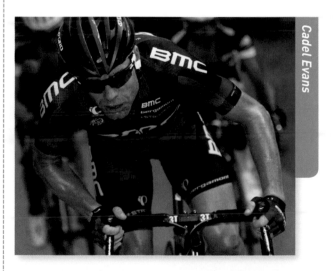

Cadel Evans

take the gold medal. It just shows how these fine lines are so important at elite level. So how do you maximise concentration and, most importantly, minimise distraction?

It's thought that as arousal increases so does our performance, but only to a point as then further increases in arousal will cause a decrease in performance. At low levels of arousal, performance is usually poor. You're not engaged in the activity. In other words, the mind wanders.

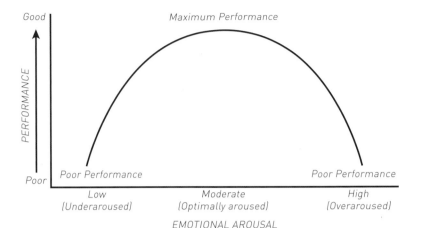

Good — Maximum Performance

PERFORMANCE

Poor — Poor Performance — Poor Performance

Low (Underaroused) — Moderate (Optimally aroused) — High (Overaroused)

EMOTIONAL AROUSAL

ABOVE Psychologists, Yerkes and Dodson created the 'inverted U' theory way back in 1908, and helps best in describing how attention shifts from broad to specific, to narrow.

We've all been there when we're plodding along, our mind elsewhere. It's usually at this time when one is most prone to mistakes and accidents.

■ 'As a stage racer, accidents happen, and you'd be surprised it's often not the 80–90 kph technical descent when they typically happen as everyone is engaged and focused,' says Cadel Evans. 'It's the times when everyone is cruising along looking at the view or whatever that they tend to crash. When racing on the bike, I deliberately don't socialise a lot and that helps me to stay focused and concentrate.'

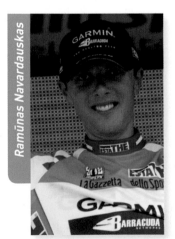

Ramūnas Navardauskas

■ 'When you come into the finale of a race that you feel you can win, you sense what the opposition is doing and at the same time you have a zen- like focus on what your body is doing, which allows you to act and react quicker than you normally would.'

As an optimal point of arousal is reached, peak performance often occurs and our concentration is focused – often the state of Cycling Nirvana – reacting to only relevant internal and external cues. This is 'the zone' you want to stay in. But beware of becoming over aroused, as this can cause tunnel vision and result in a decrease in concentration. Ever been cut up by a car and can't let it go? That's over arousal.

■ 'Staying on top of your emotions is extremely important,' says Cadel Evans. 'If you get pissed off or angry with another rider at a race as their lack of concentration has nearly crashed you or whatever, then it will stimulate your fight or flight response, and this can be a huge drain of energy, which is a waste as you need every drop of energy in a Grand Tour for example. As in life, you learn to control aggression or emotions; you need to do the same on the bike. It's going to be related to your personality or disposition and you need to control your own character and know what it takes to benefit your own training or racing.'

What can you do?

There are a number of things that can help keep you focused while riding. And yes they take practice but once mastered, they can be highly effective.

Give yourself a talking to: This can really help in both raising and lowering your arousal levels. Have you ever seen a professional rider talking to themselves on a big climb, or while they are attacking? This is self-talk and they are prompting their mind and body to focus. It's extremely important that self-talk remains positive as it can be extremely easy to talk yourself *out* of a competition. The best thing is to avoid 'over emotional' self-talk and focus on self-instructing, motivational content. When you are having doubts during a race, competition or even training, combat these with positive thoughts.

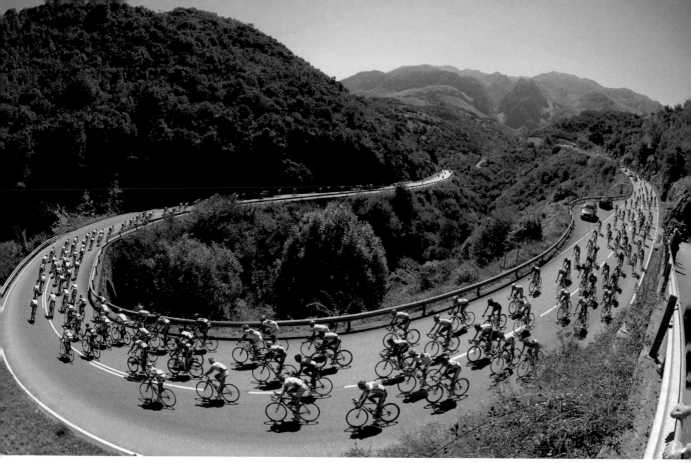

ABOVE Don't let the scenery distract you when riding

Shut out the world: You will never deal with distractions in a sportive or road race if you forever train on an indoor home trainer. Try training in locations and environments where distractions are present so you become comfortable riding in all situations and you'll become immune to the distractions.

Break it down: To keep your arousal levels constant and your attention high, many sport performers break their game into 'chunks'. In road races, sportives or long training rides, you may be in the saddle for 4–5 hours, and this no doubt will affect your attention span, as it will be extremely difficult to concentrate for so long without your mind wandering. Instead, try breaking the route into sections with appropriate changes in focus of attention at various points. This will keep your mind fresh and fully focused on each section individually.

Let it go: We all make mistakes and an inability to forget about what just happened creates an internal distraction. Stay calm, put your negative thoughts behind you and stay focused on the present. A strong-minded individual is able to accept mistakes and let them go rather than dwelling on them. Remember, you can't change what's been and gone.

Motivation and drive

Another aspect that separates the elite from the rest is their motivation and huge inner drive. Motivation goes hand in hand with single-mindedness, obsession and even selfishness.

There are two personality types: 'need to achievers' (Nach) and 'fear of failures' (Fof). People who possess a 'need to achieve' personality will thrive on challenges, they are determined and

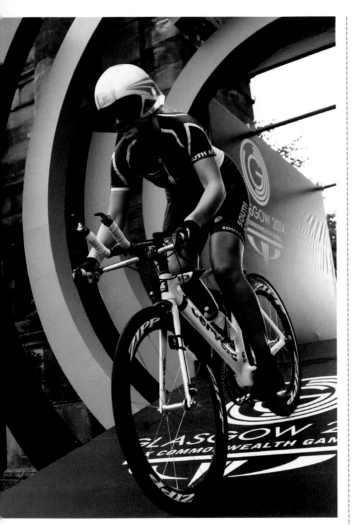

ABOVE There are no excuses if you give 100 per cent

Controlling the controllable

Remaining positive is key. Especially in cycling. Of course things can go wrong, but more often than not, they are uncontrollable factors. For example, crashing is unfortunately inevitable at some point, so learn to accept it. There are going to be stronger cyclists than you, too. That's cycling, accept it. Many cyclists also have an unhealthy fixation on others, whether they are rivals, teammates or clubmates. The moment you start focusing on others is the moment you take your eye off what *you* should be doing. You're now focusing on uncontrollable factors.

Controlling the controllable is a top-level cyclist's mantra. It's a way of coping with the stress and pressure that comes with bike racing. Yes, they want to win, but they realise that all they can do is their best, and as long as they have given 100 per cent, nobody can ask for more.

■ *'During races when your legs feel bad or someone looks like they are going better than you, it can make you think there's something wrong with you,'* says Tom Danielson. *'The number one way to combat that is to pay attention to yourself only, your objectives, your goals. What I learnt was to only base my self-confidence on what I was feeling, not how anyone else was performing and that's helped me a ton.'*

take risks and tend to think of things in terms of goals and accomplishment. These people see things in black and white; it's kept simple and follows a progressive plan.

On the flip side, people who hold a Fof personality avoid challenges and do not want to take risks. One would think that all elite cyclists naturally hold a Nach personality, but this isn't always the case. In fact, many athletes possess self-doubt, and it's this fear of failure that can ultimately hinder performance. So how do you get over this? You have two options: controlling the controllable and self-confidence.

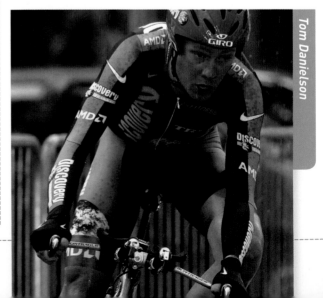

Tom Danielson

ALEX HOWES: FEAR IS NOT AN OPTION

■ *'I don't allow the fear to creep in. The only time it tries to show up is after a bad crash so I just get back up and get going again. You've got to have faith in your skills, you may be freaked out but I just let my skills as a pro come to the surface to squash it. I wouldn't recommend that approach to everyone but working hard on my bike-handling skills and technique allows me to go into autopilot in a sense when lack of confidence tries to pop up.'*

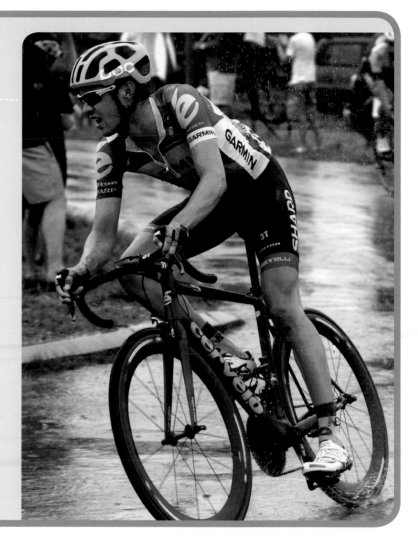

Self-confidence

Mark Cavendish epitomises self-confidence and self-belief. Some may mistake it for arrogance, but it's not. It's complete self-assurance. Confidence is one of the most influential factors that distinguish between successful and less successful cyclists. Put simply, self-confidence is the belief that you can successfully perform a desired behaviour.

Use our easy-to-follow guide to build self-confidence:

Set achievable goals: if things go well, you expect things to continue to go well. So set yourself attainable goals to build confidence. But be careful – not achieving what you set out to do can knock your confidence back. Sometimes, it's helpful to set 'easier' goals to initially build confidence. Replaying good rides from the past in your mind – maybe even your Cycling Nirvana – at night before going to sleep can help build confidence.

Copy other people: not to be confused with 'focusing on others'. This is also known as

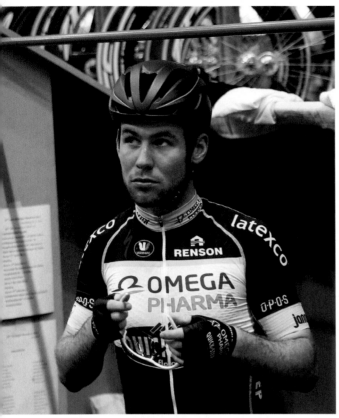

ABOVE Don't dwell on mistakes

Anxiety

Anxiety can significantly impact performance. While it's very difficult to identify it, the biggest problem is that many will accept these feelings before they start riding or racing, reinforcing them rather than combating them.

Anxiety can have three effects on the body:

Thoughts: fear, negative thoughts, indecision, lack of confidence, defeatist attitude and inability to take instructions.

Physical symptoms: sweating, increased heart rate, tension, 'butterflies' and clammy hands.

Actions: fidgeting, biting fingernails, lethargy, uncharacteristic outbursts and incessant talking, lack of performance.

So how can you control it? Firstly it's important to be able to identify the onset of anxiety and understand the symptoms. Only then will you be able to put a halt to them before they start to affect your actual performance.

Prepare the best you can: make sure you go into your race or sportive in the best shape possible. Not only will this help you to build confidence, but it will also reduce the quest to find excuses.

Be positive: it's not arrogant to think you will do well. It's confidence.

Focus on the ride and nothing else: provided that you've prepared as best you can, there should be nothing else to think about.

Deep breathing: controlled breathing (see page 159) helps lower the heart rate, as well as reducing stress levels. A focus on deep breathing will help focus your mind and prevent it from worrying about other external variables.

Mental rehearsal (aka visualisation or imagery): this is the process of creating a mental image of intention of what you want to happen or feel. By imagining a time you previously performed well, remembering what you did, how you did it, how you felt, both mentally and physically, will help you to repeat that performance by simply stepping back into that situation.

modelling. Let's say you're struggling for confidence after a crash. Finding someone who was in a similar position to you but managed to overcome it will help build confidence that you too can overcome this issue and progress. Ask them what they did, and the struggles they had to deal with. It's proof that success is achievable, and you will get over it and move on.

Take the compliments: remember nice things people have said about you and hold on to them. Having people show confidence in your ability is hugely beneficial and will make goals seems more achievable.

Don't let nerves get the better of you: learn to enjoy it and turn negatives into positives. For example, to some, an increased heart rate and sweaty palms may be a sign of nerves and apprehension. See this as your body's natural preparation for high performance.

CYCLING NIRVANA

Phil Gaimon UNITED STATES OF AMERICA | REDLANDS CYCLING CLASSIC WINNER

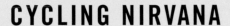

■ *'There's a ride in North Georgia about 30 minutes from where I live. I would do it every Sunday and I had a routine – I'd go to the waffle house on the way, eat as much as I could, then get out on my bike and burn it all off. The roads there are awesome; it goes up some climbs, it goes on a dirt road, all the way round a pretty lake in the mountains. It's about 180 km in total with about 3000 m of climbing.*

I never said it was easy. I've done it so many times, I know every turn, every bump, every pothole to avoid, every place to pee –

halfway, there's a country store and I'll get a fried apple pie. I do this ride alone anytime I get home. It's an amazing workout, it's beautiful, it doesn't feel like training and despite being really hard – I always burn at least 5000 kcal – it never feels like an effort. This is my absolute Cycling Nirvana.'

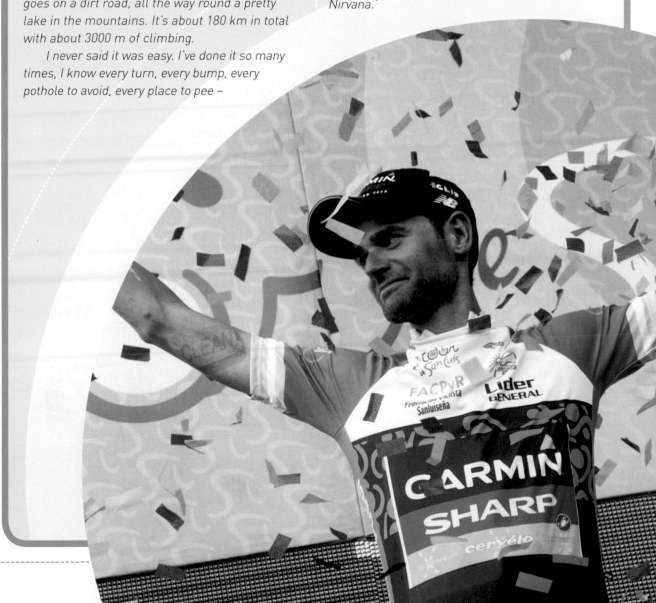

7 RECOVERY: WHEN THE CYCLING STOPS

"Nutrition, massage and sleep all play important parts in my recovery strategy. It's about the balance, timing and most importantly consistency."

Tom Danielson AMERICAN PRO CYCLIST AND TWO-TIME TOUR OF UTAH WINNER

Line up 100 pro cyclists and ask them for one piece of advice and many will talk about the importance of recovery. Without adequate rest and recuperation (R and R), you're not giving your body a chance to recover from the stresses you've placed upon it. See it as the key that unlocks the door to progression and improvement.

BELOW Pro cyclists benefit from having a support team to help them recover after races

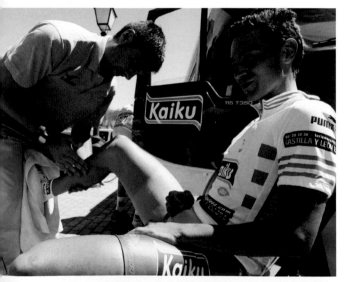

Riding a Grand Tour requires the body to remain on top form on a daily basis for three weeks, which is why pro teams employ an extensive backroom staff including everybody from physiotherapists and masseurs, to chiropractors, osteopaths, nutritionists and chefs. Without a support team, no cyclist would finish a three-week race, let alone compete in one. Just because you're not a pro doesn't mean you shouldn't take your recovery seriously. If you ride on a regular basis, you need to give your body a chance to recover afterwards.

■ *'Recovery is such an important component of cycling,'* says former Spanish pro cyclist and winner of the 2008 Tour de France, Carlos Sastre. *'If you get it wrong, you could get ill, injured and your performance will suffer. After any heavy bouts of cycling you have to recover and give your body a chance to adapt and grow stronger.'*

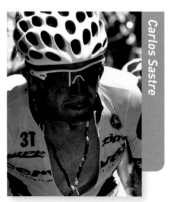

Carlos Sastre

The fundamentals

During heavy bouts of cycling, the body is under enormous strain: muscle fibres get damaged; the heart and lungs are continuously working hard; the temperature regulatory system is working flat out to keep body temperature down and manage sweat rates; endorphins are released that help to diminish your perception of pain; and the immune system is temporarily weakened. There's a *lot* going on and, don't forget, cycling also depletes the body of its glycogen stores, nutrients, minerals and fluids. It's no wonder you need to focus on recovery after each ride.

The warm-down

The initial hours immediately after cycling are important for helping to return the body to a resting state and the first step is a warm-down. This is still a relatively new topic to sports science, but, increasingly, people are starting to understand the importance of it.

When you stop cycling, the systems of your body continue to work at a heightened level, remaining at an elevated state preparing for *more* exercise. A warm-down will begin to switch your body into recovery mode by helping to gradually lower your body temperature and your body's hyper-active state, as well as helping clear the muscles of lactic acid, a by-product of exercise that can cause muscle soreness.

■ *'After a hard day's racing, the finish is uncontrolled as you may sometimes roll in easy or it may be a hard sprint or an uphill finish,'* says Canadian pro cyclist and 2012 Giro d'Italia winner Ryder Hesjedal. *'To just finish the race and pull the brakes and stop makes no sense. After most race finishes I'll jump on the rollers for 10 minutes. It allows me to wind down and ease the body temperature down, and loosens the muscles up before I stop for the day. Recovery starts immediately after you cross the finish line and the warm-down is the first part of that.*

If I'm training, I can control my own finish and I just cruise for the last 10 minutes till I get home.'

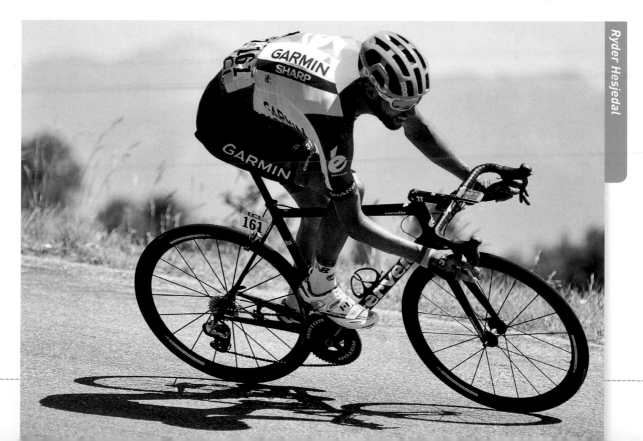

Ryder Hesjedal

A warm-down doesn't need to last long, nor does it require specific structuring. You can use the last 10 minutes of your ride to gradually slow down and ride easy *or* you can do a warm-down at home when you finish riding consisting of stretches, movements and exercises. See the pain-free cyclist warm-down on page 201 for a routine to help you recover when you get in from your ride.

To stretch or not?

A 2007 review of the literature showed that stretching doesn't prevent delayed onset muscle soreness, but it's still heavily practised and advocated because it can help you relax and simply feels good. 'When I get in from a long ride my hip flexors often feel tight so I'll spend a few minutes stretching those out.' says Australian pro cyclist, Rohan Dennis.

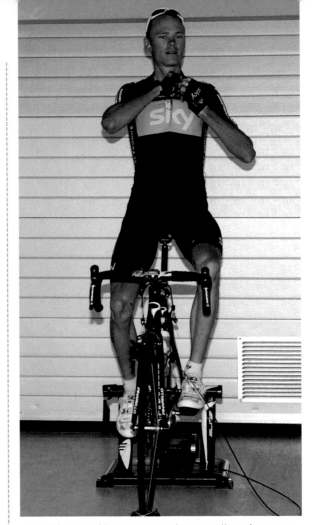

ABOVE Many pro riders now warm down on rollers after a race

> ### Delayed onset muscle soreness (DOMS)
>
> Heavy and achy legs that occur 2–3 days after a big ride, that's DOMS. Caused by either lactic acid build-up or miniscule tears to the muscle fibres, DOMS takes a couple of days to come to fruition. Effects aren't long lasting, it's nothing to worry about and shouldn't significantly affect performance. And the good news is the fitter you get, the less chance you'll get it.

Nutrition for recovery

Nutrition plays an important role in the recovery process. Inadequate nutrition has the ability to bring the strongest of cyclists to a standstill, putting an immediate halt on performance. Once you have warmed down, you should adhere to the three 'R's: Rehydrate (water and key electrolytes), Replenish (energy) and Repair (damaged muscles). The longer you ride, the more the recovery nutrition is important. If you ride at low to

medium intensity for an hour to 90 minutes, you should be aware of these strategies but they're not so important. For rides of 2–3 hours or longer, or higher intensity shorter rides, nutrition to help your recovery becomes more important.

■ Ryder Hesjedal says: *'Have your recovery drink ready when you get home so that you can start rehydrating and replenishing energy while doing your warm-down exercises.'*

Rehydrate

Water will go some way to rehydrate you, but to optimally rehydrate after longer rides it's not ideal as you need to replace the salts lost in your sweat.

Drinks containing sodium promotes absorption of water in the small intestine, encourages thirst, and helps delay the rate at which you urinate – perfect to rehydrate you. You can also include some sugars (carbohydrates) in your drink as these help replace glycogen stores and will also taste better encouraging you to drink more.

Recommendation: 1.5 litres of fluid for every 1 kg of weight loss – most sports drinks are ideal for this.

You will continue to sweat as you recover and possibly lose some fluid to urine. This is the reason for drinking more than the equivalent weight loss.

Replenish glycogen

■ *'After a long ride, I'll eat within 30 minutes of getting home,'* says British pro cyclist, Tao Geoghegan Hart. *'I usually eat porridge or rice and eggs. For me, it makes a big difference to eat right away and get my glycogen stores replenished quickly.'*

Carbohydrates will restore glycogen stores used during the ride, replacing the body's main fuel source in the muscles and liver.

The golden hour

This refers to the hour window after exercise in which the body is more receptive to the intake of fuel. This hour is when your muscles are able to soak up incoming carbohydrates and optimise glycogen stores. Waiting longer than two hours reduces short-term muscle glycogen re-synthesis by as much as 50 per cent. This is due to the role carbohydrate consumption has on insulin production, which aids production of muscle glycogen. Insulin levels peak within 40 minutes after exercise, and then fall dramatically. Failure to take advantage of this has a knock-on effect, resulting in your body taking much longer to recover.

Real foods

Real foods are recommended. However you can kill *three* birds with one stone by consuming a sports drink that contains electrolytes, carbohydrates and proteins to increase the chances of optimising your recovery in the golden hour.

Recommendation: 1 gram of carbohydrate per kg of body weight immediately after riding. Then you can go back to your normal meal strategies. This is the best way to help rebuild glycogen stores after exercise.

Repair (damaged muscle):

To help optimally repair muscle tissue that gets damaged during hard riding, the body requires protein immediately afterwards. Think of protein as the building blocks of muscles. Proteins also help stabilise blood sugar levels and strengthen the temporarily weakened immune system.

For a ride under an hour, the need for protein isn't as great as you probably haven't worked the body hard enough. Many amateur cyclists will work out for 45 minutes or so, and then consume a recovery drink, full of protein, carbohydrates and calories. It's simply not required, and they wonder why they aren't losing weight.

Recommendation: For hard rides of longer than an hour, 20 g of high-quality lean protein is advised.

Foods containing 10g protein

- 1 cup low fat milk or soy milk
- 200 g low fat yoghurt
- 40 g skinless cooked chicken
- 2 small eggs
- 4 slices bread
- 60 g nuts or seeds

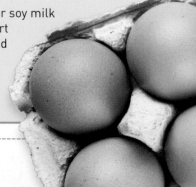

Sleep

Want to *really* enhance your recovery? Get a good night's sleep. 'Sleep is the most powerful recovery aid out there,' says retired American cyclist and 2012 US Road Race champion, Timmy Duggan. And he's right. Sleep is when your body is able to rebuild most effectively. Your body recharges, muscle repair can take place and you aren't exerting excess energy. Your immune system is also at its strongest when at complete rest.

■ British pro cyclist, Geraint Thomas says: *'Sleep is as important as any training session that you do. It is where your body adapts to the training. Getting it right will help optimise your improvement gains; get it wrong and you can end up going backwards.'*

Good sleep – anywhere between six and eight hours – is essential for this process to occur. There are a few top tips you can try to ensure you are optimising your sleep.

Good sleep habits

- Maintain a regular bedtime.
- Avoid stimulants such as caffeine and alcohol in the hours before you go to bed (yes, alcohol encourages sleep onset but as it gets metabolised in the body it causes arousal later into the sleep cycle).
- Eat your last meal at least 90 minutes before bedtime.
- Associate your bed with sleep; avoid watching TV, reading or listening to the radio in bed.
- Sleep in a dark room.
- Avoid vigorous exercise in the evening.

CYCLING NIRVANA
Cadel Evans
AUSTRALIA | 2009 WORLD CHAMPION AND 2011 TOUR DE FRANCE WINNER

■ *'I've been very lucky over my career and cycling has given me a lot of great opportunities. For me, when I think of Cycling Nirvana there are three stand out moments that I think back to.*

The first was when I was a junior still living in Australia. I was riding through the National Park near where I lived, miles away from anyone on my own and I remember chasing six kangaroos through the bush. The whole thing felt playful as I was with them following them through the park, I could hear them bounding through the park as they sped ahead and I followed in awe on my bike. At that young age it reinforced to me the opportunities you get when riding a bike, and since then, riding a bike has brought me nearly everything I have. The power and the movement and noise of the kangaroos was amazing and I was there with them, out in the middle of nowhere with nobody else around, a memory I hark back to as, after everything I've done in my career, here I am, 20 years later, still talking about it.

The last 3 km of the 2009 World Championships in Mendrisio I was riding solo at about 60 kph on a big gear. I remember it was 53–11, and I felt like I had the whole world behind me as well as 250 of the best cyclists in the world, and only the finish line in front of me. I didn't know if I was racing or if I was dreaming. It was special, and a huge Cycling Nirvana moment, as that road was about 2 km from where I live, and I've ridden that road literally hundreds if not thousands of times before. It's not as if I was thinking about how close they were behind me, I didn't know the time gaps, but that day everything came together. When I attacked up the last climb, which was 10 per cent in places, I did it in a huge gear, 53–17. I've done that same climb many times since that day and have never been able to get up the climb in the same gear. That was my day. Every time I ride that stretch of road again, I can't help but think of that day in 2009 and it gives me a great feeling. That was my day.

The last 6–10 km of the final time trial of the 2011 Tour de France, I couldn't feel my legs. Normally by that point in the final TT of a Grand Tour your legs are on fire and burning up. My director was in my ear on the radio telling me to slow down, not to risk it, which meant I knew I was going well, but I felt focused, in a trance, in my own world.

As I crossed the finish line I had come second in the TT by two seconds, I think, but I had all but won the Tour de France. A moment like that stays with you forever. I'd been to the Tour for seven years and been second twice and now I had won it. Does Cycling Nirvana get any better than that? I think it took me six months to even realise what I'd done. I was driving alone six months later and I remember having to pull over in the car as it had just hit me that I had won the Tour, what it really meant. I guess I relived that Cycling Nirvana moment in my car all alone that day all over again.'

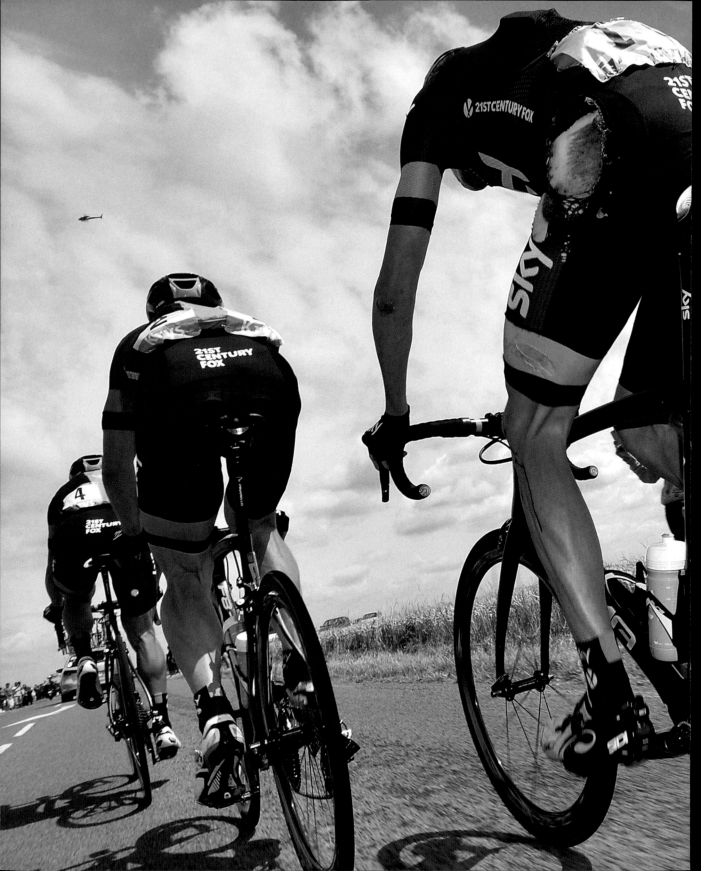

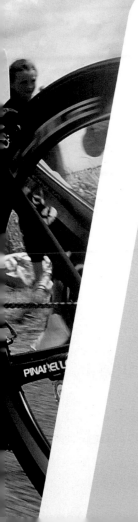

There's so much information and misinformation out there, it's hard to know what to trust. For cycling injuries, it's simple – start with this book. Find out what you need to know, apply it, put the injury behind you and get back out on the bike.

Andreas Klier RETIRED GERMAN PRO CYCLIST AND GENT-WEVELGEM WINNER

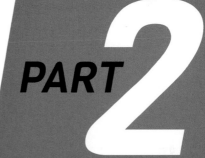

PART 2

INJURIES

Wouldn't it be nice if you could guarantee a pain-free ride every time you went out on your bike? If you could avoid crashes or scrapes and instead concentrate on polishing your performance on the open road. Unfortunately, however fastidious you are about bike fit, however rigidly you stick to your core strength programme and however dedicated you are to your nutrition, you will get injured from time to time. That's just the nature of cycling.

Cycling might not be as aggressive as boxing, or as high impact as running but the repetitive action involved in pedalling combined with the unnatural position maintained on the bike – we weren't designed to be supported on all fours – mean overuse injuries are almost inevitable. The other danger point is, of course, crashing. Potholes, bad weather, other road users and lack of concentration all create a dangerous cocktail that can get the better of even the most experienced of riders.

Glossary of terms

It can be tempting to ignore aches and pains; after all, they often mean time off the bike, frustrating for any keen cyclist. But pain is your body's red light – the warning sign that something isn't right. Learn to act on the correct signs quickly, and you'll be back on the bike in no time. Ignore the warning signs and you risk lengthy periods off the bike, recurring injuries and significant periods of pain.

Before we dig into the ten most common cycling injuries themselves, we're going to give you some really useful background on the advice and treatment options that we'll be prescribing – from the first checks you should do when you feel an injury, the correct dosage of painkillers should you need to take them, how and why different treatments work, and which practitioner is best for which problem. It'll give you an instant head start, stop us repeating ourselves as we tackle the injuries later on and, most crucially, gift you with the tools to pinpoint your injury super-quick. Below we have compiled an index of all things injury related that we will refer to as we discuss the injuries. From foam rollers to hands-on treatment, from medication to recovery rides, it's all here spelled out to navigate you out of pain and into Cycling Nirvana.

First aid for injuries

REDUCING THE PAIN

You're probably familiar with the acronym 'RICE', (rest, ice, compression and elevation), as you've probably had it drilled into you at a young age if you were keen at sports. But familiarity and understanding are two separate things. We'll let you know the specifics of application of each of these when we go through the injuries individually

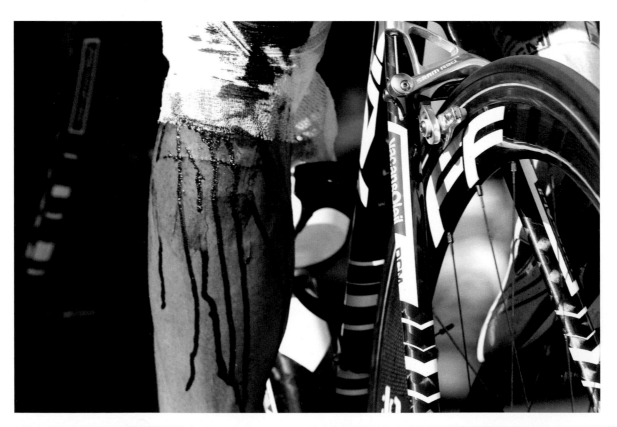

as many are still relevant today, but for now it's important you know *why* we'll be telling you to do them and how they work. The objective is to swiftly reduce the pain and discomfort, which is even more important when symptoms persist off the bike.

REST

Gone are the days when rest means putting your feet up and lying in bed while you wait for your symptoms to resolve. Nowadays, when we're talking about rest, it means reducing, or preferably stopping, any activity that causes the symptoms you're suffering from being aggravated. Basically, if what you're doing is making the symptoms worse off the bike, then it should be avoided. For example, if you're getting knee pain when you ride, but you don't when you're walking or swimming, then these are fine. If you get the same knee pain when you're running, then running should be avoided. Pain is your friend, remember. Listen to your body and avoid any activities such as specific exercises in the gym that are irritating your symptoms. Rest essentially means reducing the load on the injured part of the body to provide an optimal environment for healing to take place.

ICE

Applying ice reduces the temperature of damaged tissue, causing the local blood vessels to constrict, which will help reduce the swelling that occurs when tissue is damaged. As this starts to happen, pressure is alleviated around the site of the injury, helping to reduce symptoms. Yes, swelling is the body's natural first line of defence following injury, but the response is usually slightly over the top, like sending a whole fire brigade to put out a fire in a waste paper basket. Excess swelling can actually delay the healing process. By applying ice, the body is better able to organise its healing response. Ice is the easiest and safest form of anti-inflammatory and painkiller there is and can provide great relief from symptoms such as sprains of joints or muscle strains in their acute stage, for example, the first week of an injury and sometimes even longer in certain circumstances.

We'll discuss the best application method for each injury; but you won't go far wrong applying ice for 10–20 minutes to the site of injury up to three times a day. Always remember to cover the ice in a cloth/tea towel to avoid ice burns.

Heat rubs, creams and sprays

e.g. Deep Heat, Tiger Balm and Rock Sauce
These rapidly absorb into the skin, and act in
a similar way to heat treatment although the
effects aren't as penetrating. They're most
effectively used to help reduce symptoms in
tight muscles, although again, not advised in the
first week following injury. These should never
be applied to broken or irritated skin. In some
cases they may also promote skin reactions
such as rashes, burns and blisters, so testing
it on a small area of skin first is advised.

Compression and elevation

Traditionally, compression meant apply some
form of elastic bandage around an injured area
to help limit and decrease the swelling to aid
recovery. While elevation referred to keeping the
injured area of the body raised (typically above
the level of the heart) to also help limit swelling
by reducing the effects of gravity on the injured
area and helping the return of blood flow to the
heart.

While there's still some merit in the use of
compression and elevation for many injuries,
it doesn't much apply in the classical sense
to the common cycling injuries that we'll go
through. You won't often see many cyclists using
'Tubigrip' or other compression bandages while
riding as freedom of movement is all-important
and they're too restrictive to provide any benefit
for the majority of injuries that relate to cycling.

As we see it, Kinesio tape covers the
compression and elevation element of the RICE
mnemonic as there's both a compressive and
elevative element to it.

RIGHT Pro riders are keen advocates of kinesio tape

Kinesio tape

Kinesio tape, kinesiology tape, or RockTape
– whatever you call it, or whatever brand you
choose, the adhesive flexible tape, when applied,
can help support and protect vulnerable, painful
and possibly injured parts of the body either away
from the bike or as you start to integrate back
into cycling following injury.

The next time you watch a pro bike race,
look closely at the riders on your screen, you'll
likely see some colourful strips of tape running
down the front of their legs, or poking out from
under their jersey. You don't even need to look
that far as the use of this tape has trickled down
to mainstream use with everyone from weekend
warriors to sportive riders reaping the benefits.

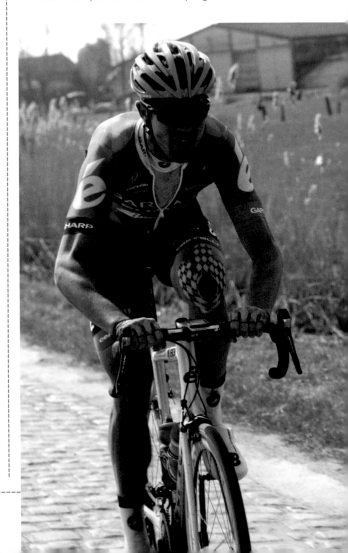

Kinesio tape was invented by Japanese chiropractor, Kenzo Kase, in the 1970s. He claimed that the tape could help alleviate pain, reduce inflammation (by elevating the skin away from the damaged tissue and improving drainage of the swelling), relax muscles, help with rehabilitation by getting muscle to engage and even enhance performance. It's worth noting that there hasn't been a lot of substantial evidence to back up all these claims but that hasn't stopped athletes, including pro cyclists, from using it.

In our rehab toolkit you'll find all the kinesio tape applications we recommend under the region of the body that they relate to, see page 175–200. We'll show you how to apply it to specific areas of the body and advise you when it might be applicable to use it as we go through the relevant injury recommendations.

 When you see this icon you may want to consider using the tape for support.

MATT SAYS:

'Yes, there's little evidence that the tape does what its creators claim and there's certainly no magic in the tape. However, for a low impact sport like cycling, it offers support when applied to certain parts of the body to help reduce symptoms while you ride (or even help manage symptoms off the bike). It's not a fix, it's not a cure, but when used alongside other forms of injury management it definitely has a part to play.'

TIPS ON KINESIO TAPE APPLICATION
Kinesio tape is relatively simple to apply on yourself, but like anything it takes a little practice to get right. After five minutes you'll barely notice that it's there. If you find you're using the tape on a regular basis just to get

you through, go back through the section of the book that relates to the related injury and work through the appropriate rehab programme to get the injury fully resolved.

- Apply to clean dry skin.
- Rub the tape after you've applied it for a minute or so as warming the area will help the glue stick better.
- If you can shave the hair around the area you're applying it to, it will stick better.
- Once applied be careful putting on clothing (jersey, socks, etc.) to not peel the tape off before you've headed out!
- If you round the edges of each piece of tape, it will reduce the chances of the edges peeling up.

 A small proportion of people will have a mild skin reaction to the tape; if this happens, you should avoid using it.

GOAL OF USING THE TAPE
Your objective if you use the tape to help you integrate back into cycling, is three consecutive pain-free rides wearing the tape before continuing to ride without it. If the pain returns when you stop using the tape, continue to support the injured area when you ride with the tape for the next couple of weeks while you work through the exercises we recommend in each section before reducing the usage. You can use the tape off the bike for support and to help provide relief from symptoms as you see appropriate.

Over-the-counter medication

We ideally want your ride to be pain free through natural intervention rather than with the use of pain killing tablets, or anti-inflammatory pills or gels. However, when pain gets too much, you might find yourself reaching for the medicine cupboard, so it's good to know what you should be reaching to grab.

PARACETAMOL

 This is a mild painkiller (analgesic), one of the most widely used medications in the world, and a go-to medicine for relieving common aches and pains. How it actually works still isn't fully understood but it's thought that it acts by stimulating a protein on nerve cells that interferes with communication and reduces the transmission to the brain of information from pain-sensing nerves in damaged or irritated tissue. Remember, this means you will 'sense' there's less pain, but the problem almost certainly still exists, you're just not getting the painful reminder.

Paracetamol won't have much of an effect on severe pain, but for mild to moderate pain such as sprains, stiffness in the joints and muscles, and headaches, for example, it can help ease the discomfort. Paracetamol can also help to reduce the mild aches and pains associated with the common cold and has been shown to help reduce fever.

Most people can take paracetamol without any problems, but you should speak to your doctor or pharmacist before taking it if you regularly drink large amounts of alcohol or you have known liver or kidney problems as they can suppress functioning.

Dosage: For adults: 500 mg to 1 g (one dose) every 4–6 hours. Do not take more than four doses of paracetamol within 24 hours.

> Paracetamol is often combined with other ingredients in over-the-counter medications. For example, it can be combined with a decongestant medicine and sold as a cold and flu remedy. So always read the label.

NON-STEROIDAL ANTI-INFLAMMATORY DRUGS (NSAIDS)

 e.g. aspirin and ibuprofen 'COX' enzymes help to make other proteins called prostaglandins at the site of tissue damage and injury, and these prostaglandins are involved in the production of pain and inflammation, which typically leads to local swelling. Prostaglandins also protect the lining of the stomach from the damaging and corrosive effects of certain stomach acids. NSAIDs work by blocking the effects of these COX enzymes meaning a reduction in prostaglandin production which in turn reduces pain and inflammation.

For injuries that are severely painful, NSAIDs won't do much, but for mild to moderate pain such as the majority of cycling injuries they can be effective at reducing both pain and inflammation.

The two most commonly used NSAIDs are aspirin and ibuprofen taken orally. Aspirin affects the blood clotting system, leading to a slight thinning of the blood that could cause increased bleeding within the damaged tissue and delay the recovery process. Ibuprofen doesn't affect blood clotting to the same extent as aspirin.

While NSAIDs reduce pain and inflammation they can have a negative effect on gut health by reducing the COX enzymes that protect the stomach's lining from the acids that digest food. Continued use of NSAIDs can lead to ulcers and bleeding as the lining of the stomach becomes vulnerable.

Of course, we're all different so medications can affect us differently, and using a coated aspirin may work for some people to reduce stomach irritation.

NSAIDs may help reduce pain and discomfort of an injury, but if you can do without them, you are encouraged to try to, as pain will be your guide to which activities could further damage

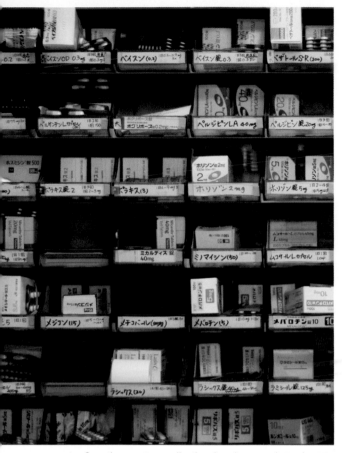

ABOVE Over the counter medication does have a role to play

the injured area. Also, there's not a lot of evidence suggesting they will make you heal any faster; in fact, prolonged use for several days after injury can actually slow down your body's natural healing response.

Dosage: Every NSAID has its own dose and interval for how often to take the drug. It's very important you don't exceed the recommendations.

If they are being prescribed, the GP will give the lowest effective dose for the shortest period of time necessary.

- Ibuprofen: 200–400 mg of ibuprofen, 3–4 times daily if needed.
- Aspirin: 1–3 (300 mg) tablets every 4–6 hours when needed, but you should not take more than 4 g (13 tablets) in a 24-hour period.

TOPICAL NSAIDS

e.g. Voltarol
These come in the form of gels, creams and patches and are applied directly onto the skin over the injured area. They absorb through the skin exerting their effects only on the area they're applied to rather than on the body as a whole as the orally taken ones are. They work by the same mechanism as the oral NSAIDs but because they don't pass through the digestive system, they're less likely to cause side effects, such as irritation to the stomach lining, making them better tolerated for individuals sensitive to oral NSAIDs. However, some will naturally enter the bloodstream so if you have a history of disorders affecting the stomach or intestines, you should consult your doctor and limit the amount you apply.

Topical NSAIDs are particularly advantageous when the injury is superficial to the surface of the body as it's more likely to get absorbed right to the site of the injury, for example, the Achilles tendon.

Dosage: Depending on the size of the painful area and the type and brand you use, you should apply approximately a pea size blob (2–4 g) to the affected area and rub it in until it's absorbed 3–4 times a day or as per the instructions on the packet. In some cases they can cause skin irritation, so always test on a small area first and they should never be applied to broken or already irritated skin.

 Choose between oral or topical NSAIDS, never use both to avoid overdosing. If you need to reduce symptoms before you ride by using medication (not that we would encourage you to do so), then at least use topical NSAIDs as the orally taken version is more likely to irritate your stomach and cause discomfort when you ride.

Foam rollers

As we continue to dig down into practices that can make a difference as you attempt to banish your injury, there's one piece of kit a keen cyclist should invest in: a foam roller. When used correctly this inexpensive tool will help release tension and tightness between the muscles and the fascia (the tissue that surrounds the muscles) and help your recovery when you get back from cycling.

'After most training sessions I'll use the foam roller,' says German road cyclist, Fabian Wegmann. 'It's easy – I can sit in front of the TV, unwind, use my roller and this helps my muscles recover. It's a worthwhile investment.'

Ok, it might not be a substitute for a thorough massage in skilled hands, but there's no doubting that it's quicker, easier, cheaper and can be performed almost anywhere, and most importantly can be used as and when the time is right for you. See it as 'self massage', your portable therapist ready and on hand whenever you need it.

Many cyclists use foam rollers to aid the recovery process, as research has shown it can help ease muscle tension and reduce muscle soreness after high intensity exercise. By also helping to improve range of motion it can help return tightened muscles to their appropriate functional length, which will also increase comfort both on and off the bike.

Foam rollers aren't just a recovery tool though, they can also help with your warm-up, as they aid blood flow to the muscles and increase muscle temperature.

In our rehab toolkit you'll find all the foam rolling routines we recommend under the region of the body that they relate to, see page 190–91.

HOW TO USE AND CHOOSE A FOAM ROLLER

There are many variations of foam roller on the market, ones to suit you whatever your budget may be, from relatively cheap lightweight rollers, ones covered in nobbles and bobbles to get stuck into muscles, and the more elaborate, expensive branded ones. The type we recommend is simple, go for the cheap and cheerful lightweight version that is about the 15–20 cm in diameter and smooth, and looks a bit like no.1.

Or if your budget extends to it, a worthy investment is to get a quality roller such as the TPT therapy roller that they call 'The Grid' (no.2). This too is a lightweight robust roller, and attempts to closely mimic the 'feel' of a firm hand against the body when rolling, making it more closely resemble a 'real' massage.

Having a tennis ball or a specialist massage ball such as the TPT massage ball (no.3) is also useful to target specific focal muscles that you can't reach with a foam roller and we'll explain when and how to use it as we go through the individual injuries in the rehab toolkit.

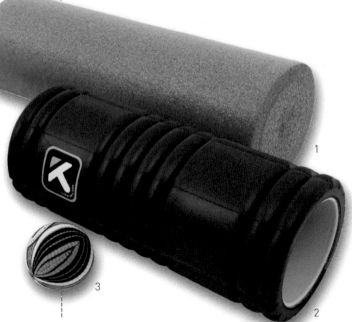

MATT SAYS:

'The Grid is always the roller I recommend people to get if their budget extends to it. Foam rollers may all look the same but how they perform is key. Having spent time with the "inventor" of this piece of kit, I have no problem endorsing its use, as I've consistently got great feedback from many pro cyclists who use it on a daily basis.'

Tips for using a foam roller

- Rolling muscles in a rush is a waste of time; use the roller when you have at least five minutes to focus on a particular area.
- Use the foam roller to help scan your muscles because getting to know your troublesome areas will better assist your ability to target its use for your particular needs.
- Remember it can be used as part of your warm-up as well as for recovery.
- Take it slow to begin with and you'll get more out of the rolling.
- It *will* hurt, but this is a good pain and it will get easier as the muscles become looser.
- Start at one end of a muscle and work to the other end and back again to ensure you get all the tight spots.

 See the rolling routines we recommend explained under the area of the body you are trying to target in the rehab toolkit.

Rehab Exercises

Once the initial pain and discomfort has settled, the aim is to chase the injury further away, keep it away and prevent it from coming back. This is where your rehabilitation *really* begins. We'll explain the exercises you need to perform and when you should start them as we go through each injury in turn – exercises will help to further settle down discomfort, mobilise problem areas and increase strength in weak muscles, to help give you the support you need to move you to the next level. You'll find all the exercises laid out by regions of the body in the rehab toolkit (see page 157–203).

GETTING BACK ON THE BIKE

 We'll let you know how much time we recommend to take off the bike for each of the 10 injuries in our 'injury at a glance' section. This will give you a rough idea of how long you can expect to be sidelined from cycling.

BELOW Getting back to bike riding is your goal

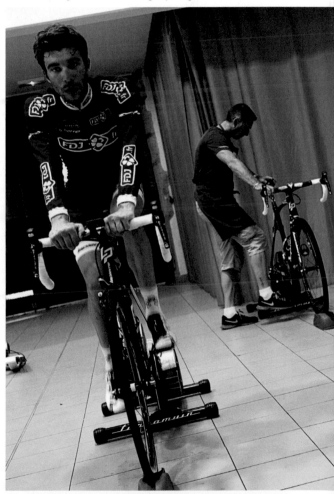

THE HOME TRAINER

Depending on the injury, we may suggest your first few rides back from injury are in the comfort of your own home on the home trainer. This will have a much lower impact on the body so is less likely to cause irritation of your recovering injury compared to riding on the road. This is for a number of reasons: you don't need to balance; you won't have a pedestrian potentially stepping out in front of you; there's no braking required; the ride is smoother as you won't have the vibrations coming from the road; there are no potholes; it'll be less stop and start; you won't need to unclip at traffic lights, etc. Eliminating these factors means a reduced load and stress on the body as you come back from injury, which we will recommend for certain injuries.

When we recommend the home trainer, see it as part of your rehab back into cycling and you should only return to the road once you feel totally comfortable riding and handling the bike and have no problem or discomfort getting on and off the bike. As a general rule you should spend a week or two riding the home trainer before you get back out onto the road when recommended.

When you see this icon, it means we suggest you start riding the home trainer before returning to the road.

RECOVERY RIDES

Once you progress to the road, it's important that the first ride back from injury is a 'recovery ride'. By this we mean an easy ride of low to medium intensity and not longer than 90 minutes duration. Riding on roads familiar to you is also recommended as you'll know where possible obstacles, such as road furniture and potholes, may lie. Riding flatter roads when possible will put less stress on your recovering injury and is also advised. This ride is designed to let your body feel its way back into cycling while you monitor for any discomfort from your injury.

BELOW Take your recovery rides easy

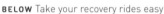

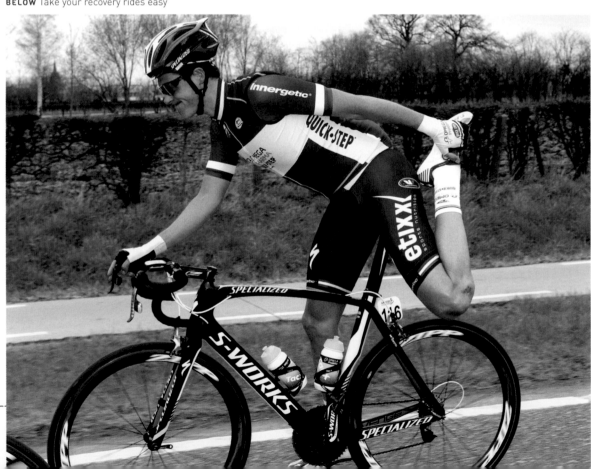

MONITORING YOUR RETURN TO CYCLING
It's not unusual to feel some mild discomfort from your recovering injury as you start riding again. If the discomfort builds or the pain persists after 20–30 minutes of riding once your body is fully warmed up, then there's no point in pushing it, your body may not be quite ready. Stop and take a few more days off before trying again. Apply some ice to the injury when you get back and run through any exercises we recommend for that particular injury.

Warming-up and warming-down

We've discussed the benefit of a good warm-up. As you get back to cycling following injury, it's even more important to get your body properly warm and loose. This is the time to put a thorough warm-up into practice. We've chosen a selection of exercises from our rehab toolkit to help prepare your body for the rigours of cycling. Each exercise works on specific parts of the body – either warming up key muscles that are essential for cycling or loosening up the spine and joints that will help support both symmetry and flexibility on the bike, getting you ready to perform.

As we've stated earlier in the book, when the pedalling stops, the recovery starts. After the ride is when the real work begins and it starts the moment you unclip from the pedals. Throughout the duration of your ride, the muscles have been working damn hard and have become tired and are in desperate need of some tender loving care. You may also find that certain joints will have stiffened and tightened as well. Don't worry, this isn't unusual, and providing you follow some simple post-cycling exercises, this will ease, and your body will thank you for it.

However, ignore a good warm-down and the body could take longer to recover and even make simple tasks like sitting at a desk, or getting out of bed uncomfortable. You've been out riding your bike for hours; don't ignore these last 10–15 minutes. It can make the world of difference. We've selected a handful of exercises from our rehab toolkit specifically designed to help your body unwind and recover when you get off your bike.

Core stability

We've already told you we think it's worthwhile to start a core exercise routine for cycling, but as you come back from injury, when should this begin? As we go through each of the 10 injuries, we'll let you know the best time to start your routine alongside any other rehab work we've recommended for you. We've selected some exercises from our rehab toolkit as a fundamental core exercise programme to help you become more stable, comfortable and robust on the bike and prevent the likelihood of another overuse injury occurring – see page 202. We also ramp up the difficulty of these exercises once you have mastered the first programme, so there's enough to be getting on with to move you towards Cycling Nirvana.

By the time you're ready to start your core work, you may well be familiar with many of the exercises as there's a lot of crossover between exercises we recommend for rehab of specific injuries and those we recommend as part of our core routine. We'd love to help prevent traumatic injuries too, but Aussie pro Steele Von Hoff tells it how it is: 'I didn't crash in the whole of 2013 which was my first year as a pro whereas by April in 2014 I had already crashed five times. You unfortunately never know when a crash will be around the corner.'

 When you see this icon you know it's the week to start your core exercise routine.

Expert help

Hopefully it's not required often, but from time to time you may need outside help from an expert, but as everyone is an 'expert' these days, where do you start?

Not too long ago practitioners such as physiotherapists, osteopaths and chiropractors were seen as a luxury, available only to elite athletes, but over time people have become more knowledgeable about the body and the benefits these practitioners can give us might afford us. The need to optimise performance and minimise injury applies to anyone taking their cycling seriously – and has resulted in huge demand for sports practitioners.

For years, physios were the 'go-to' for help treating injuries. Chiropractors and osteopaths were always a secondary option. Now that education has been standardised for these professions and both chiropractors and osteopaths are nationally registered as protected titled professionals this now means that, if you visit one, you can at least be certain they're qualified as it's now illegal to call yourself either without the appropriate qualifications.

In years gone by, a doctor would normally only refer you to a physio but nowadays there are plenty of practitioners to choose from, each with different ideas and treatments that can help identify and treat your injury and help you get back on the mend. Don't limit your choices.

So let's take a look at what's on offer, and how they can help. When it comes to the 10 most common cycling injuries we'll direct you to which practitioners are most appropriate for your problem, plan A, and those that you might consider as plan B options, suitable but probably not the first port of call.

PHYSIOTHERAPY

Sports physios specialising in musculoskeletal injuries can help to restore normal balance and function of the body by correcting biomechanical issues, weakness, stiffness and asymmetry. They typically promote independence and self-management and don't just focus on rehab. In fact, for the modern sports physio, a lot of attention concentrates on 'prehab', a pro-active way of addressing weakness and imbalances before they become injuries.

A physio with an understanding of cycling can be extremely beneficial as they can often help to assess the function of riding positions and issues within the musculoskeletal chain. Physios will usually focus on strengthening the body through specific exercises as well as possibly tweaking the bike set-up (some bike fitters may actually be physios) to optimise position for comfort and performance. Physios would be the first choice to go to when recovering from surgery as their rehab skills are particularly well suited to this environment, above and beyond that of other approaches.

What to look for:

- Physios registered with the Chartered Society of Physiotherapists (CSP).
- A post-graduate qualification such as an MSc in Sports Physiotherapy or Sports and Exercise Medicine will mean they'll be well suited to help you.

OSTEOPATHY

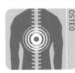

Osteopaths tend to examine the body as a whole, paying particular attention to the spine, and will aim to develop optimal function of the body through treatment. Osteopathy uses a variety of hands-on treatments, excluding the use of drugs or surgery, such as manipulations, soft tissue work and trigger point massage to help injuries improve.

They can be extremely advantageous to cyclists both for injury prevention, treatment of injuries and helping performance. Osteopaths with an interest in cycling will focus on the biomechanics of riding, ensuring the body is functioning at its peak, to maximise performance and minimise injury.

An osteopath will both try to prevent injuries from occurring and treat cyclists recovering from injuries as they can help where there's stiffness in the muscles or joints and begin to loosen them with specific manipulations, some slow and rhythmic and others fast.

What to look for:

- All UK osteopaths should be registered with the General Osteopathic Council (GOC).
- You can search for a UK osteopath at osteopathy.org.uk.
- Osteopaths with an interest in treating sports injuries are likely to be members of the Osteopathic Sports Care Association (OSCA).

CHIROPRACTIC

Chiropractic is a hands-on profession that treats biomechanical problems to do with joints, muscles and tissues predominantly of the spine without the use of drugs or surgery. Chiropractors will find out what is wrong with the individual biomechanically – meaning to do with the joints or muscles – and help to improve the range of motion of restricted joints, mobility and stability, addressing these issues in order to get the body working back at its full potential.

If you're riding a bike and you feel pain or if you get off the bike and something doesn't feel quite right, then a chiropractor with a sports emphasis could help identify the cause of the problem and improve it through manipulations and stretches, releasing tight muscles and prescribing exercises to help increase flexibility and reduce muscle tension and stiffness. If you have constant niggles, aches or pains that you cannot shift yourself or long-term reduction in range of movement in particular joints, a chiropractor can help ease these issues and improve function.

What to look for:

- All UK chiropractors should be registered with the General Chiropractic Council (GCC).
- You can search for a UK sports chiropractor at chirosport.org.
- Ideally look for practitioners holding the ICCSD qualification if possible, but not essential. The International Chiropractic Sports Science Diploma (ICCSD) programme produces chiropractors qualified to work at sporting events throughout the world. It's the minimum qualification required to be part of an official chiropractic delegation at international events such as the Olympic Games.

DOCTOR

Your doctor will be able to identify whether there's something they can help you with, or whether they need to refer you to someone else more appropriate. It will typically be your doctor you need to see if you feel you need stronger painkillers than can be purchased

MATT SAYS:

'What's the difference between chiropractors and osteopaths? A question I get asked on an almost daily basis. There are more similarities than differences between chiropractic and osteopathy than there are similarities between both professions and physiotherapy. As far as I'm concerned each profession simply offers a different door to the same house. We all treat the same things but go about it using different methods. Which is "better" is an impossible question to answer as it lies in the skills of the practitioner themselves.

Don't get too caught up in the "profession" that's treating you. Find out more about the specific person who's treating you, how they approach your injury, what techniques they use, etc. It's better to go and see a good practitioner than a bad one whatever their profession is; so not getting caught up in the "I need to see a chiro" or "I must see a physio" will keep you open to all of them and hopefully allow you to find the best person to treat you for your problem. One approach may work for some and not others, that's life. The most important thing is to find someone you can trust and that you have confidence in and, if you do that, you're on to a winner. Any decent practitioner knows their limitations, and if they can't help you, they'll often be well placed to recommend someone within their network of colleagues that can, and that for me is the essence of good practice.'

over-the-counter. While they may not have the same depth of knowledge of cycling injuries as the other professions we mentioned, if you're undecided on who to see, then, as your primary healthcare provider, they offer a suitable segue to find out more about your injury. Don't necessarily expect them to have an in-depth knowledge of your cycling injury, but for certain problems they may well be the chosen expert to seek help and assistance from.

SPORTS MEDICINE PHYSICIAN

A sports medicine physician is a specialist doctor whose role is to assess and treat injured athletes or those experiencing medical problems due to a wide variety of sports. They'll often be able to help with injury prevention through specific training techniques, paying particular attention to your biomechanics when cycling and when off the bike if it's relevant. They're qualified to offer medical advice and will understand the pressures placed on you from cycling and can often offer advice on training programmes that are safe and effective for your recovery.

Sports medicine physicians can help diagnose many conditions and refer you to other practitioners where appropriate. For other problems, such as chronic fatigue, fractures or heart palpitations for example, that may have developed through cycling, it would be appropriate to see this group of doctors, which you can often either do directly or as a referral from your regular doctor.

Get a recommendation

There's no better recommendation than one that's come through word of mouth, rather than trawling the internet trying to find someone, but at least if you *have* to do that, then we've told you what to look out for to help find the most suitable person.

BIKE FITTER

You may well be able to kill two birds with the same stone here, as your bike fitter may well be a physio, chiro, osteo or even a sports doctor. At certain times it can be beneficial to return to your bike fitter to get their opinion on your injury – even more so if they're one of the professionals mentioned.

You've initially had a bike fit so it's not necessarily recommended to continue to move components around on your bike as it can leave you frustrated and chasing shadows. That said, there's a time and a place when going back to your bike fitter for a reassessment may well be recommended and we'll let you know when this is the case.

MASSAGE

In the hands of a skilled massage therapist, getting rid of knots in and around tight muscles can help offload certain muscle groups and fascia – the connective tissue that surrounds the muscles. Changing the tension on muscles can help relieve areas of discomfort and allow you to feel looser and move with more freedom on the bike. There's not a lot of evidence to support massage *curing* injury, but there's a reason a pro rider will have one after every race, because it can help with recovery and significantly help you *feel* better.

When you see this icon it is when we feel it could be recommended to have a massage to help as part of your recovery from injury.

ACUPUNCTURE

Physios have held the key to the treatment door of athletes and the athletic population for a long time and only more recently are chiropractors and osteopaths being accepted. This is because the sporting population can now trust in some consistency as both chiropractic and osteopathy have levels of standardised education, are government regulated, and are protected titles as we mentioned before. In fact, the advances of these professions lead to them both being offered as part of the core medical services in the athlete's village for the first time at the 2012 Olympic Games in London.

Acupuncture originated in the Far East and has been used by the Chinese people for thousands of years. Nowadays 'acupuncture' is a general umbrella term that encompasses many different approaches and philosophies of inserting fine, solid (yet flexible) needles into the body for pain relief and healing or general well-being. Traditional Chinese acupuncture (TCA), medical or western acupuncture, electro-acupuncture and dry needling may all be familiar terms, but it can make it confusing as to what 'acupuncture' really is.

Generally, TCA is performed by a practitioner of Traditional Chinese medicine (TCM), which includes the use of traditional Chinese medicine assessment methods such as checking the pulses of the wrist or observing the tongue to gauge general health and make a diagnosis. Needles will then be inserted along 'energy lines' of the body known as meridians to help balance the energy flow ('qi', pronounced 'chee') on the body and help restore health. Needles are often placed superficially in the skin as this is where it's believed the qi is reached for treatment.

When western professions like physiotherapists, osteopaths, chiropractors or even orthodox doctors, adopt the practice of acupuncture it will be used in context to reduce pain as part of an overall management approach following clinical reasoning and a working diagnosis. In this framework the traditional Chinese explanation of 'flow of energy' and 'meridians' is largely abandoned in favour of consideration of the anatomy and physiology of the area being treated and how this will be affected by inserting needles. Typically needles will be inserted more deeply – up to 5 cm or more – into areas of muscle spasm or trigger points to help reduce the tension and pain coming from these muscles and the structures they're affecting. In these cases it will more commonly be referred to as dry needling, medical or western acupuncture. This dry needling form of acupuncture can assist as part of the management of cycling injuries and will often be used by a practitioner with post-graduate training specifically in it.

Technically, in the UK anyone can call themselves an acupuncturist as it's not a government regulated profession or a protected title yet. However, if a physiotherapist, osteopath, chiropractor or doctor performs it having done the appropriate clinical reasoning and thinks it will be beneficial, then you can be reassured it'll be used in a suitable context to help improve your condition often alongside other approaches to maximise the benefit.

Getting started

Over the next 10 chapters we'll shine a light on the 10 most common injuries that affect cyclists. We'll tell you everything you need to know about that injury – how to spot it, the symptoms, causes and, most importantly, how to treat it with the least time away from the bike possible. All of these injuries affect everyone from weekend warriors to the elite of the sport, so we've quizzed the pros about when they had the injury, how it affected them and what they did to get through it.

HOW TO USE THIS SECTION

For those who like to be prepared, read through each of the 10 injuries now and you'll be fully equipped to spot an injury next time you crash or experience a niggling pain. Alternatively use it as your 'pain encyclopaedia', tapping into it after a fall or when you feel problems developing.

Every injury follows the same format we've discussed and we've tried to make it easy to understand. You'll notice some similarities across the injuries with regards to recommended exercises and rehabilitation programmes. This is because, as we mentioned earlier, many muscles are interconnected and required for cycling, and these are responsible for causing many different issues when they go wrong. This makes treatment for one injury and muscle group often apply to others. After all, it'll be similar muscles which become weak, short and tight due to overuse, and eventually break down causing injury, and these need to be addressed.

Injuries are a nuisance; they can kill morale, wreck entire seasons and keep you off your bike for months at a time. But providing you follow our advice, you should be able to put them behind you quickly and efficiently.

8 PATELLOFEMORAL PAIN SYNDROME

Sharp pain in the front of the knee every time you increase effort or shift into the big ring? A dull ache ringing from behind the kneecap towards the end of the tamest of rides that you just can't shake? Chances are your knee pain could be patellofemoral pain syndrome. There are many factors that can underlie the problem but it all comes down to poor tracking of the kneecap when you pedal, which can irritate the joint, cause pain, and frustrate any cycling enthusiast. So let's get it sorted.

The lowdown

Knee pain is common among cyclists. In fact you'll struggle to find any pro or keen amateur that hasn't succumbed to it at some point, and patellofemoral pain syndrome (PFPS) is the No. 1 culprit. With every turn of the pedals and with the feet anchored to the cleats, the knee flexes and extends; a motion it's not necessarily designed to perform so repetitively.

The good news is this common overuse injury can, with the right approach, disappear as quickly as it came. However, ignore it and your bike could be sitting in the garage gathering dust for 2–3 months or longer.

PROFESSIONAL INSIGHT

Chris Sutton AUSTRALIAN PRO AND VUELTA A ESPAÑA STAGE WINNER

■ 'It was on one of the first few stages of the 2012 Tirreno Adriatico. I'd never really had knee problems before but in the middle of the stage I started to get some pain at the front of my left knee seemingly out of nowhere. It wasn't that bad but I knew it was there and it was annoying.

As I got towards the end of the stage the race went up a mountain and then the pain started to feel sharper. I got to the finish and followed up with some physio and acupuncture that evening and started the race again the next day. I eventually pulled out of the race two days later

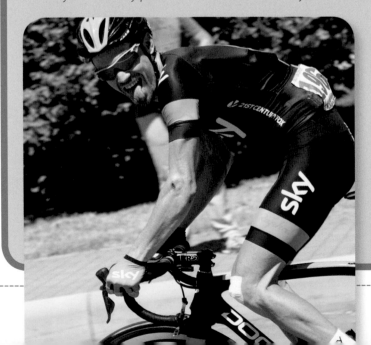

Symptom checker

- Dull ache at the front of the knee that comes on for no apparent reason.
- Pain may begin as mild awareness and increase to become searing in nature as it progresses.
- Discomfort during power phase (down stroke) of pedal stroke.

- Increased pain with increased effort – for example, climbing or extended time in the large chain ring – and less pain with less effort.
- Pain may come and go throughout the ride.
- Often associated with lower back stiffness and discomfort.
- Knee not usually swollen or tender to touch.
- Pain often relieved once you get off the bike.

as the pain was getting worse not better. I went home and had a few days rest off the bike and started training lightly a few days later. My bike got checked to see if the fit had altered in any way from racing, but that was all fine.

Off the bike the knee was no problem but when I got back on the pain would build soon after riding. I also noticed some mild discomfort in my back at the same time but didn't think it was relevant. The knee pain lingered around for about six weeks and I was getting frustrated as all the tests I had done said there was "nothing wrong with my knee".

I was at home still training lightly and I got recommended to see a local physio in Girona. When I told him my story he immediately thought the knee problem could be the result of a back issue. He was right, and it turned out that we had been looking at my bike and my knee as the problem when the whole time it was my back that was the issue. As soon as I started getting my back treated the knee pain disappeared and never came back! Now I've learned if I get an injury out of the blue it's just as important to look for where else and what else might be causing the problem rather than looking just at the site of the pain itself.'

The science bit

The knee basics

- The knee connects the bones of the upper and lower leg and consists of two joints. One connects the thigh bone to the shin bone and is the 'knee' joint as we know it – and the other is the joint between the kneecap (patella) and the thigh bone – the patellofemoral joint.
- The knee is a hinge joint, meaning it pretty much works in a straight line as it bends and straightens.
- The kneecap is located within the large thigh muscle tendon (quadriceps muscle) over the front surface of the knee joint.

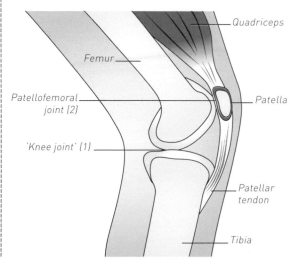

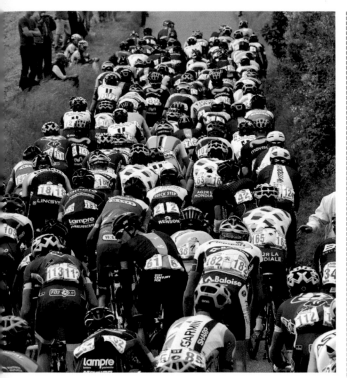

ABOVE Climbing puts more stress on the knee joints

Cause of injury

To understand how and why PFPS develops, the joints either side of the knee, which are the hip above and ankle below, need to be looked at.

The hip is a ball and socket joint and can move in multiple directions. The ankle joint is unique; it too can move in many different directions because it's actually made up of three joints very close together that almost act as one, allowing multidirectional movement. This multidirectional movement that occurs at the hip and ankle means they're well suited to absorb forces from many different directions. However, the knee with its single direction of motion can only really deal with forces that occur up and down in a straight line – the movement of the knee. The forces through the leg won't always be in a straight line when cycling and while the ankle and hip can buffer the non-linear forces, the knee is poor at doing this and this is where problems occur.

Pedal stroke and Q-angle

The knee is a weak link, but there's more to the story when it comes to PFPS, and it's all to do with the Q-angle.

When cycling, the kneecap glides over the front of the knee as it bends and straightens (like a train on a track) following a specific line known as the 'tracking' of the patella. The direction of tracking will be determined by what's known as the Q-angle. This angle is established by forming a line between the direct pull of the thigh muscle and the direction of the patella tendon.

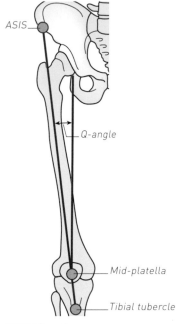

ABOVE Q-angle

The smaller the Q-angle, the better the kneecap slides up and down in a straight line, which creates less stress on the patellofemoral joint. The larger the Q-angle then the greater the opposing forces that are acting on the tracking of the kneecap. This increases stress on the muscles and soft tissue around the knee, making an individual more prone to developing patella tracking which contribute to PFPS.

Women have a larger Q-angle than men because they naturally have a wider pelvis that increases it. However, it isn't widely accepted that women suffer from increased prevalence of PFPS and this may suggest Q-angle change *for* the individual rather than *between* individuals could be the important factor in the tracking of an individuals' kneecap which leads to symptoms developing.

So any functional changes to the pelvis, for example, muscle imbalance, back symptoms or following a fall, could alter your Q-angle away from the norm by creating torsion (a 'twist') in the pelvis. This dysfunction could lead to the kneecap

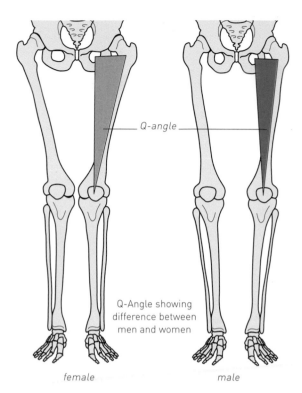

Q-angle

Q-Angle showing difference between men and women

female　　　　　*male*

not running ideally on its track during the pedal stroke. Multiplying this poor function with hours of cycling, a vulnerable joint and the consequent increased stresses that occur in and around the knee with faulty patella tracking, and, you guessed it, the symptoms of PFPS have the perfect storm to develop.

Treatment

Injury at a glance

Pain scale	Mild to moderate
Time off bike	1–2 weeks
Call in the professionals?	Not for now
Surgery?	No

First action: bike and equipment check

When you get off the bike the pain will often subside, making it easy to forget there's an issue until the next time you ride. This is key to remember as pain has a short memory, meaning that when you stop riding and the knee stops hurting you may think you are OK – wrong! To combat this potential slip-up, go through the following checklist the first time you get anterior knee pain and deal with them quickly if they're issues:

Saddle height: If this has dropped, it will reduce the angle of your knee at the top of the pedal stroke putting more strain on the front of the knee – patellofemoral joint – which can lead to symptoms in this area.

Cleats: If these have moved, it can alter how your kneecap glides over the knee as your foot is in a slightly different position, putting different stresses on the knee that could lead to anterior knee pain.

Clothing: Not obvious or common but PFPS may occur during the winter simply due to the type of clothing you are wearing. For example, wearing tight leggings or knee warmers could compress the kneecap against the knee causing irritation and pain of the patellofemoral joint.

MATT SAYS:

'Saddle height matters, and the more you're in tune with your body the more this is the case. I've been in countless races where a pro has dropped back to the follow car to have their seat changed by 1–2mm. If you develop pain in the knee, saddle height dropping is the first and most obvious place to look.'

Week 1

THE NEXT STEP

The bike is set-up how it should be, so it's now time to address the pain and the problem, which in the case of PFPS may not be the same thing. By this we mean, where you are experiencing the pain – the knee – firstly needs to be addressed. Then the reason you got the pain in the first place, the *cause* of the problem, can be dealt with afterwards to try and ensure PFPS does not return.

Ice the area 2–3 times a day for 10–20 minutes each time.

Continue to ice for three days or continue otherwise for as long as you have knee pain if you're still getting the discomfort off the bike. You shouldn't need to ice for longer than a week.

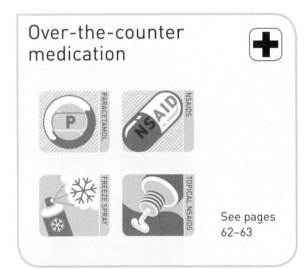

Over-the-counter medication

PARACETAMOL

NSAIDS

FREEZE SPRAY

TOPICAL NSAIDS

See pages 62–63

MOVING ON

Throughout the first week of rest off the bike avoid any other exercise or activity that aggravates the knee such as running or squatting, as this will slow your recovery. During this time be careful of leaping and bounding up and down stairs as it's an activity in everyday life that may irritate the injury.

This week is all about getting to work on the joints and muscles that are tightened and weakened that have likely contributed to the injury. Using the first week to loosen up certain muscles will also improve your symmetry for when you get back on the bike.

Continue to ice your knee as appropriate and start working through the following routines and exercises.

RECOMMENDATIONS
Foam roller

Begin by rolling the key muscles that may be implicated when you develop PFPS. These muscles can affect how the kneecap tracks and how the knee functions when you're cycling.

Four to work on:

REHAB TOOL KIT EX.	EX. NO.	PAGE
The quads	6.9	199
The glutes and piriformis	5.19	190
The tensor fascia latae	5.20	191
The calf	6.7	198

Reducing tension in these muscles and getting them the appropriate length, free from knots and working properly will allow you to get more return for the exercises you will do afterwards.

Now move onto these exercises:

REHAB TOOL KIT EX.	EX. NO.	PAGE
1. Lumbar spine movement	5.1	182
2. The cat and camel	5.2	182
3. The stand tall and reach stretch	3.1	175
4. The child's pose	5.3	182
5. The bridge	5.10	185
6. Patella tracking sit to stand	6.3	193

Weeks 2 – 4

 It's time to get back on your bike.

 Now's the time to start a core exercise routine, see page 202.

Kinsesio tape

 Kinsesio tape can help offload tissues around the knee and help manage any remaining symptoms as you integrate back into your riding and should be considered if you feel you need the extra support. See page 200.

Week 5

STILL HAVE KNEE PAIN – WHO SHOULD YOU CALL?

If four weeks have passed and you've not made significant progress, are still getting pain at the front of the knee when you ride and have followed the above advice, it's time to seek expert opinion.

PLAN A

 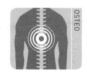

PLAN B

Knee dingers: banged your knee on the handlebar?

A classic issue that happens time and time again. The annoying thing is, you won't pay it too much attention at the time and will probably dismiss it. Then a few days later or the next time you ride, there it is, causing pain on the muscle above the kneecap and affecting your pedal stroke. Well, the message is simple, when you do it, get ice on it as soon as you get home and continue this a couple of times a day for three days, more if you have to. Take 2–3 days off the bike too and you'll find the problem will resolve, rather than dragging out as it otherwise can.

9 NONSPECIFIC (MECHANICAL) LOWER BACK PAIN

Getting lower back pain is no fun at any time, least of all when you're cycling. That heavy aching sensation, the boring and burning sharp stab you feel in the small of your back as you grind at the pedals, it feels as if you're cycling with a 50 kg weight on your shoulders. Lower back pain can also affect the amount of power you can get out of your legs and it will make you feel older than your years, quickly. Immediately you question: will it ever get better? And as the pain lingers, it feels like it never will. But trust us, it will; and providing you follow our advice, lower back pain will be banished, and before you know it, you'll be cycling again, feeling strong and pain-free.

The lowdown

Everyone has either experienced lower back pain or knows somebody that has, as it affects 85 per cent of the population at some time in their life. The good news is that in the vast majority (90 per cent) of cases it will naturally improve over a three-month period. On the other hand however, almost half of lower back pain sufferers will get at least one recurrent episode, so how should you approach it?

As soon as you clip into your pedals and reach for your handlebars, your lower back is put into a somewhat compromised position. As the spine is flexed forwards, the weight of the body becomes uncharacteristically and unevenly distributed through the lower back. Did you know that almost all of the muscles that provide stability on the bike and help turn the pedals attach in the lower back region? During every pedal stroke, these muscles continually contract and relax so it's quite clear that there's a lot of stress placed on the lower back when cycling. After riding for several hours, generating hundreds of watts of power from the lower back, hips and legs, the result can unfortunately be the development of lower back pain as the body breaks down when it can no longer compensate and adapt to the stresses thrown at it.

Nonspecific lower back pain (NLBP), also known as mechanical lower back pain, is a catch-all term that encompasses pain originating from one of several structures of the lower back, notably the joints or the lumbar discs. It can also occur due to muscle spasms in the area.

Symptom checker

✔ Dull ache/burning pain in the lower back that builds.
✔ Can feel like the lower back is throbbing.
✔ Pain can be central or more to one side.
✔ Discomfort often continuous once started.
✔ Sharp pain on certain movements or going over bumps in the road.
✔ Difficulty generating normal power or maintaining normal speed.
✔ 'Blocked' sensation in lower back.
✔ Pain into buttocks or groin.
✔ Pain into legs, often no further than the knee.
✔ Secondary issues such as pain in the knee can develop.

PROFESSIONAL INSIGHT
Dan Martin
IRISH PRO AND WINNER OF THE OLDEST RACE IN PROFESSIONAL CYCLING, LIÈGE-BASTOGNE-LIÈGE

■ 'A lot of people, professional cyclists included, underestimate the amount of power produced from your posterior chain – the muscles in the back and back of the legs. As soon as there is a problem in the lower back, it's not only uncomfortable but your optimal power output and, therefore, performance is compromised.

I work very hard to create a stronger lower back that can cope with the torque put on it because of racing and bring greater stability to my pedal stroke. It's inevitable there will be occasions when I get occasional lower back pain as I ride so many miles. I know what I need to do when it comes on, simple stretches and exercises I can do to settle things down quickly. If I need to get the problem sorted properly, for immediate relief if I'm in the middle of a race or important training block, then I know an adjustment from a chiropractor or some osteopathy will get me right.

The most important advice is to strengthen the lumbar area to cope with the stresses exercise puts on the body so you don't need to get extra help that often as your body is strong and robust enough to cope with riding as much as you want.'

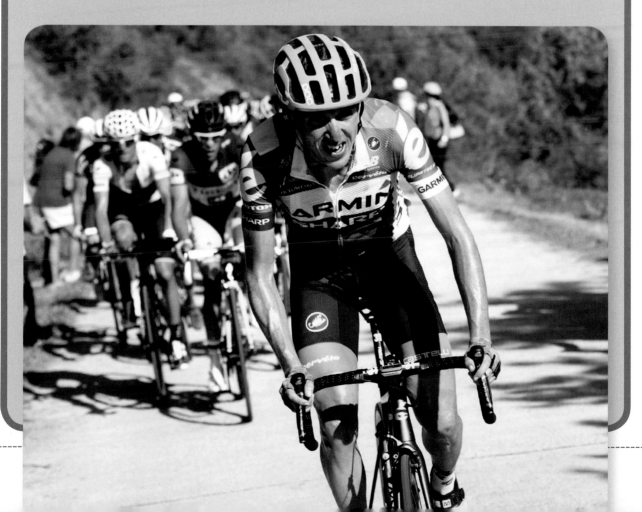

Half of all recreational cyclists are reported to get lower back pain at some time and you will be hard pushed to find any pro cyclist that hasn't been affected by it at some point in their career or even at some point during each season.

It's often one of those injuries you 'feel like you can ride through' but you must get on to this early if you want to prevent it from developing further. Letting it fester will not only cause increased prolonged pain, but could progress into leg pain and numbness, and even secondary knee problems can develop. However, by treating it early, you will have an excellent chance of resolving it and being out on your bike inside a couple of weeks.

The science bit

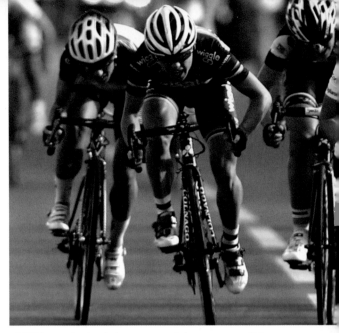

ABOVE Lower back pain is a common injury among cyclists

The lower back

- The lower back supports the weight of the body and extends from the bottom of the rib cage to the creases of the buttocks.
- The skeleton portion consists of the lumbar spine (five lumbar vertebrae) and pelvis.
- The lumbar vertebrae are the largest, able to support the weight of the body above.
- The vertebrae are joined at the front by large discs that act as shock absorbers for the body and at the back by smaller (facet) joints that allow movement between them to occur.
- An extension of the spinal cord runs through the lumbar spine providing nerve supply to the organs of the abdomen, muscles and sensory supply of the legs.

- The sacrum is attached to the lumbar spine and the pelvis, the latter at the sacroiliac (SI) joints. These are large joints that play an important role in controlling the torsion/rotational movement through the pelvis – the motion you see when the pelvis 'rocks' from side to side while cycling.

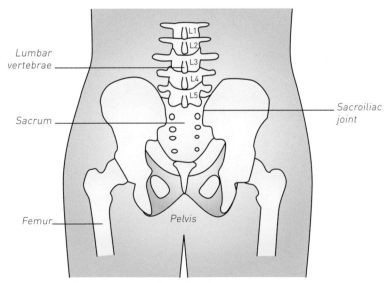

Posterior view

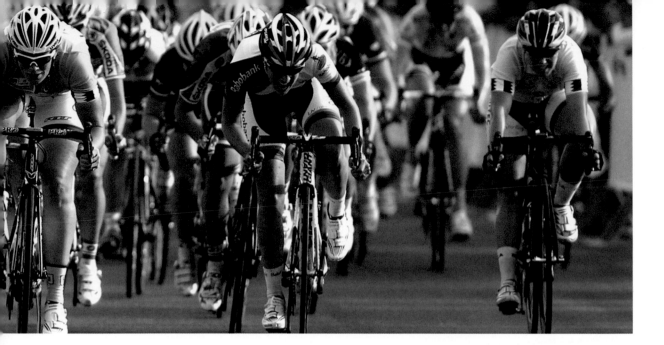

On the bike stability

Stability on the bike is important. It allows you to be more comfortable while cycling for longer periods of time, improves the transfer of energy through the body into the pedals making your riding more efficient, and protects the lower back, helping prevent injury in this area. Muscles that provide stability in the lower back can be broken down into local and global stabilisers.

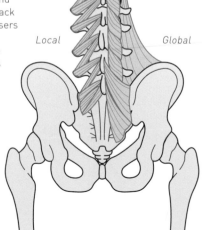

RIGHT Local and global lower back muscle stabilisers (multifidus, erector spinae and quadratus lumborum)

Local

Global

Local stabilisers

The local stabilising muscles are small muscles that provide stability in the lower back allowing a solid foundation for other movement. In fact, these 'core' muscles engage first to support the spine before *any* other movement of the body takes place. When these muscles don't automatically contract prior to movement it's a problem and is a common thread among chronic lower back pain sufferers. Examples of local stabilisers are the transverse abdominus – the deepest layer of abdominal muscle – and the multifidis muscles.

 Whenever core strengthening is referred to, it's these muscles that are ultimately targeted through exercises.

Global stabilisers

Global stabilisers are larger, longer muscles that sit closer to the surface. They're responsible for producing large forces for controlled movement of the torso such as twisting or turning the body or sitting up from lying down and are also engaged throughout the pedal stroke. These are also postural muscles that help keep you standing upright all day and will help support you in your cycling position. Examples of global stabilisers are the erector spinae and quadratus lumborum muscles.

If stability of the lumbar spine is reduced, it leaves the lower back vulnerable to injury and there are four primary areas that generate pain causing the problems of NLBP.

Pain generators

1 **Lumbar facet joint:** small joints of the lower back that allow movement to occur, which can get irritated and sprained causing pain.
2 **Sacroiliac joints:** large weight bearing joints at the base of the spine that come under constant continuous stress and can become irritated, sprained and cause pain.
3 **Lumbar disc:** shock absorbers of the lower back can become overloaded, damaged and cause pain.
4 **Muscle spasm:** large muscles that support the lower back can go into spasm preventing further damage by restricting movement of an area but will be painful at the same time.

These structures can all cause pain when injury to them occurs. It's likely for any given incidence of back pain that it'll be more than one of the above structures that's causing the discomfort, for example, muscle spasm can occur secondary to lumbar facet sprain.

There are three main causes for the common incidence of NLBP in cycling: one is traumatic and the other two are through overuse. While it's self-explanatory that the consequences of a crash from the bike can cause lower back problems, the two overuse causes of NLBP are less so, and these are due to 'creep' and 'shearing' forces.

OVERUSE CAUSE 1: CREEP
Cyclists usually adopt one of three positions when riding, on the drops, on the hoods or the bars, and each position changes the stress on the lower back. The drops are the most aerodynamic position, but means you're reaching the furthest of the three positions and stretching the most, putting the lower back under the greatest stress. Riding

the bars is the least aggressive, most upright position and puts the least stress on the lower back while riding the hoods is between the two.

Changing between these riding positions alters the tension in the lower back, but ultimately as you are leaning forwards your lower back is in 'flexion'. Prolonged and repetitive lower back flexion coupled with the vibrations from the road causes stretching in tissues of the lumbar spine which is known as 'creep'. When this happens, the muscle of the lower back can spasm as the body attempts to protect the area and prevent further irritation. The muscle spasm as well as the tissue creep will affect the joints and discs of the lower back, which will contribute to NLBP.

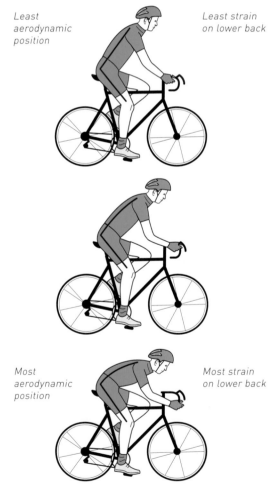

Least aerodynamic position

Least strain on lower back

Most aerodynamic position

Most strain on lower back

ABOVE Lumbar spine angles while in three different riding positions

Lumbar spine creep and bike fit

Lumbar spine creep only starts once the body is totally warmed-up and relaxed, which is why NLBP often doesn't come on immediately. So whenever you're doing a bike fit it's extremely important (and often overlooked) that it's done once the body has fully warmed-up as only then will you get a true reflection of the function of the individual's lower back. If you do a bike fit prior to a proper warm-up, then what might look like an ideal fit could functionally turn into a bad one once the person is properly warmed up and out on the bike for longer periods of time.

OVERUSE CAUSE 2: SHEARING FORCES

The sacroiliac (SI) joints sit at the base of the lower back. They're weight bearing joints absorbing both the body weight from above as well as the force through the pelvis from the ground below. The transfer of force from the lower back into the legs goes through the SI joints while pedalling. They're unlike many other joints as they're so strong yet there's only a limited amount of movement that actually occurs in the joint; in fact, up until the 1930s it was thought they were fused and had no movement in them at all.

Look at any cyclist from behind on the bike and you'll notice a rhythmic rocking of their pelvis from side to side, as the weight is transferred from one side of their body to the other with every pedal stroke. The SI joints are responsible for limiting and controlling some of this torsion force. This creates a shearing stress of the SI joints themselves.

With fabulous core strength, the perfect bike set-up and an immaculate pedalling action, the shearing force is minimised and it might not be a concern. For others, the repetitive nature of pedalling over different terrain with the ground reaction forces being felt through the body can mean eventually a time comes when the body is no longer able to compensate and adapt to the shearing force through the SI joints, making them become irritated, resulting in pain and

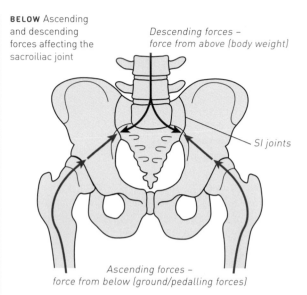

BELOW Ascending and descending forces affecting the sacroiliac joint

Descending forces – force from above (body weight)

SI joints

Ascending forces – force from below (ground/pedalling forces)

contributing towards NLBP.

Pain coming from the SI joints can be referred down the leg with pain felt into the hamstring, the outside of the leg or even into the groin region. Symptoms related to SI joint problems won't usually extend past the knee; if they do, it usually means a different issue is causing the pain.

Progressive issues

In some cases, NLBP can progress and over time can cause other issues to develop. If you're experiencing leg symptoms, such as numbness, pins and needles, and tingling, the problem has moved on beyond a mechanical lower back pain cause, as it is indicative that there's a 'trapped nerve' somewhere.

There are two common culprits related to cycling where compression of the nerves that form the sciatic nerve *or* the sciatic nerve itself can become compressed: the first is a lumbar disc herniation and the second is at the piriformis muscle in the buttock.

Progression from simple mechanical lower back pain to a lumbar disc herniation can occur when increased stresses on the lumbar disc cause the disc to herniate backwards and either bulge or leak fluid. This places direct pressure on the spinal nerves of the back (that supply the legs), which will result in symptoms down the leg and even into the foot.

If you have mechanical back pain it can develop into something called 'piriformis syndrome'. Poor and faulty mechanics of the lower back can lead to tightness and weakness of the piriformis muscle which is one of the lower back stabilisers found in the buttock. The sciatic nerve that comes from the lower back and travels down the leg can get irritated because it either passes through (as occurs in 17 per cent of people) or passes extremely close to the piriformis muscle. When this happens, symptoms down the leg such as numbness and pins and needles would be seen.

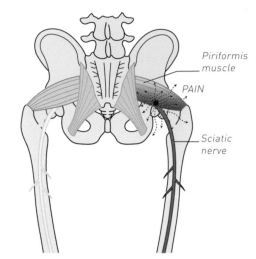

ABOVE Piriformis syndrome (muscle pinching sciatic nerve)

If you get pain down the leg, pins and needles or numbness in the foot when you ride that doesn't disappear when you rest for a week or two, it's important to seek expert opinion. Whereas with NLBP you have a great opportunity to get to work yourself, when nerves are involved it's important to seek an opinion sooner rather than later so the problem doesn't get worse.

Treatment

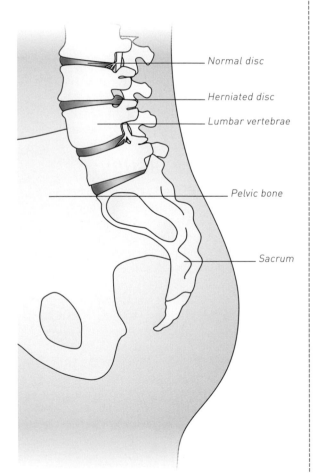

Injury at a glance

Pain scale	Mild to severe
Time off bike	1 week
Call in the professionals?	Not for now – unless you have any referred pain down the leg
Surgery?	Not likely

First action: bike check, anything moved?

Saddle height: If this has dropped, it will alter the angle of your lower back, putting different stresses through the spine than you're used to. Abnormal stresses placed on the back when riding due to a dropped saddle can contribute towards developing NLBP.

Saddle position: If the saddle slides backwards or tilts, it will also change the angle of your lower back making you reach further, putting different stresses on the lower back and potentially creating symptoms of NLBP. Knowing your saddle position beforehand will help you see if there's been any movement on your ride that contributed to the NLBP.

These slight alterations may not be the cause at all, but it's good to tick them off your list, and from here you can delve deeper into what's causing the pain. If you didn't have a good bike fit, or bought the wrong sized bike because you got a great deal, this too can actually cause back problems. Head back to your fitter first if this is the case.

The next step: once you get off your bike

Lower back pain may linger when you get off the bike but it will generally subside and ease within a few hours, but sometimes it can remain there for the rest of that day or even the next couple of days. When you get back from a ride, run through the following procedure to help reduce the discomfort:

FIRST AID TO REDUCE LOWER BACK PAIN

Ice the area 2–3 times a day for 10 – 15 minutes at a time. Continue to ice for the first week or for as long as you have pain off the bike. You shouldn't need to ice for much longer than a week but you can continue to do so if you need to. These two exercises will allow some swift relief to the lower back discomfort.

MATT SAYS:

'I often get asked about using heat for lower back pain. I usually always recommend ice as it will have a painkilling effect as well as help any local inflammation. Heat is recommended for muscle strains, which in the lower back will often be secondary to another issue. Alternating between ice and heat – 10 minutes of ice followed by 10 minutes of heat – can offer improved relief and help relieve symptoms once you're through the acute injury phase after four or five days.'

REHAB TOOL KIT EX.	EX. NO.	PAGE
The lower back relief position	5.22	191
The knees to chest hug	5.4	183

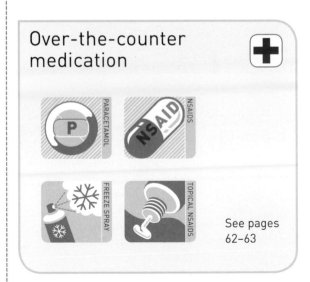

Over-the-counter medication ➕

PARACETAMOL   NSAIDS

FREEZE SPRAY   TOPICAL NSAIDS

See pages 62–63

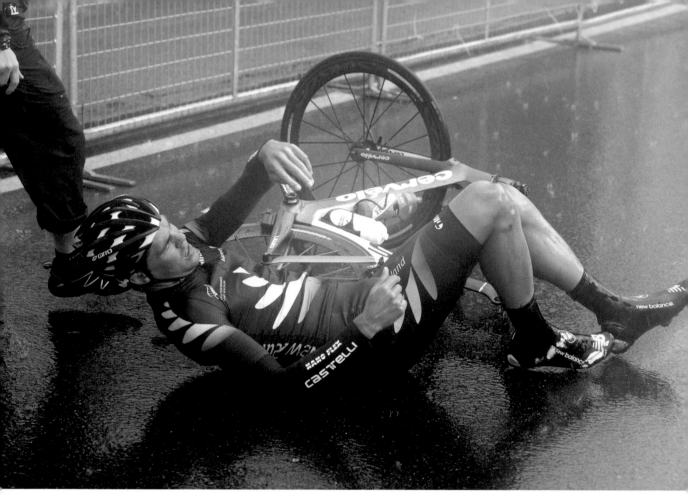

ABOVE Crashing can be a cause of back pain

Massage

A lot of cyclists who experience back pain will often go and see a massage therapist. However, the majority of NLBP has some relationship to the underlying joints and massage only really deals with the muscular component so the evidence to recommend massage as a form of stand-alone treatment for lower back pain really doesn't exist to support it. Don't get a massage expecting it to fix your lower back problem, but if you find it helps you to relax and loosens the muscles to give some temporary relief, then we're all for it.

Week 1

MOVING ON

During the first week, rest and avoid any other exercise or activity that aggravates the lower back. However, it's important to maintain a balance so try and keep mobile and active – walking for example. Being sedentary is not advised in the early stages of mechanical lower back pain as it can cause the back to seize.

If you have a deskbound job, avoid sitting for longer than 30 minutes at a time as the lower back doesn't like this. Even if you get up and touch either wall of the office or walk to the water cooler and back, this can be enough mobility to reduce 'creep' and avoid stiffening up. The following exercise can help provide relief from discomfort while at the desk too:

Brugger relief position

- Sit forwards and upright on your chair with your chin gently tucked in making your neck long.
- Hold your arms down by your side, with your backward palms facing forward. Push your hands down while gently squeezing between your shoulder blades.
- Remain in this upright posture, breathing deeply for 10 – 30 seconds.
- Reps – Every hour at the desk or whenever you feel yourself slouching.

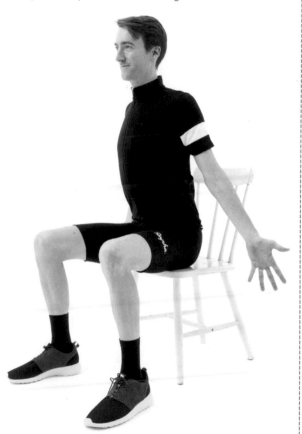

RECOMMENDATIONS

During the first week, you want to reduce the symptoms by loosening the lower back, getting the lumbar spine and pelvis moving appropriately, and working on muscles that may be weak or shortened causing asymmetry and contributing to the back pain when you ride. This will help improve comfort, stability and symmetry both on and off the bike. These exercises will help:

REHAB TOOL KIT EX.	EX. NO.	PAGE
1. The sphinx	5.5	183
2. The cat and camel	5.2	182
3. Lumbar spine movement	5.1	182
4. Stand and reach stretch	3.1	175

 Continue on a daily basis for as long as discomfort persists.

Sleeping positions to alleviate lower back pain

a Sleeping on your side with a pillow between slightly bent knees will help keep the pelvis in a neutral position and keep your spine straight reducing the chances of experiencing back pain at night.

b Sleeping on your back with a pillow under your knees will help relieve tension in the lower back when you sleep.

a
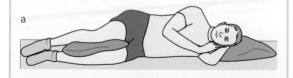

b
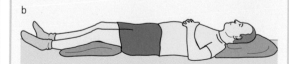

Sleeping position with back pain

Getting out of bed with back pain

- Roll over on to your side and draw your knees up towards your chest.
- Let your legs move over the edge of the bed and use your arms to sit upright.
- This will reduce the chances of straining the back when getting out of bed.

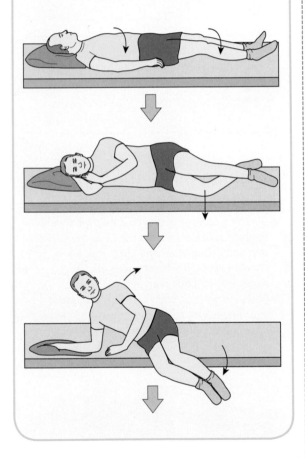

Weeks 2 – 4

Time to get back on your bike.

Time to start a core exercise routine, see page 202.

Kinesio tape

Kinesio tape can help support the lower back as you come back to riding, you'll need someone else to apply this tape for you. See the rehab toolkit page 191.

Week 5

STILL HAVE PAIN: WHO SHOULD YOU CALL?

If after four weeks you've not made significant progress, are still getting pain in the lower back when you ride and have followed all of the above advice, it's time to seek expert help, or rest a couple more weeks without riding and continue with the exercises.

PLAN A

 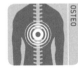

PLAN B

CYCLING NIRVANA

Magnus Bäckstedt SWEDEN | 2004 PARIS–ROUBAIX WINNER

■ 'One day above everything else – Paris–Roubaix 2004. In the morning when I left the bus my soigneur casually said "T minus one hour till your day". I looked back and said "yeah, definitely", as if I knew it would be a special day.

The first 100 km of the race were panicky and stressful but I was well looked after by my teammates. As we went through the Arenberg Forest, a key point in the race, it was a big group but I was in the front. We kept riding hard. With 60 km to go, I jokingly said to my teammate, "Can you check my bike as I don't think I've got a chain". It was hard but it didn't feel it. From then on a teammate covered every attack so I could just sit in looking out for the three race favourites to attack.

In one attack I followed Johan Museeuw, but it wasn't as hard as I thought it would be to follow his move. We got out the end of the infamous Carrefour de l'Arbre cobblestone sector and I can remember every left and right turn. By this time there were only five riders left, me included. Going through the last section of difficult cobbles, I was on the front. It was a twisty section, bike handling was tough as the bike was bouncing all over the place. I shifted across the road and just missed a huge stone and thought to myself how lucky I was. I remember vividly thinking "if nobody hits that stone it's a miracle". Well, Museeuw hit it and punctured and with only six or seven kilometres to go, we weren't gonna wait.

Then there were four of us left as we headed into the velodrome. I remember everything: I went in third; it was Fabian Cancellara, Roger Hammond and then me as we headed in. I felt good and was backing myself. We entered into a complete wall of noise. You couldn't hear a single thing – except I was so focused I could hear our tyres on the track and the boys changing gears. It was strange, it was so loud but I also remember hearing my three-year-old daughter shouting "Go Daddy".

I launched my sprint and I got boxed in and strangely didn't panic at all. I knew as soon as Hammond went outside I could go inside. I waited. As I had thought, as we turned the final corner I dived into the opening inside and two pedal strokes later I was in the lead and crossed the line. I crossed the line in disbelief: "is there anyone in front of me?" I had won Paris-Roubaix. Sheer Cycling Nirvana. A moment I had dreamed about my whole life leading up to that day and have thought about every day since. It doesn't get much better than that.'

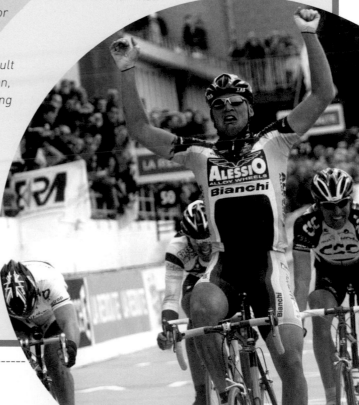

10

ACHILLES TENDINOPATHY

You've been working towards that sportive, upping your training and you finally think you've nailed it, but it hasn't come without a price. Now with every pedal stroke you feel a nagging, sharp sensation at the bottom of your leg where the strong thick tendon meets the heel – the Achilles (tendon). It won't shift, it's getting annoying and the more you ride the worse it gets. It's that painful that when you pinch the tendon between your finger and thumb you almost yelp with pain. Yep, you've irritated the tendon due to overuse and have probably developed Achilles tendinopathy. This is an injury to heed or you could be off your bike for weeks or even months.

The lowdown

You can't ride a bike without force going through the Achilles tendon with every pedal stroke. The calf muscles contract during each spin of the pedals and every time they do they transfer their force through the Achilles. The force may be relatively small compared to running or even walking. However, this force accumulates to be a significant load when each pedal stroke is multiplied by the hours of time spent cycling. It's the continued repetitive strain on the tendon that can lead to overload and consequent Achilles tendinopathy developing.

As this injury develops, microscopic damage of the fibres of the Achilles tendon is seen. When the breakdown of the tendon from overuse is occurring at a faster rate than the body can repair the damage, then Achilles tendinopathy will be the outcome.

This injury can affect you whatever level of cycling you're at, from weekend warriors, cat 2 and 3 riders all the way up to the pros. Dutch pro Lars Boom competing in his first Grand Tour at the 2009 Vuelta a España reported Achilles pain on stage five and he ended up finishing second to last that day, 194th of 195, such was the pain. In fact, Boom was one of the fortunate ones as the

Symptom checker

- ✔ Symptoms may begin as awareness or stiffness in the Achilles.
- ✔ Dull ache of the Achilles tendon throughout pedal stroke (about 2–6 cm from the bottom usually).
- ✔ Sharp to searing local Achilles pain as it progresses, worse when climbing or in a big gear.
- ✔ Pain almost always on one leg only.
- ✔ Stiffness in Achilles on walking when you get off the bike and first thing in the morning as it progresses.
- ✔ Pain may come and go during a ride in early stages, becoming more continuous as it progresses.
- ✔ Tender to touch – 'pinch test'.
- ✔ Tight calf on affected side sometimes noticed.
- ✔ Pain can spread into lower calf or heel bone while riding.

PROFESSIONAL INSIGHT

Daniel Lloyd RETIRED BRITISH PRO CYCLIST
AND TOUR OF QINGHAI STAGE WINNER

■ 'Back in 2008, I was riding for the An Post team.
It had been a good year already, but I was always
motivated for the Tour of Britain, and went into it
with hopes of a high placing overall or a stage win.

   During stage 4, I noticed a small twinge in my
left Achilles. It had been a long, cold and wet day,
and it was a very minor niggle which I didn't really
give a second thought to at the time. I didn't do
anything in the way of treatment that evening.

   The following day it had got worse. I could feel it
when I got up in the morning to go to breakfast and also
as soon as I got on the bike. I thought it would go off as
I rode myself in and warmed my body up, but it didn't.
I tried pedalling at a higher cadence to put less pressure
on it, and then started favouring my other leg more.

   I managed to get through that stage, and that
night I took some anti-inflammatories and put ice on
it. We didn't have a physio, chiro or doctor on the team
so I couldn't really get any professional advice.

   The next day it was worse still, and I only managed
about 30 km before I decided to call it a day and step into
the team car. I was very disappointed, I wasn't the sort
of person to give up and I rarely packed a race in.

   Once I got home I simply rested it for two days
and continued to use ice and anti-inflammatories,
plus doing some stretching. This seemed to do the
trick, and when I got back on the bike three days later,
it was all but gone and I was able to do some more
racing at the end of the season.

   I learned a lesson: treat Achilles injuries
immediately, and they won't cause you much harm.
Leave them alone and the consequences could be
hugely detrimental.'

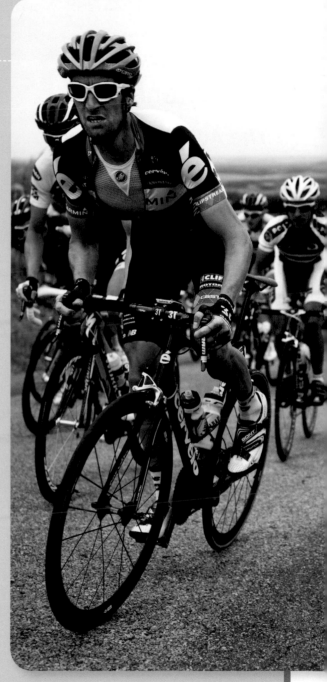

injury recovered and ten days later he went on to win stage 15! If a professional rider with all the support, advice and treatment can be affected by this injury, what hope is there for the rest of us? That's why it's important to know how to tackle it should it rear its head.

The science bit

The Achilles tendon

- The two large muscles of the lower leg, the gastrocnemius and soleus, merge around halfway down the calf and extend to form the Achilles tendon inserting into the middle of the back of the heel bone.
- The Achilles is the largest, thickest and strongest tendon in the body and is roughly 12–15 cm in length.
- It's surrounded by a layer of connective tissue fascia that helps reduce friction forces when it's under stress.

- At its narrowest point just behind the ankle it is easily palpable as it stands prominently where it can easily be pinched between your finger and thumb – which will be painful when it's injured.
- Fibres of the Achilles run in a spiral fashion – like a coiled spring – allowing the tendon to optimally transmit the energy from muscle to bone and efficiently release the energy stored in it during movement.
- The tendon can increase its stress load almost four times your body weight during walking alone and almost eight times your body weight during running. During cycling the loading is notably less although the nature of the pedal stroke sees the tendon under stress almost continuously.
- The Achilles has a notoriously poor blood supply making it a slow healer when it gets injured.

Causes of injury

The joints of the foot and ankle allow the foot to paddle up and down and turn in and turn out. When the foot paddles upwards and moves into dorsiflexion it places the Achilles under tension.

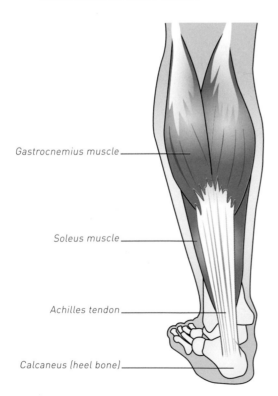

Gastrocnemius muscle

Soleus muscle

Achilles tendon

Calcaneus (heel bone)

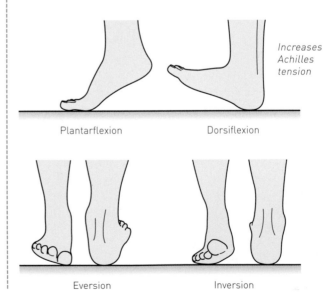

Increases Achilles tension

Plantarflexion

Dorsiflexion

Eversion

Inversion

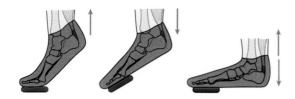

ABOVE Heel moves up on an upstroke (left), heel drops on downstroke (middle) and the maximum Achilles tension is at the bottom of the pedal stroke

During the pedalling action of most cyclists, the toes will point down on the upstroke and the heel will drop slightly on the power phase down stroke, increasing tension on the Achilles. Depending on the amount of pedal float, if any, and tightness of the shoes, there'll also be small

amounts of natural foot movement inwards and outwards (pronation and suppination) during the normal pedalling action, which will add to the stress on the tendon.

The primary action of the calf muscles was first thought to perform the 'toe-off' motion, putting the foot into the toes down position and *initiating* the power phase of the pedal stroke, but this isn't the whole story.

It's now understood that the most important role of the calf muscles during pedalling is to prevent the heel from dropping too much at the bottom of the pedal stroke. The calf muscle engages, preventing too much heel drop by putting a brake on this movement like a coiled spring stretching (an example of strong eccentric contraction) and, as the heel drops, this action pulls hard on the Achilles tendon.

When a spring lengthens, more 'stretch' occurs in the middle of the spring than at either of the ends. This is the same in the Achilles too, meaning more load goes through the middle portion of the tendon (also its weakest point), making the middle part of the tendon the common area to become injured while cycling.

Weak muscles in the calf mean too much pronation (rolling in) of the foot can occur, meaning the Achilles tendon is more likely to become overloaded. This results in an exaggerated stretch and whipping motion of the Achilles as the heel drops and the tendon absorbs this extra force (see overleaf).

Concentric and eccentric muscle firing

Concentric firing (below left) involves the muscle shortening as it contracts. Eccentric firing (below right) involves the muscle legthening as it contracts.

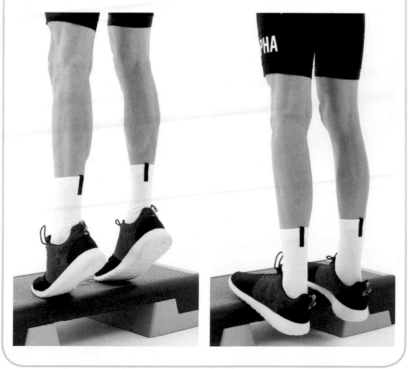

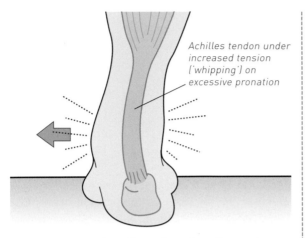

Achilles tendon under increased tension ('whipping') on excessive pronation

The cumulative effect of weak calf muscles (that are also likely to be shortened, tightened and have trigger points in them), poor pedalling action and faulty foot mechanics coupled with the volume of repetition of force through the tendon that occurs when cycling can cause overload and injury of the Achilles tendon. This is especially likely to be seen when there's not enough time between bouts of cycling for the tendon to rest and heal. The result will be development of local pain and even swelling as the tendinopathy gets worse. This needs to be managed appropriately to prevent it progressing – which could lead to a lengthy spell off the bike.

Stages of injury

When the tendon becomes irritated from overuse, it progresses in stages along an injury continuum. When overload occurs too much for the tendon to repair at a suitable rate, this is called the **reactive phase**. At this early stage the tendon will be painful while riding and if it continues can become swollen. This happens because the increase in load activates cells of the tendon causing them to produce a painful substance and release proteins that causes fluid to be drawn into the tendon causing it to swell. This makes the tendon painful, alerting you there's a problem and hopefully encouraging you to ease off. The majority of pain experienced in the Achilles while cycling will be in this reactive stage.

Continued load during the reactive phase can lead to the second stage developing as the tendon has moved past the attempt to manage the load and is now trying desperately to heal itself. This is known as the **stage of disrepair**.

Continue riding at this stage and you'll continue to load an already aggravated tendon and it's possible to move into the third stage. Once you create damage to the point the body can't actively repair the tissue, you enter **the degenerative phase**. You don't want to let your Achilles problem progress past the reactive phase as this is the time when it has the best capability to heal. It's the most important phase and it's vital you manage it properly then.

Treatment

Injury at a glance

Pain scale	Mild to moderate
Time off bike	2–6 weeks
Call in the professionals?	Not for now
Surgery?	Not likely

Treatment of Achilles tendinopathy is a complex subject with multiple approaches and many different factors that make no two cases the same. This can make it a tricky injury to design a rehabilitation programme for. However, many of the current thoughts on how to manage the injury have been curated for you to follow and get the problem sorted.

First action: bike and equipment check

Saddle height: if this has dropped, it will slightly change your pedal stroke meaning your calf muscles will be used in a slightly different pattern, which could lead to changes in the pull on the Achilles.

Cleats: if your cleats have moved from their fixed position on the shoe plate, it can lead to different leverage on the Achilles while riding, which can contribute to injury.

Clothing: certain shoes or shoe covers you might wear in the rain or cold may be tight causing mild compression on or around the Achilles at the back of the foot, which could restrict the tendon's ability to slide and cause irritation.

Pedal spindles/axles: riding in the wet and on dirty roads can lead to a build-up of grit in the spindle of the pedals, this may affect the smooth movement of the pedal on the spindle causing resistance in smooth movement of the foot, potentially putting more stress on the Achilles leading to discomfort.

Chain: if the chain movement is restricted because of a lack of lubrication or getting clogged up in bad conditions, it will increase the natural resistance of its movement, which could affect the Achilles tendon leading to pain.

A quick fix?

Try moving your cleats back 2 mm on your shoes. This will reduce the leverage placed on your Achilles tendon during the pedal stroke, which may be enough to reduce the load and relieve symptoms when you ride. If it doesn't, then move on to the next step.

Week 1
THE NEXT STEP

If your Achilles pain persists, now's the time to attack it from two directions. The first thing is to reduce the local pain; the second is to try to fix and improve any secondary issues contributing to the problem such as shortened or weakened calf muscles.

Catch it early while it is still in the reactive phase and you won't usually have many symptoms thereafter.

FIRST AID FOR ACHILLES TENDINOPATHY

Ice the area 2–3 times a day for 10–15 minutes at a time. Continue to ice for the first week or for as long as you have pain. Start on these excercises to relieve Achilles pain.

Start on these exercises to relieve Achilles pain:

REHAB TOOL KIT EX.	EX. NO.	PAGE
1. Calf stretches	6.4	193
2. The calf muscles foam roll	6.7	198
3. Achilles isometrics	6.5	194

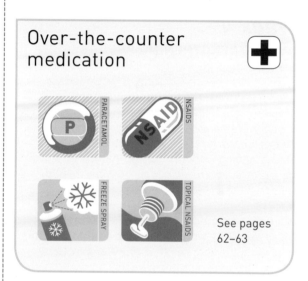

Over-the-counter medication

See pages 62–63

The first week after suffering suspected Achilles tendinopathy is all about rest. The aim is to reduce the pain and the key to this is managing the load on the tendon. This means avoiding anything that excessively causes stress on the tendon and would include refraining from activities that involve rapid loading and stretching the calf muscles, for example, running.

Tendons need some load in order to maintain function; walking around, as you typically would, will provide sufficient loading to help normal function and the first aid routine you've started should be continued as it will continue to help reduce symptoms.

Week 2

Time to start some core exercise work.

Week 3

If you are free from symptoms off the bike, now's the time to get back to cycling.

Week 4

CALF-STRENGTHENING PROGRESSION

If everything is back to normal and you're riding pain free by now, that's great; it may not have been a calf muscle weakness underlying your problem. If not, then alongside the strengthening of your core you've been doing for a couple of weeks, now's the time to advance the specific strengthening work of your calf muscles that will help provide improved support of your Achilles tendon.

The isometric exercises you've been doing will have improved strength in the calf a little and these exercises will increase the strength, further improving the chances that your Achilles issue doesn't become a problem again.

If this is the second or third time you're getting an Achilles problem, then you can jump straight into these exercises as it's a sign that perhaps the calf muscles need to be strengthened.

REHAB TOOL KIT EX.	EX. NO.	PAGE
1. Calf strengthening	6.6	194

Week 7

STILL HAVE PAIN – WHO SHOULD YOU CALL?

If after six weeks having gone through all of the above you are still not comfortable on the bike and are experiencing Achilles pain, you should seek help.

If you have patience, you can wait a little longer as it can take around eight weeks – or sometimes up to 12 – to significantly increase calf strength with the rehabilitation programme we have laid out to strengthen your calf in the rehab toolkit.

PLAN A

PLAN B

 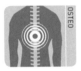

MATT SAYS:

'This can be a frustrating injury and the approach that fixes one person can be very different to what helps the next. My advice is always to give it the suitable rest it deserves. During this time you can put the wheels in motion to get to the underlying cause that will typically need to be worked on. This is not normally one of those injuries that just 'gets better on its own' once it's been there for a few weeks, so taking an active approach to your recovery can mean a swifter resolution to the problem.'

Advances in treatment: shock wave therapy

Shock wave therapy is nothing new; in fact, as long ago as 1980, it was first used to treat kidney stones. More recently, however, it has evolved to become a non-invasive approach for the management of Achilles tendinopathy. A device is used that passes shock waves through the skin to the affected area of the tendon. The actual mechanism as to how it works is still relatively unknown, but it's thought to somehow stimulate the body's healing response by irritating the tissue. Yes, this treatment is therefore often painful. There's evidence to suggest there's some benefit, however, and if done alongside a good rehabilitation programme, the evidence becomes stronger. The other consideration is cost, you'll need to consult either a physiotherapist or a sports doctor for this treatment and will typically need multiple visits so weighing up the cost/benefit of the approach is important. A miracle cure or a guarantee for success it certainly is not, but it should be considered prior to more invasive procedures such as surgery, although we are hopeful that you don't let your injury get to that stage.

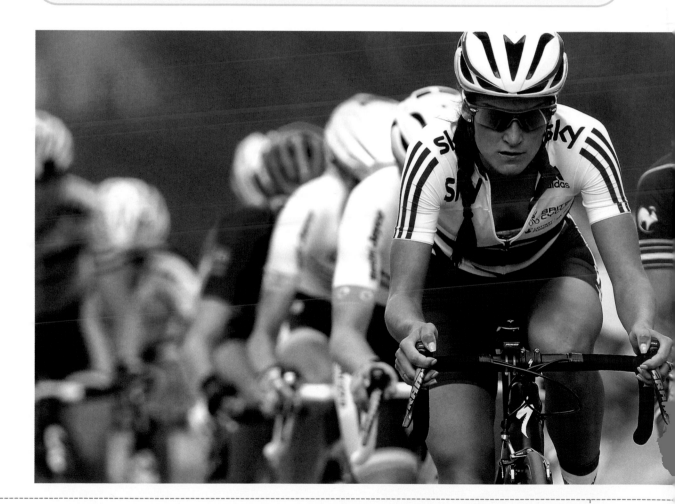

11 ILIOTIBIAL BAND FRICTION SYNDROME

Cycling was once effortless, but now with every turn of the pedals you can feel a sharp pain on the outside of your knee; it feels like someone is sticking a hot knife in there with every revolution. It wasn't always like this, but it came out of nowhere and now it's only getting worse. Time to get off the bike and rest up as you've probably developed iliotibial band friction syndrome. Be warned: irritation and inflammation at the iliotibial band as it attaches near the outside of the knee can be a problem that can go on for months, or even years, if it's not dealt with.

The lowdown

Iliotibial band friction syndrome (ITBFS) is the most common cause of pain to the outside of the knee in cyclists of all levels. This injury accounts for between 15–24 per cent of all overuse injuries in cycling.

BELOW Know the symptoms of ITBFS

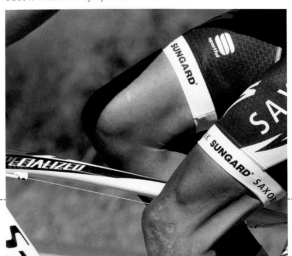

ITBFS is caused by both friction – and compressive forces as we'll describe. The continuous repetitive bending and straightening of the knee that occurs when pedalling can lead to irritation between the iliotibial band (ITB) and the femur (thigh bone) near the outside of the knee causing local inflammation and pain to develop.

Whether you're a commuter cyclist, sportive rider or professional, the pain can build with this injury and keep you off your bike for a lengthy spell. If you're lucky, it will just disappear as quickly as it came, but once this injury has developed and you're getting symptoms, they usually need to be addressed. The good news is that there are things you can do to chase the pain away, resolve the injury and get you back flying on the bike.

Symptom checker

- ✔ Dull pain on the outside of the knee.
- ✔ Progresses to sharp pain on bigger gear efforts or climbing.
- ✔ Once pain presents you will often feel it throughout the ride.
- ✔ Can become searing in nature and feel like a hot poker is stabbing in the knee.
- ✔ May feel a 'clicking' sensation on the outside of the knee when cycling.
- ✔ Outside of the knee can become swollen and tender to touch.
- ✔ The hip and lower back on same side of the knee pain can become painful too as the problem gets worse.

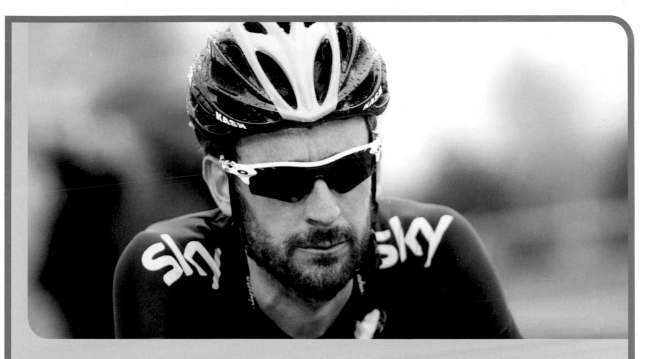

PROFESSIONAL INSIGHT

Sir Bradley Wiggins BRITISH PRO AND TOUR DE FRANCE WINNER

■ *'My knee pain came on during the 2013 Giro d'Italia. From being fine on one stage, all of a sudden on the next it started to flare up and became painful on the outside of my left knee early during the stage. As the stage wore on the pain started to build and in particular any small climbs we had to do that put more torque on the knee only made the pain worse.*

I could feel my whole left iliotibial band getting tighter throughout the day and I couldn't get out of the saddle without pain. I made it to the end of the stage and that evening began having the knee treated by the physio, which involved loosening off some of the muscles and icing it.

Our team doctor gave me some anti-inflammatory medication to try and ease the pain too. In a three-week tour it's always a challenge to try and recover for the next stage and my team did

an excellent job to keep me in the race for the next few days. Unfortunately, as soon as the harder mountain stages begun and we started climbing more, the pain became too much. I could tell it wasn't going to get better if I continued the race and I ended up withdrawing.

I had scans and tests and all my bikes were re-checked to see if it was a bike fit issue. I ended up having a steroid injection under ultrasound guidance, which took the pain away, but only for a few days. Eventually I went to see Matt who helped fix my lower back and improve the function of my pelvis, which in turn made a quick difference to the symptoms in my knee. I started a rigorous specific core routine and used the foam roller daily, and between this and the chiropractic work, I was back on my bike pain free within a week.'

The science bit

The iliotibial band

- The ITB is a connective tissue band that runs down the outside of the leg and attaches to the outside of the shin bone just below knee.
- The band of fascia is thick, strong and fibrous and is actually an extension of the buttock muscles, gluteus maximus, gluteus medius and tensor fascia latae (TFL).
- Contraction of these muscles controls the tension in the ITB.
- The main role of the ITB is to provide sideways stability of the knee during movement at the knee joint especially during knee straightening.
- The ITB helps provide stability to the knee during the pedal stroke and also helps stabilise the hip by preventing it turning in too much during pedalling (stopping the knee hitting the cross bar while riding).

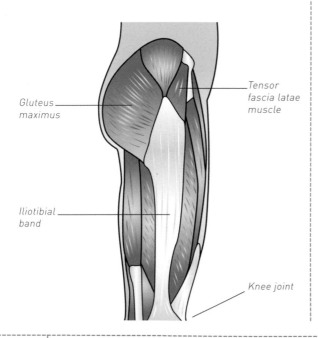

Gluteus maximus

Tensor fascia latae muscle

Iliotibial band

Knee joint

Causes of iliotibial band friction syndrome

The pedal stroke

Cycling is a low-impact sport, however, the overall load on the knees can be significant purely due to the number of repetitions of the pedal action that sees the knee bend and straighten continuously. For the average cyclist, who rides five hours a week, it will mean the knee is flexing and extending over one million times per year. No wonder the knee can become overworked, overused and break down.

When the knee is bent to 30 degrees – as it is going from flexion to extension and vice versa – the shin-bone (tibia) is mildly turned inwards (internally rotates) as part of normal function. This 30 degree knee flexion is known as the 'impingement zone'. As the shin bone turns inwards it gently pulls the attachment of the ITB with it, causing the end of the ITB to become compressed against the outside of the thigh bone.

Between the ITB and the bottom of the outside of the thigh bone there's a layer of fat that has both good nerve and blood supply. The most recent theory suggests that repetitive knee flexion and extension causes this layer of fat to

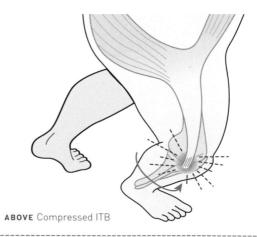

ABOVE Compressed ITB

get repetitively compressed by the ITB moving over the widening at the bottom of the thigh bone femoral near the knee at 30 degree knee flexion. It's the repetition of this mild compression in the impingement zone, rather than the actual *force*, that leads to the fat layer becoming irritated, inflamed and symptoms of ITBFS developing. Bearing this in mind perhaps ITB *compression* syndrome might be a more appropriate name!

ITBFS is an overuse injury like many others and, although there are many factors that contribute to it, poor function of the pelvis and legs also play a significant and detrimental role in the process. Anything that can either influence pelvic mechanics and change the 'pull' on the gluteal and TFL muscles that control the ITB (or even weakness of these muscles), or change the mechanics of the lower leg causing increased internal rotation of the shin bone, could potentially make an individual more prone to developing this injury.

Q-angle and pelvic mechanics

The directional pull of knee tracking is determined by what's known as the Q-angle. Taking a line between the direct pull of the thigh muscle and the direction of the patella tendon forms this angle.

It's thought that the larger the Q-angle the more vulnerable an individual will be for knee injuries because the knee is moving further away from working up and down in a straight line. Any force that isn't helping the knee move directly up and down in a linear fashion will increase the tensile stresses on the soft tissue around the knee and can contribute to the development of ITBFS. Women have a

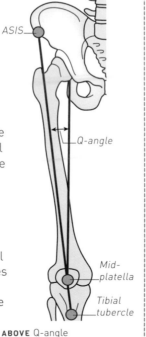

ASIS

Q-angle

Mid-platella

Tibial tubercle

ABOVE Q-angle

Q-Angle showing difference between men and women

female *male*

larger Q-angle than men because they naturally have a wider pelvis meaning their knees 'squint' inwards slightly, which is why women may be more susceptible to ITBFS as research suggests.

Anything that can cause functional variance of the pelvis, for example, muscle imbalance or a fall from the bike, can influence or alter an individual's Q-angle away from their norm. This imbalance can lead to a subtle difference in leg length between the left and the right legs, which is known to be a contributing factor for ITBFS.

Overpronation of the feet

There are 52 bones in the feet, almost a quarter of all the bones of the body. The feet have an intricate role and important function in absorbing forces and releasing this energy when walking, running or cycling. During cycling, when the leg moves into the down stroke, the initial role of the foot is to absorb and help dissipate some of the impact. At this point the foot rolls inwards absorbing the force like a coiled spring, known as pronation of the foot, and stays like this throughout the down stroke as the knee extends.

As the foot is pronated, there's a natural internal rotation of the shin bone at the same time. The more the foot pronates, the more the shin will internally rotate and as the ITB is attached to the top of the shin bone, the more tension there will be placed on the ITB as it passes the widening on the outside of the thigh bone in the impingement zone at 30 degree knee flexion. Overpronation is a condition where the arches of the feet have flattened, increasing the internal rotation of the shin bone, putting more stress on the ITB during the pedal stroke and consequently making an individual more prone to developing ITBFS.

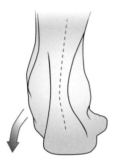

LEFT Overpronation of the foot

Treatment

Injury at a glance

Pain scale	Moderate to severe
Time off bike	2 weeks
Call in the professionals?	Not for now
Surgery?	Not likely

First action: bike and equipment check

Saddle height: if the saddle has dropped, there'll be increased knee flexion during the pedal stroke while the leg muscles aren't working at

their appropriate optimal lengths during the pedalling action. Both of these scenarios change the mechanics of the pedalling action and can contribute to ITBFS developing.

Cleats: if these have moved slightly, there'll be a slight and subtle change in the energy transfer from the feet all the way through the legs while cycling. This might be enough to lead to symptoms of ITBFS starting as the muscles aren't used to working and firing in that particular way.

Once your bike is set up correctly, it's time to address the pain and the problem. The pain experienced on the outside of the knee will normally reduce quickly after getting off the bike but you may feel it under stress, for example, walking up or down stairs. The first concern is to reduce the pain and discomfort locally at the site of the injury, but at the same time you want to begin to work on the lower back and pelvic muscles and are closely linked with the function of the ITB which have probably contributed to the development of the injury. Getting these muscles stronger and more readily engaged will help to reduce the likelihood of this injury returning.

FIRST AID FOR ILIOTIBIAL BAND FRICTION SYNDROME

 Ice the area directly over the painful area 2–3 times a day for 10–20 minutes at a time.

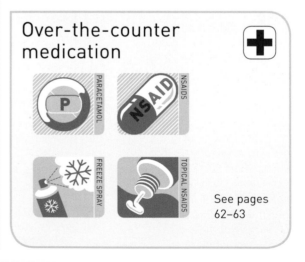

Over-the-counter medication

PARACETAMOL

NSAIDS

FREEZE SPRAY

TOPICAL NSAIDS

See pages 62–63

Weeks 1–2: the next step

Resting and avoiding any other activity that causes repetitive knee flexion, such as running or rowing, are key at this time. Exercise in general is best avoided. Spend this down-time loosening up the lower back and reducing tension in some of the pelvic muscles while also getting the stabilising muscles and buttock muscles working properly to improve the function of the muscles that control the ITB. This will help comfort, stability and symmetry on the bike. These exercises will help:

RECOMMENDATIONS

REHAB TOOL KIT EX.	EX. NO.	PAGE
1. The glutes and piriformis foam roll	5.19	190
2. The tensor fascia latae foam roll	5.20	191
3. Lumbar spine movement	5.1	182
4. The cat and camel	5.2	182
5. The stand and reach stretch	3.1	175
6. The child's pose	5.3	183
7. The bridge	5.10	185
8. The clam shell	5.6	184
9. The sitting gluteal stretch	5.7	184

Massage

Can help to release tension in the buttock muscles that control the ITB, but stay away from the painful area to avoid irritation.

Week 3

Time to get back on your bike.

Time to start a core routine.

MATT SAYS:

'It's vital to take care of the site of the pain and ice does this extremely well and is important to reduce pain and inflammation. However, the key to reducing symptoms of ITBFS swiftly and consistently is recognising that while the pain is felt low down near the outside of the knee, it is usually the muscles up in the buttocks that are short, tight and have trigger points in them whose function has been affected that can be the underlying cause of the injury. When I'm treating cyclists for this injury, an emphasis on these muscles and getting them to work better and improving pelvic function is at the heart of my approach.'

Week 5:

STILL HAVE PAIN – WHO SHOULD YOU CALL?

If after four weeks you've not made significant progress, are still getting pain on the outside of the knee when you ride and have followed all of the above advice, it's time to seek expert help:

PLAN A

 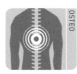

PLAN B

A medical approach

If you don't respond to the above, often the medical treatment of choice is a steroid injection into the site of the pain. This will help by greatly reducing the local inflammation and often the pain, but remember it won't solve the *reason* the problem developed in the first place.

CYCLING NIRVANA

Charly Wegelius

GREAT BRITAIN | BEST PLACED BRITISH FINISHER 2007 TOUR DE FRANCE

■ 'My Cycling Nirvana was at the 2008 Giro d'Italia on the Passo Giau climb. There had been a few climbs before and the whole peloton had stayed together. A few of my teammates looked at each other, and we just said, "Shall we do it?". We started riding as hard as we could. At the bottom of the climb there were loads of switchbacks, it kept going up and we kept pushing on.

When I was racing, I was always happiest when I was on the front of the peloton and I could just "ride my bike". So I got to the front, and just started riding. I went to what I thought was my limit, sat there a while and then pushed on some more. It was like an experiment I was having with myself, as the whole peloton sat on and rode behind me. I kept riding and then I noticed it had gone all quiet. I was in my own head, I didn't really feel anything. It felt as though my body stopped at the waist and my legs were part of the bike. It didn't matter if I was in the saddle or seated, it felt like the hairpins were sling-shotting me faster, not slowing me down.

There were TV crew on motorbikes and helicopters but I was totally oblivious. My teammate was talking to me and it felt like a whisper, telling me everyone was hurting and could I do more. I kept pushing. All those days I had been pushed against the ropes and been on the receiving end of someone pushing on, now it was my turn and I rode and rode. The whole Giro peloton was whittled away. When I had first got on the front there

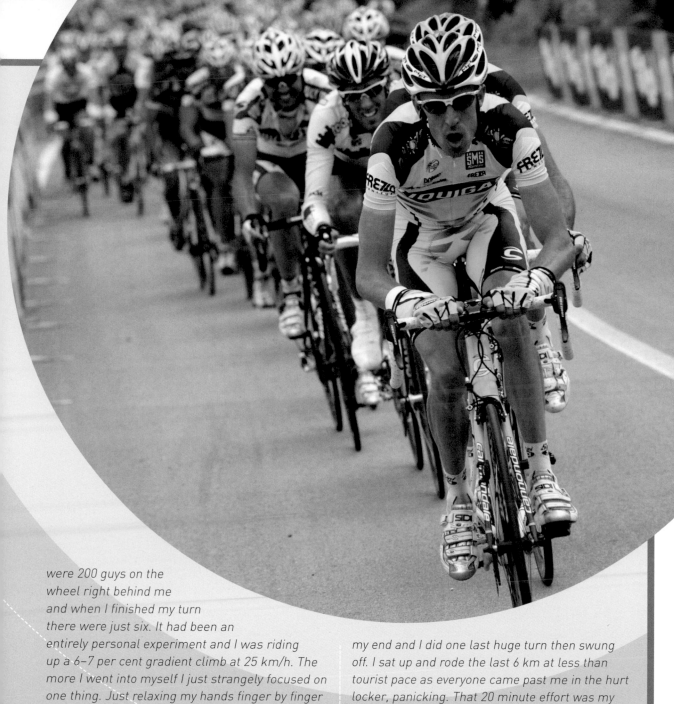

were 200 guys on the wheel right behind me and when I finished my turn there were just six. It had been an entirely personal experiment and I was riding up a 6–7 per cent gradient climb at 25 km/h. The more I went into myself I just strangely focused on one thing. Just relaxing my hands finger by finger and focusing on that allowed my body to do what it wanted to do without the mind interfering.

As we went through a tunnel, I knew I was at my end and I did one last huge turn then swung off. I sat up and rode the last 6 km at less than tourist pace as everyone came past me in the hurt locker, panicking. That 20 minute effort was my Cycling Nirvana. The rest of the day before that I had no idea I was going to do that well. It was that moment when everything just comes together.'

12 CERVICAL FACET STRAIN (MECHANICAL NECK PAIN)

You can be riding along innocently, commuting to work or out having a Sunday spin, you've turned your head to look for traffic the same way you have a thousand times before, but this time you've felt a 'twang', a slight pain on one side of your neck that gets worse when you move your head and feels better when you keep it still. Now it's hard keeping your head upright while riding to see where you're going and the vibrations of the road only make it worse. If this is the case, you may have strained one of the cervical facet joints, the small joints in the back of your neck, and now the neck muscles have gone into spasm protecting you from injuring it more, resulting in a hot intense focal pain. This injury is very common and will hamper your cycling, have no doubt about it: time to get it sorted.

The lowdown

Neck pain is an occupational hazard for most keen cyclists at some time or another. Blame it on the bike: the standard cycling position sees the head tilted back, putting the neck into extension, causing a compression of the small facet joints in the back of the neck making them more likely to become irritated and painful. The neck wasn't designed to be held in this position for hours on end; throw in the fact it's constantly moving and adjusting as your head moves while you're riding, and it's almost inevitable something might give at some point and that's usually what happens when you strain your neck.

But it's not just the bike position. A fall from the bike can cause a whiplash injury, which is a sure way to fast-forward and create neck strain too as the facet joints brace a lot of the stress from the fall.

While neck strain can hamper the comfort of your cycling, it shouldn't affect your performance as the pedal stroke isn't affected – many professionals have ridden for days in Grand Tours with this injury. But who wants to ride in pain? Getting this pain in your neck sorted quickly should mean minimal time off the bike and minimal loss to fitness.

Symptom checker

- ✓ Rapid onset of local dull ache at back of the neck, usually to one side.
- ✓ Sharp pain with certain neck movements, rotation restricted in one direction worse than the other.
- ✓ Difficulty keeping head upright on the bike, meaning you want to hold your head lower than normal.
- ✓ Mild ache into the shoulder and arm can sometimes be felt.
- ✓ Headache at back of the head that may extend behind the eyes on one side or both while riding is not uncommon.
- ✓ Pain always noticeable when on the bike, eases off the bike, but still present on movement.
- ✓ Neck muscles feel in spasm and are sore to touch.

PROFESSIONAL INSIGHT

Rohan Dennis AUSTRALIAN PRO AND TOUR DOWN UNDER 2015 WINNER

■ *'I've had a few neck problems over my cycling career. They are usually the results of the number of miles I do on the bike, with the neck always in extension. I have to get on top of it quickly, which I can usually do with some exercises and stretches and, if I need it, I'll make sure I get some massage and see a chiropractor.*

Every now and again I'll be aware the neck is about to get tight as I'll possibly wake up with a mild headache or one would pop up at some time during the day. This wasn't too bad to deal with, as often, if I need it, I take a paracetamol or ibuprofen and it will be gone. I know this isn't a fix so I also step up my neck mobility exercises and stretches and that will keep things sorted.

The headaches would normally affect me mainly while in the TT position on the track as you spend so long with your neck in extension tucked in to be as aero as possible. With such an extreme position, the neck would get irritated as it would put a bit of strain on there and the shoulder muscles. Again, frequent massages and chiropractic work along with stretches, and simple

exercises help to keep everything working properly and sort out the pain. The key is I've learned to listen to my body and have learned what I need to do whenever I strain my neck.'

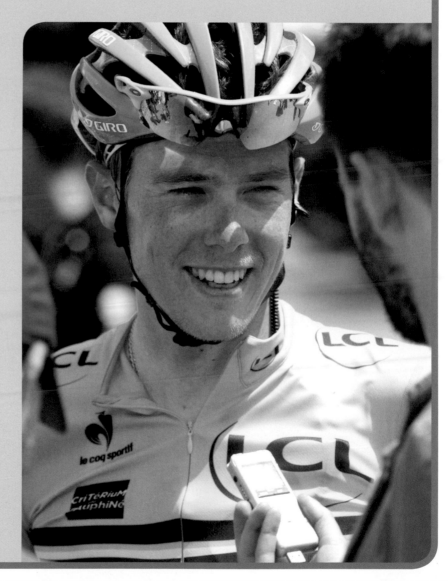

The science bit

THE NECK

- The cervical spine runs through the neck and is made up of seven vertebrae stacked on top of each other.
- The vertebrae are separated by discs that act like shock absorbers providing cushioning to vibration forces that travel through the neck.
- From the side, the cervical spine has a natural curve in it (lordosis) and this allows better weight distribution of the head and improved mobility.
- The spinal cord that comes from the brain stem above runs straight through the cervical spine that protects it.
- At the back of the cervical spine are the small facet joints that link each vertebra to the one directly above and below it. These joints allow motion between each segment, letting the neck move forwards, backwards, laterally bend and rotate.

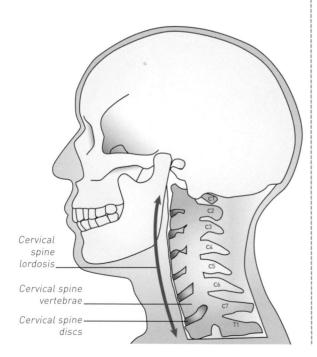

Cervical spine lordosis

Cervical spine vertebrae

Cervical spine discs

Causes of neck strain

Standing upright is the posture nature intended; adopt the cycling position and we begin to move away from it. As soon as the feet are clipped into the pedals and the hands are on the handlebars, the cervical spine is put in a compromising position. Why? Well, in order to keep your eyes forwards on the road, the neck extensor muscles are engaged, lifting the head up and putting the neck into extension. As this happens the facet joints slide over each other and overlap. Not only is the neck extended, but the chin often naturally sticks out too.

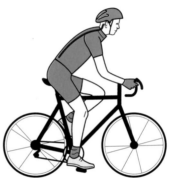

ABOVE The cycling position puts the neck in extension increasing stress on the joints compared to standing

For every inch your head is held forward, the muscles of the neck have to work that much harder just to maintain this posture, plus the weight distribution of the head on the shoulders becomes uneven, putting increased pressure on the small joints of the neck. So you can see how once you've got on to your bike, even before you've turned the pedals, the neck is under increased stress.

If you have an aggressive position on the bike or are on the drops, there's more extension in the neck, jamming the facet joints even closer. Unfortunately, most roads are far from 'glass smooth' (if only!). The small vibrations that are felt while riding over rough roads, travel through the whole body and up through the neck. Yes, the cervical discs absorb much of this shock, but not all.

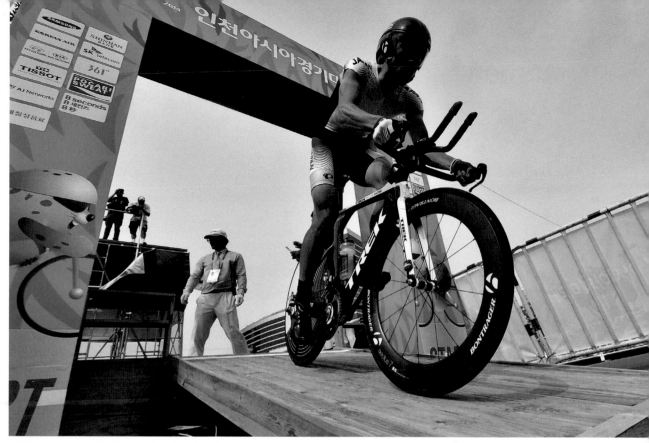

ABOVE During any ride the neck is put under a lot of pressure

While riding you're constantly looking out for the next corner, the next person to step out on the road, the lights to change, the next pothole to avoid; you are consistently on alert swivelling the head looking out. The neck joints never get a moments rest while riding.

Joint receptors

Small receptors called mechanoreceptors, found in all the joints of the neck, give constant feedback to the brain on the movement occurring in the joints. These receptors are also responsible for detecting when the joints have become stretched more than they should. After hours of riding, the cumulative compounding effects of the continuous vibration, the constant movement of the neck, and an overworking of neck extensor muscle contractions just to keep the head upright can become too much and something gives.

When normal movement of the facet joints is momentarily exceeded, the receptors fire and the muscles kick in, but this time it's too late: the joint's been stretched further than it should be and the facet joint's been strained, causing local tissue damage. Now pain receptors are stimulated, causing the neck to become painful, while the body starts a local inflammatory response, working to heal the damaged tissue. The neck muscles go into spasm, causing reduced and painful head movement, the aim of which is to prevent further damage to the aggravated neck joints.

In the case of a whiplash type injury where the facet joints are strained, it's more common to strain the lower cervical vertebrae as the neck hinges at around the 5th and 6th cervical vertebrae level. Aside from cases of traumatic whiplash, cervical facet strain are generally caused by overuse.

Knowing how it got there is one thing, recognising it and knowing what to do to sort it becomes the challenge.

Treatment

Injury at a glance

Pain scale	Mild to severe
Time off bike	1 week
Call in the professionals?	Not for now
Surgery?	No

First action: bike and equipment check

The cycling position impacts the cervical facets in the back of the neck and the more aggressive your position, the more you'll irritate your complaint.

Handlebars slip: if these have rolled forwards, you'll be in a slightly more aggressive position as you reach further and extend your neck more, putting increased pressure on the joints of your neck. This may be all that's needed to irritate the joints and strain them.

BELOW Check your bike, but once you get off

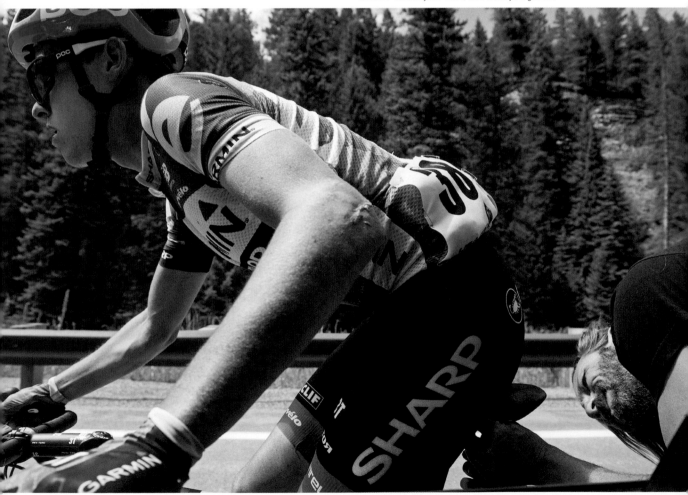

Week 1

THE NEXT STEP

Your bike is set up correctly and you still have neck symptoms when you ride so it's now time to address the cervical facet strain specifically.

FIRST AID FOR NECK STRAIN

 Ice the area for 10–15 minutes over the painful area 2–3 times per day. Continue to ice for 3 days or continue for as long as you have pain off the bike. You shouldn't need to ice for longer than a week but you can continue to do so if you need to.

MATT SAYS:

'I often get asked about using heat for (mechanical) neck pain. I usually always recommend ice at first as it will have a painkilling effect as well as help any local inflammation. After 3–4 days, if you want to introduce heat once the acute stage is over, then alternating between ice and heat – 10 minutes of ice followed by 10 minutes of heat – can help further relieve symptoms.'

Over-the-counter medication ➕

See pages 62–63

Stay off the bike for seven days after the onset of neck pain, or at least drastically reduce the amount of hours you ride. Avoid any activity that will further aggravate your neck: for example running because the vibrations can aggravate neck pain; weights can increase the strain in the neck; and swimming too is best avoided (although backstroke may be comfortable). Now's the time for recovery.

 Run through the following exercises to help reduce the discomfort and increase mobility:

REHAB TOOL KIT EX.	EX. NO.	PAGE
1. Improve your breathing	n/a	159
2. Neck rotation	1.1	163
3. The shoulder roll	2.1	169
4. The sphinx	5.5	183
5. Upper back mobility	1.2	164
6. The neck stretch	1.3	165
7. Upper back tennis ball release	1.9	168

 Neck pain accompanying cervical facet strain will often still be felt when you're off the bike, especially when you turn your head in one direction or tilt your head backwards.

When the head is held straight in a neutral position, the neck will often feel better as symptoms subside. Pain is a sign to tell you there is a problem so addressing it swiftly will normally mean a quicker recovery.

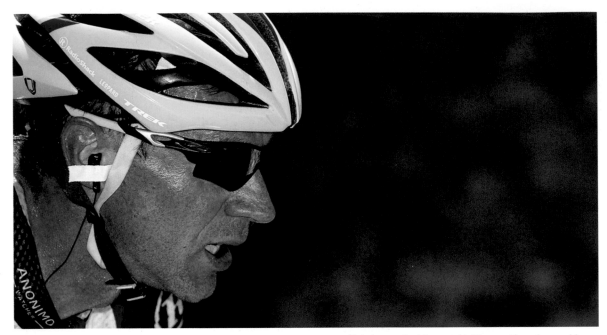

Week 2

Time to get back on your bike after a week's rest.

Time to start your core exercise work. Continue the exercises you have been doing that are specifically related to the neck and upper back.

RECOMMENDATIONS

Tag on the following exercises to the regular core exercise programme in the rehab toolkit as they will help to engage the deep neck flexor muscles, which are the 'core' muscles for the neck region.

REHAB TOOL KIT EX.	EX. NO.	PAGE
1. Deep neck flexor activation	1.4	165
2. Deep neck flexor strengthening	1.5	166
3. Scapular stabiliser activation	1.6	167
4. The wall angel	1.7	167

Week 5

STILL HAVE PAIN – WHO SHOULD YOU CALL?

If after four weeks you've not made significant progress, are still getting neck pain when you ride and have followed all of the above advice, it's time to seek expert help:

PLAN A

 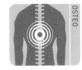

PLAN B

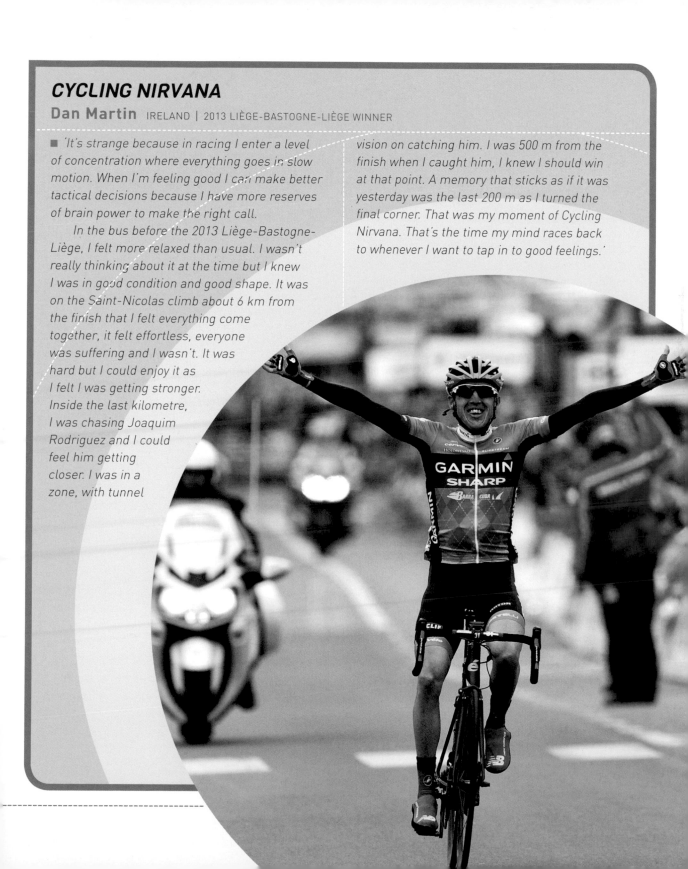

CYCLING NIRVANA

Dan Martin IRELAND | 2013 LIÈGE-BASTOGNE-LIÈGE WINNER

■ 'It's strange because in racing I enter a level of concentration where everything goes in slow motion. When I'm feeling good I can make better tactical decisions because I have more reserves of brain power to make the right call.

In the bus before the 2013 Liège-Bastogne-Liège, I felt more relaxed than usual. I wasn't really thinking about it at the time but I knew I was in good condition and good shape. It was on the Saint-Nicolas climb about 6 km from the finish that I felt everything come together, it felt effortless, everyone was suffering and I wasn't. It was hard but I could enjoy it as I felt I was getting stronger. Inside the last kilometre, I was chasing Joaquim Rodriguez and I could feel him getting closer. I was in a zone, with tunnel vision on catching him. I was 500 m from the finish when I caught him, I knew I should win at that point. A memory that sticks as if it was yesterday was the last 200 m as I turned the final corner. That was my moment of Cycling Nirvana. That's the time my mind races back to whenever I want to tap in to good feelings.'

13 EXTERNAL ILIAC ARTERY ENDOFIBROSIS

You may well have never heard of this tongue twister, so you also probably won't know that it affects approximately 20 per cent of top-level cyclists and, if you do enough miles, it could potentially affect you too. But what is it? Well, quite simply, it's a limitation of the blood flow through one of the main arteries in the leg often caused by something called kinking. This occurs when the artery becomes twisted and can result in pain and a powerless sensation in the leg when riding at high intensity.

The lowdown

Limitation in the blood flow through the external iliac artery is caused by endofibrosis of the artery wall which is a narrowing that may be caused by compression, stretch or kinking of the artery or a combination of them.

The unique posture and action of cycling where constant repetitive hip flexion occurs and is continued for lengthy periods of time creates the perfect storm for external iliac artery endofibrosis (EIAE) to develop. This injury is hugely frustrating because it robs you of your ability to cycle flat out at high intensity and so your riding performance is significantly affected. Having EIAE and trying to ride hard is like having a Ferrari but being limited to second gear; all the power is there under the bonnet but the ability to use it isn't, because the blood flow to the muscles that provide the power is limited.

Another reason for frustration is because it normally takes so long to get properly diagnosed.

Symptoms can mimic other injuries and your doctor is more likely to expect artery narrowing in older, unhealthy smokers or ex-smokers, rather than younger fit and healthy cyclists.

Most cyclists that develop the injury have ridden between 14,500–20,000 km in the previous

PROFESSIONAL INSIGHT
Mike Friedman
RETIRED AMERICAN PRO AND TOUR DE KOREA WINNER

■ *'In 2011 I began noticing on a more regular basis that my left leg was not functioning properly or normally compared to what I was used to. When I was riding hard my left leg felt as if it was loaded up with lactic acid and working significantly more than my right.*

As I started to ride harder my left glute would seize up, then my left quad and my whole left leg would become painful. It would then be sore for the rest of the day. It started gradually but got more consistent when I rode hard. When it got to the point that I couldn't pedal properly I knew it was serious. It started as cramping generally but then on the drops or aero bars of the TT bike it was always worse and very painful so I started to think it could be the artery getting choked.

year, which is quite a lot for amateurs. This, however, works out at under 300 km a week. It's not just your total kilometres ridden that can cause EIAE to develop; if you have suddenly and significantly increased your training load, you could be more vulnerable too.

Symptom checker

✔ Pain, burning, weakness or numbness experienced in the leg usually the thigh or calf areas during high intensity cycling that backs off as soon as intensity drops.
✔ Pain is almost exclusive to high intensity cycling.
✔ Symptoms often in one leg only.
✔ May notice a colder foot on the affected leg immediately after riding.

The science bit

Blood supply to the legs

- The aorta is the main blood vessel taking freshly oxygenated blood from the heart to the rest of the body.
- A branch of the aorta passes into the abdomen and divides into two branches at its lower end, the common iliac arteries.
- The pair – left and right sided – of common iliac arteries continue to descend and lower down divide again into the internal and external iliac arteries.
- The external iliac artery provides the main blood supply to the muscles and tissues of the legs.

I eventually saw a doctor and he immediately suggested it could be the artery and referred me. I had tests and that confirmed I had significant reduction in blood flow into the left leg. On testing in the lab, leg pain came on within two minutes of riding hard! Further testing revealed I had a 90 degree kink in one of my arteries and an endofibrosis had developed. I was told that I had reduced blood flow in the artery to almost a trickle rather than a good flow; no wonder I was getting symptoms. The reduced blood flow was causing the leg to load up with lactic acid leading to the intense burning pain. Cycling didn't cause it but it definitely made the symptoms worse. I eventually had the surgery to repair the problem and it was a success, although it's been a slow recovery. I feel much better now and the symptoms have all but gone.

I'm grateful the problem didn't affect me reaching the highest levels of the sports or riding at the Olympics.'

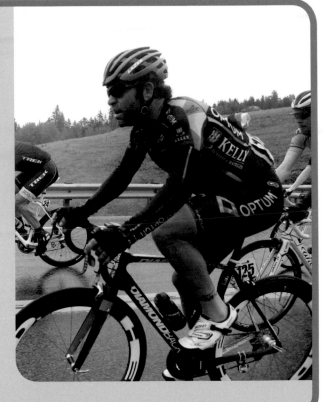

- Each branch of the artery travels through the pelvis and into the lower abdomen, becoming the femoral artery as it enters the leg.

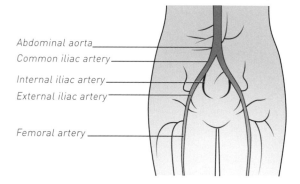

Abdominal aorta

Common iliac artery

Internal iliac artery

External iliac artery

Femoral artery

Causes of external iliac artery endofibrosis

Kinking (like drinking through a straw that's been bent) can stretch and damage the blood vessel wall and is believed to be a precursor to endofibrotic (scar tissue build-up inside the artery) lesions developing. But why should it kink? Depending on the position of the blood vessel in the abdomen, the artery can become stuck to the local muscles. Another reason is that it's thought that the repetitive hip flexion movement of cycling can also cause the artery to become kinked in cyclists that naturally have longer blood vessels.

The external iliac artery is long enough to adapt, compensate and stretch to the different leg positions that occur in normal everyday activity. However, cycling causes the hip to be repetitively and continuously flexed *beyond* its normal everyday range of motion. The excessive continual 'hyperflexion' of the hip causes additional bending and stretching of the artery and it's thought this too can occasionally cause damage to the artery wall, which along with the artery kinking leads to the development of endofibrotic lesions that narrow the artery.

A combination of stress on the artery wall from repetitive pedalling, tethering of the artery to local muscles, compression of the blood vessel against the larger hip flexor muscles that keen cyclists naturally have and excessive kinking of the artery is thought to result in damage to the wall of the artery leading to endofibrosis. Kinking of the artery alone has been shown to cause *some* blood flow limitation through the artery but it's the endofibrotic lesions that develop, usually between 2–6 cm long, which are the real culprits, significantly narrowing the artery and leading to symptoms.

Cycling requires constant blood supply to the legs so freshly oxygenated blood can get to the working muscles. Exercise at high intensity increases the demand of the blood supply to the legs. As the heart rate increases, the blood flow to the legs increases to meet the demand. Only, with EIAE, the amount of blood flow through the artery *supplying* the legs is limited, like stepping on a hose. Now the ability of the muscles to continue to work properly is reduced as the oxygen supply is reduced. Continue to ride at high intensity and the muscles struggle to function properly and this leads to intense pain and a cramping sensation of the leg muscles, especially in the upper thigh area. At the same time, performance drops because of reduced power output from the muscles as function is compromised. This isn't usually a problem with low and medium intensity cycling as enough blood can get through the narrowed artery to supply the demand of the working leg muscles. Also, likewise at rest and away from the bike, the blood flow through the narrowed artery is sufficient enough that it's not a problem and no cause for concern.

Is cycling the culprit?

Outside of cycling, EIAE is not such a prevalent injury. Why? The unique posture and action of cycling, maintained for lengthy periods of time, creates the ideal environment for this injury to develop. There aren't many sports aside from cycling, rowing and speed skating where constant repetitive hip flexion occurs and therefore it's understandable that outside of these sports the problem is largely unheard of.

Treatment

Injury at a glance

Pains scale	Moderate to severe
Time off bike	No
Call in the professionals?	Yes
Surgery?	No, unless you're a pro

First thought

You'll normally only get symptoms with high intensity cycling. So the good news is if you knock back the intensity and ride at a level where you're not giving it your all, you probably won't even notice there's a problem. However, if you do notice symptoms, don't panic. The good news is it's unlikely to get much worse regardless of the training you do, but unfortunately the not-so- good news is it's unlikely to get much better. This means you don't really need to take any time off the bike though, just continue to ride at a level and intensity that doesn't cause symptoms to come on, while you try and get a diagnosis to find out if EIAE is to blame.

The next step

PLAN A

PLAN B

There's little point spending time or money calling on other health experts as a sports doctor should be able to help make the diagnosis or likewise your doctor should be able to make the necessary referral to move you towards a diagnosis. The surgical repair for this problem is a big operation and carries significant risk, and if you're not an elite cyclist, there's little point in having it done as this injury will not cause problems during any aspect of your everyday life.

MATT SAYS:

'This injury sucks, there's no two ways about it. The main reason is because there is nothing much you can do about it. Surgery isn't necessary unless you're a pro. The good news is, once you know what's going on, you can continue to ride knowing that you're not going to make things worse and as long as you're careful you'll never know you have the issue.'

Ankle brachial index test

This is the least invasive test to help get an early diagnosis. A doctor compares the blood pressure in your arms and legs. This is measured before and immediately after riding a stationary bike. The ankle brachial index (ABI) is calculated by dividing the (systolic) blood pressure at the ankle by the (systolic) blood pressure in the arm to provide a ratio. Anything from 1 to 1.1 is considered normal and when performed at rest this will often be the case. The post cycling measurement in patients with EIAE will see a notable reduction in blood pressure in the leg and consequently a drop in the calculated ABI to below 0.9 (0.9–1 is borderline abnormal). This indicates there's a restriction of blood flow to the legs during exercise, which may indicate EIAE. When both legs are compared you would only expect to see changes in the ABI after exercise in the symptomatic leg.

14

ACROMIO-CLAVICULAR JOINT SPRAIN
(SHOULDER SEPARATION)

Falling off your bike at speed will instinctively force your body to tuck and roll as the momentum throws you forward, often over the handlebars. As you catapult from your bike it becomes a lottery as to which part of your body bears the impact. If you rotate enough in the air, you may be lucky and avoid banging your head, but the chances are you may land on your shoulder, right on top of your acromioclavicular joint, causing a momentary separation of the joint, damaging the ligaments. This frustrating injury can result in a slow recovery and while you can be back on your bike usually in a couple of weeks, it can take far longer before you feel totally comfortable riding again. Sustain this injury and it's important to take action right away to speed up your recovery.

The lowdown

The problem with this injury is that there are no large muscle groups covering the acromioclavicular (AC) joint. It's a superficial joint that's not well protected. Although there are strong ligaments that hold the joint together keeping it in place, when these ligaments get damaged in a crash the stability of the joint becomes compromised. This is a problem while cycling as the upper body weight is braced through the hands and arms and into the

shoulder partly through the AC joint. The support of the upper body, coupled with the constant vibration forces from the road, can cause the joint to be extremely painful while riding as you recover from the injury.

The ligaments that stabilise the joint are naturally slow healers so the pain can go on for weeks or even months as they can get repetitively aggravated in everyday life and with cycling. This makes it even more important to follow certain steps to allow the best recovery in the shortest possible time.

Symptom checker

You've crashed, landed on your shoulder, could it be the AC joint?
- ✔ Sharp pain on tip of shoulder with possible swelling.
- ✔ Difficulty moving the shoulder, feels like it is grinding and clunking.
- ✔ Once back on bike, throbbing pain at top of shoulder.
- ✔ Arm on the affected side feels weak.
- ✔ Pain almost constant throughout the ride in the shoulder after the crash.

PROFESSIONAL INSIGHT

Johan Vansummeren BELGIAN PRO AND PARIS-ROUBAIX WINNER

■ 'I separated my right shoulder a couple of weeks before the Worlds in Salzburg in 2006. Many of the Belgian national team had decided to go to the Ardennes to do our last proper training ride and get together five days before the race. We were all relaxed riding next to each other, catching up, and then I remember hooking the handlebar of my teammate. The next thing I know I had landed on my right shoulder. (My teammate crashed too and broke his collarbone). Immediately it was agony. I couldn't move my arm for the pain. I knew it was separated and I later found out it was a grade II (see page 121) and it was PAINFUL.

Luckily the season was over so I could rest, but I was annoyed as it meant I couldn't represent my country at Worlds that year. I remember it being really painful for the first two weeks which was frustrating because you are just waiting for it to get better, whereas with a collarbone fracture I could've had an operation and been in less pain and back on my bike in a few days.

There wasn't much I could do, other than tape it and ice it. I couldn't sleep on my right side for weeks. I went to physio regularly to help with treatment and did exercises to get my shoulder working properly as quickly as I could. I personally didn't bother with a sling and I only took painkillers for the first few days but did continue to ice it.

As it was the end of the season I was in no mad rush to get back, which was a nice stress not to have, so I took my time and did everything right. Within a month I was back training again, pain-free and had no problems. I could've probably ridden sooner but I wanted to enjoy the off-season!'

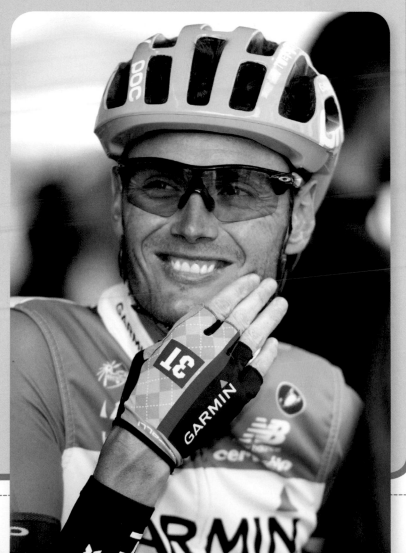

Road side test

Think you've damaged your AC joint?
- Place the hand of the injured arm on the front of your opposite shoulder, as shown.
- Now try and lift your elbow to the horizontal. If this causes obvious significant pain, you've probably injured your AC joint.

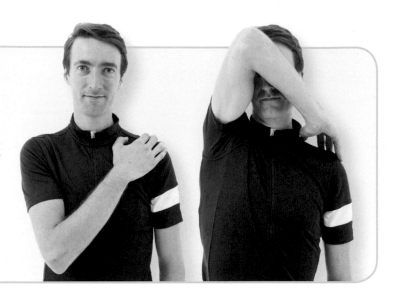

The science bit

The acromio-clavicular joint

- The AC joint is a small joint found at the top of the shoulder formed at the junction between the scapula (the acromion) and the end of the collarbone (the clavicle) – hence its name 'acromioclavicular joint'.
- There are no muscles responsible for voluntarily moving it unlike the majority of other joints in the body.
- The joint is held in place and stabilised by three short and strong ligaments (acromioclavicular①, coracoacromial② and coracoclavicular③ ligaments) and the joint capsule.
- The joint can vary significantly in size and form between people but its function remains the same and this is to allow the arm to be moved over the head when it acts as a pivot allowing the increased shoulder rotation to occur.

Coracoclavicular ligament ③

Acromioclavicular joint

Clavicle

Acromion process

① *Acromioclavicular ligament*

② *Coracoacromial ligament*

Glenohumeral joint

Humerus

Subscapularis muscle

Scapula

Degrees of separation

When you land on the tip of the shoulder at force, usually something will give and it will normally either be the collarbone or the AC joint that takes the brunt of the impact. Tuck your head in and get enough momentum and you can end up rotating over and landing on the back of the shoulder on the scapula (shoulder blade) itself which is painful but usually won't cause as much damage.

However, land on the tip of your shoulder and it becomes very easy to 'separate' the shoulder, more specifically the AC joint. This is not to be confused with a dislocation that occurs in the shoulder joint proper that sees the large head of the shoulder pop out of its socket.

When the shoulder is separated you stress the ligaments holding the AC joint stable by creating a shear force between the two ends of the joint. Depending on the severity, force and angle of impact of how you land, there are six different types of AC joint injury that are diagonsed. The grading is based loosely upon the amount of separation of the joint in addition to the ligaments that are damaged:

Grade 1: Corresponds to a sprain of the ligament capsule that surrounds the joint and is characterised by localised tenderness and pain on movement. Moving the arm forwards in front of the body past the horizontal will usually be painful. There'll be slight displacement of the joint but not enough to be seen on an X-ray.

Grade 2: Correlates to a complete tear of the ligament that bridges the end of the joint together – the acromioclavicular ligament – as well as a slight strain of the other ligaments that stabilise the joint. With the shirt taken off, you'll often see some deformity of the joint, like a bump where the two ends of the joint have been slightly separated and are barely overlapping (see below, centre). In these cases there's often been a separation of the joint of more than 5 mm (under 4 mm is normal) so you can often see this on an X-ray. This is extremely painful and can often feel like the shoulder is grinding, cracking and rubbing when the arm is moved.

Most shoulder separations that occur in a fall from a bike would come into these first two categories when you land on your AC joint.

Grade 3: When you completely tear all three of the main stabilising ligaments of the AC joint, you'll sustain a grade III AC joint strain. When this happens, deformity is obvious when compared to the other side as there's complete separation (dislocation) of the joint meaning the collarbone often sticks up and can be seen poking against the skin. There's often significant swelling that occurs with this injury (above that of a grade I or II strain) and it will be extremely painful to move the arm much at all in the first few weeks after sustaining the injury.

Grades 4–6: These are far rarer luckily but can occur following a crash at high speed. If you get anything above a grade III, then the deformity, pain and damage to the joint and surrounding area are usually obvious and make these injuries a medical emergency.

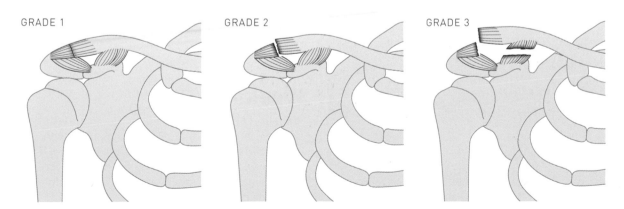

GRADE 1

GRADE 2

GRADE 3

Treatment

Injury at a glance

Pain scale	Moderate to severe
Time off bike	2–3 weeks
Call in the professionals?	Probably
Surgery?	No

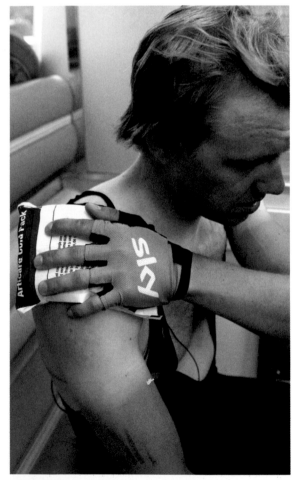

ABOVE Ice will help reduce local inflammation

First thought

If the injury is bad enough you'll usually end up in hospital having an X-ray. If they tell you that you haven't broken your collarbone but have, in fact, separated your AC joint, it's time to take action.

First action

Ice the area 2–3 times a day for 10–15 minutes at a time. Continue to ice for the first couple of weeks or continue for as long as you have significant pain.

Over-the-counter medication

 PARACETAMOL

 NSAIDS

 FREEZE SPRAY

 TOPICAL NSAIDS

Apply these with care as irritating the joint will be painful! See your doctor for stronger pain medication if it's needed.

See pages 62–63

Weeks 1 – 2

When the AC joint is injured the function of the shoulder is affected. Shoulder range of motion is reduced and 'normal movement patterns' of the shoulder get altered. There's not much you can really do besides rest and avoid putting the shoulder into painful positions.

During the first two weeks off the bike work should begin on the rehabilitation of the shoulder. This time is focused on reducing symptoms at the same time as trying to maintain and improve general shoulder function. Attempt to do the exercises five times a week initially, pain allowing. Following this, you can increase the number of repetitions and range of motion of the exercises as you see fit as recovery resumes, although three times a week is a good maintenance recommendation from when the shoulder feels more comfortable up until about 6–8 weeks.

RECOMMENDATIONS

The exercises can be started as soon as you feel comfortable to do so and can be repeated 2–3 times a day. Understand that they might be a little uncomfortable to do, but if one specifically increases the pain, you should skip it and move on to the next one. Try the next day to see if the exercise has become any easier. These are all designed to preserve and maintain shoulder function while you heal and improve the function as you start to recover, so do what you can, even if it's only minimal, as it's better than keeping it immobile in a sling all day which *will* only slow down and draw out your recovery. These exercises should be continued even as you get back to cycling.

REHAB TOOL KIT EX.	EX. NO.	PAGE
1. The shoulder swing	2.2	169
2. Scapular stabiliser activation	1.6	167
3. Isometric shoulder activation	2.3	169
4. Passive shoulder movement	2.4	170
5. Active shoulder range of motion	2.5	172
6. The wall angel	1.7	167
7. One-sided scapular stabiliser	1.8	168
8. Pectoral muscle tennis ball release	3.8	179

 Go slowly to begin with and only do what doesn't make the pain worse.

To sling or not to sling

If you're in agony, the chances are you'll end up in hospital where they might put you in a sling to help keep the AC joint stable, reducing the irritation of movement. Here's how to make a sling if you need to:

- Cut a piece of cloth, such as a pillowcase, about 40 square inches, then fold it in half to make a triangle.
- Slide one end of the sling under the arm and over the shoulder.
- Bring the other end of the sling over the other shoulder cradling the arm.
- Tie both ends of the sling together.
- Tighten the edge of the sling near the elbow.

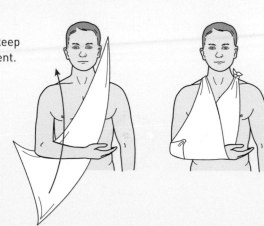

Week 3

Pain too much? Start on the home trainer

Don't worry if you are still feeling some discomfort off the bike, this would be normal and expected and can actually go on for 2–3 months in some mild form. It will be OK to get back on the bike as long as the discomfort is only mild and assuming you can bear it. Don't try and be a hero though and push through if you're not ready. Pain is there for a reason and if you're having to grit your teeth to ride your bike, then it's probably too early.

As you get back to riding, adopting a less aggressive position, such as riding on the handlebars and avoiding the drops, will mean you're able to ride more comfortably as there'll be less of the weight of your upper body going through the injured shoulder.

Kinesio tape

You'll need to get someone else to apply the tape and you'll be surprised how much support you will get from just three small pieces of tape.

See page 175 for this tape application.

Week 4

Time to begin a core exercise programme. Continue alongside your other excercises for the shoulder exercise routine. See page 202.

Week 7

STILL HAVE PAIN – WHO SHOULD YOU CALL?

If after six weeks you're still getting significant pain over the AC joint or are having difficulty moving your shoulder properly even having followed our advice, it's time to seek help.

PLAN A

You may have been under the care of a physio since the outset of this injury as your doctor may have referred you. Either way, now's the time to return to them or find one to help you.

PLAN B

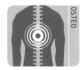

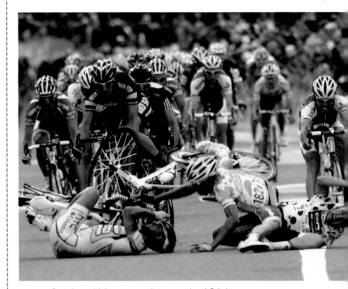

ABOVE Crash and it's easy to damage the AC joint

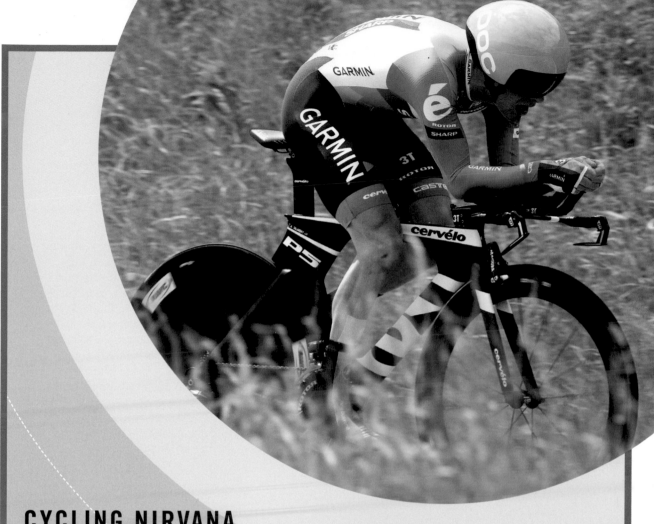

CYCLING NIRVANA

Andrew Talansky UNITED STATES OF AMERICA | 2014 CRITERIUM DE DAUPHINE WINNER

■ 'When I'm fit enough to absolutely bury myself on my time trial bike in a race it feels like Cycling Nirvana. Instead of fighting the pain, I am embracing it because I'm so focused on the present, like at the 2012 Tour of Romandie TT.

I nearly always hate the start as I need to find my rhythm and that can take a little while, but that day the course started with a rise and a descent and I was going fast, launching myself into corners and all sorts.

I remember a 4 km climb in the middle where I felt so dialed-in and had a crazy, almost zen-like focus, I even closed my eyes momentarily.

I got to the finish and I had gone that deep it took me 5–10 minutes to feel remotely normal again. On that finish line, the relief and satisfaction knowing the effort had gone exactly how I wanted it to was my moment of Cycling Nirvana.'

15 ULNAR NEUROPATHY AT THE WRIST (HANDLEBAR PALSY)

You've been out riding and began to notice pins and needles in your hand, most notably your ring and little fingers. This sensation is gradually building and now those fingers and half of your hand are numb. It started out more annoying than painful but that's changing and you try to shake it out while riding which helps a bit but it keeps coming back. You may well have developed an ulnar neuropathy at your wrist, which is when the ulnar nerve that travels down from the shoulder can get stretched and compressed at the wrist as it enters the hand. This can occur when too much pressure is placed on the hands due to lengthy spells riding. This frustrating injury will not only restrict your freedom to ride in comfort but can affect your bike handling if it gets worse. Time to get it sorted.

The lowdown

This injury is so specific to cycling that it's also known as 'cyclist's palsy' or 'handlebar palsy'. Somewhat surprisingly, approximately one third of all cycling overuse injuries involve the hands and a large proportion of those are down to this injury.

There'll come a time during your ride when you find yourself on the drops. Riding this position for hours at a time puts significant pressure on the hand at the ulnar nerve, which can cause it to become irritated, stretched and, ultimately, damaged.

For the amateur cyclist, the good news is that symptoms are often alleviated almost immediately by moving the hands into different positions on the handlebars, coming off the drops and on to the hoods or the top bar for example. However, if the condition progresses, time off the bike becomes the right approach. Luckily usually no more than a week would be needed assuming you didn't let it get too bad and there are things you can do to help you get better during this down-time which we will tell you later. If you push through, it won't really affect your cycling in general because your legs are unaffected, but your comfort will be significantly compromised if you carry on without the appropriate rest.

Symptom checker

- ✔ Pins and needles in hand, ring and little finger.
- ✔ Numbness of the bottom of hand, ring finger and little finger.
- ✔ Dull ache or sharp pain into hand, ring finger and little finger.
- ✔ Weakness and clumsiness of hand, difficulty shifting gears and braking.
- ✔ Temporary relief of symptoms as you shake your hand out.
- ✔ Symptoms made worse when riding the drops.
- ✔ Mild symptoms reproduced when tapping over Guyon's tunnel (see diagram 128).

PROFESSIONAL INSIGHT

Pete Stetina AMERICAN PRO AND TOP TEN TOUR OF CALIFORNIA FINISHER

■ 'I had intermittent numbness and tingling in the two smallest fingers of my left hand for about three seasons, which is almost three years, a long time. It comes on in race situations when I stay on the hoods for extended periods of time. It gets noticeably worse in cold or rainy weather when I think circulation becomes more challenging but I've been told that it's probably a nerve issue. I never crashed on that side or had any injury to my knowledge beforehand, it just kind of appeared from nowhere during the 2011 spring racing campaign.

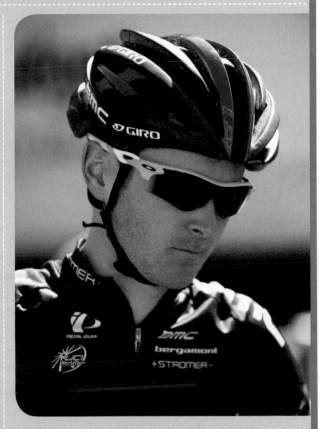

With my team of doctors, we deduced that it's most likely a compression of the ulnar nerve, probably at the wrist and is due I think to so many hours being spent in the hunched bike position and the increased tension and pressure put on the nerve when I ride the hood and drops. It's been hard to rectify as the ulnar nerve could be pinched in a number of places other than the wrist, as I understand it, like the elbow, shoulder, neck, or any combination of the above.

I've tried everything I can think of: different ergonomics of different hood companies didn't help. Bike fits didn't help. Massage didn't help. Even chiropractic didn't seem to help despite being adjusted and treated in all of the above areas. One thing that surprisingly helped was the practice of "neural flossing" which consists of sets of exercises meant to "stretch" the nerve and prevent it from snagging. When I do these exercises before I race the symptoms are usually much better. Of course the best and most simple way to combat this is to continually switch my hand position on the bars between hoods, drops, and tops. Unfortunately this isn't always possible during crunch times of a race that I endure as a pro, but for an amateur I'd definitely recommend it, that, and the exercises. It never seems bad enough to get further investigation done on it, it's more of an annoyance and luckily it's not painful and I never have a problem with braking or bike handling, but if it gets any worse than how it has been, that will be my next step. I am sure that a decent amount of rest would help I've been told, but for now I've just found my way to manage it as, luckily, it doesn't affect me all the time.'

The science bit

The ulnar nerve

- The ulnar nerve starts in the neck and extends from the cervical spine, runs into the arm and down the inside of the elbow along the inside of the forearm.
- It then passes through the wrist where it enters the palm of the hand through Guyon's tunnel – a tight tunnel formed between two small bones of the wrist and the ligaments holding these bones together.
- The nerve lies close to the surface as it travels down the arm, making it the largest exposed nerve of the body as it has little protection from either bone or muscle.
- The nerve supplies a few muscles in the forearm and many of the small muscles of the hand, including those that move the ring and little finger.
- The nerve also provides sensory supply to part of the fourth and fifth fingers as well as the part of the palm under these fingers.

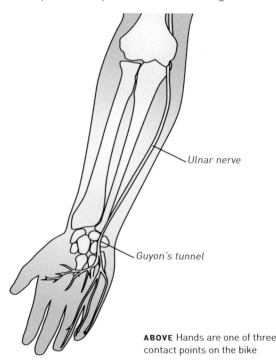

Ulnar nerve

Guyon's tunnel

ABOVE Hands are one of three contact points on the bike

Causes of ulnar neuropathy

Compression and stretch

The hands are one of three contact points on the bike when cycling, along with the pedals and saddle. While riding, the upper body's weight is largely absorbed through the arms and hands. The more aggressive the position, as determined by the saddle to handlebar height ratio (the larger this ratio, the more aggressive the position), the more pressure is placed on the hands while cycling. Riding on the drops only increases this pressure. A good bike fit aims to limit the pressure on the hands so weight is more evenly distributed at the bike contact points, but this doesn't always prevent handlebar palsy from occurring.

As the hands grip the bars, the wrists naturally become extended, putting the ulnar nerve under tension. Depending on hand position, the focal pressure and weight of the upper body through the arms is placed on the muscle of the padded area of the hand, which is the area beneath the fourth and fifth fingers. With the weight on this part of the hand, both stretch and direct pressure is placed on the ulnar nerve within Guyon's tunnel. A study in 2011 demonstrated that the loading patterns and pressure placed on this part of the hand while cycling are enough to cause ulnar nerve damage if maintained for long periods. It's an obvious mechanism for injury for the keen cyclist who spends cumulative hours in the saddle.

NERVE DAMAGE

In addition to the compressive and stretch forces on the nerve, the constant continued vibration coming through the hands from the road can focally damage the ulnar nerve, causing a condition known as neuropraxia. A neuropraxia is focal damage to the protective coating of the nerve. Impulses travelling along the nerve can't get past this point of damage (like treading on a hose and stopping water flow) affecting nerve function further along its path and causing the symptoms of handlebar palsy. Depending on where specifically or how the nerve becomes irritated, symptoms will vary from person to person from numbness and tingling in the ring and fifth finger and hypothenar area, to pain, persistent weakness and clumsiness of the hand which can create havoc when trying to shift gears or brake at high speed.

Other sites of ulnar nerve compression

The ulnar nerve is long, superficial and some-what exposed as it travels from its origin in the neck down to the hand. The nerve is therefore vulnerable to becoming entrapped at more than just the wrist at Guyon's tunnel. Symptoms can be similar in other areas of entrapment although there'll be subtle differences that allow the site of compression to be distinguished. The two other common areas that can irritate the nerve while cycling are the thoracic outlet at the neck and the cubital tunnel at the elbow.

THORACIC OUTLET
The thoracic outlet is a 'triangular space' in the neck bordered by the anterior scalene muscle at the front, the middle scalene muscle at the back and the first rib and collarbone below. The brachial plexus is a collection of nerves that starts from the cervical spine and passes through the thoracic outlet as it leaves the neck where some of its branches become the ulnar nerve. The nerve can get compressed as it travels through the thoracic outlet as cycling posture naturally puts the nerve under tension in this area. Once the

structures get stretched and compressed as they pass through the thoracic outlet, symptoms can develop, including pins and needles, numbness and pain along the distribution of the nerve into the upper arm, forearm and hand. Although symptoms can be similar with this 'thoracic outlet syndrome', mild neck discomfort and stiffness may also be experienced, differentiating it from ulnar neuropathy at the wrist.

CUBITAL TUNNEL
The cubital tunnel is a channel that contains the ulnar nerve as it passes the elbow joint. It's found underneath the bump on the inside of your elbow.

The nerve passes through, close to the surface, where it can easily get knocked, causing a shock like sensation into the forearm and hand. Riding an aggressive position with the elbows flexed for hours at a time can cause an increase in stretch on the nerve. Nerves don't like to be stretched and when they are it can cause cubital tunnel syndrome – ulnar nerve entrapment at the elbow – with symptoms including pins and needles, numbness and pain in the inside half of the forearm and into the hand. A crash that damages the elbow joint can irritate the ulnar nerve and also cause these symptoms. This is the least common of the three compression sites.

With thoracic outlet and cubital tunnel syndromes the ulnar nerve gets compressed higher up, closer to where the nerve begins which usually makes symptoms more extensive whereas with handlebar palsy symptoms are normally isolated to the hand.

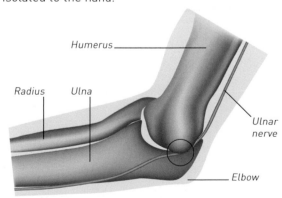

Humerus

Radius　Ulna

Ulnar nerve

Elbow

ABOVE Ulnar nerve impingement

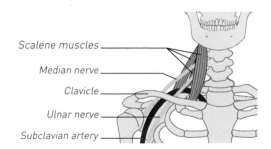

Scalene muscles

Median nerve

Clavicle

Ulnar nerve

Subclavian artery

ABOVE The thoracic outlet

Treatment

Injury at a glance

Pain scale	Mild to moderate
Time off bike	1 week
Call in the professionals?	Not for now
Surgery?	No

Pain, pins and needles, and numbness may continue for a short period when you get off the bike but usually not for very long as symptoms are often transient and cycling specific. In mild cases symptoms will normally only be present on the bike but occasionally you can be left with symptoms for a few hours after finishing your ride. This injury can mimic other injuries, as mentioned, in addition to a nerve entrapment at the neck. If your symptoms extend beyond the hand and wrist area and are persistent you should seek help to make sure you have the right diagnosis. If it looks as though you have handlebar palsy, the following routine will help relieve your symptoms.

A quick fix?

Regularly moving between the different hand positions while riding is the quickest way to alleviate symptoms. The bar will normally be the most comfortable position over the hood and drops as there's least pressure on the hands. Try different pairs of gloves as the padding between them will vary in both placement and thicknesses. You may find a pair you get on with that cushions the area, protecting the ulnar nerve from pressure and relieving the symptoms, rather than focally *increasing* the pressure and making the symptoms worse.

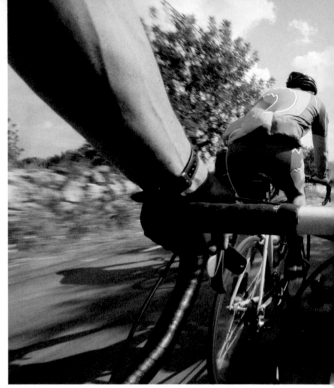

ABOVE Constant weight on the hands can cause ulnar neuropathy at the wrist

FIRST AID FOR HANDLEBAR PALSY

 Ice the area 2–3 times a day for 10–15 minutes at a time. Continue for 3 days or until the pain and symptoms ease. You may feel like you only need to ice the hand on the first day as the symptoms will often be minimal off the bike, but ice for at least the next day or two to help reduce any local inflammation.

Over-the-counter medication

See pages 62–63

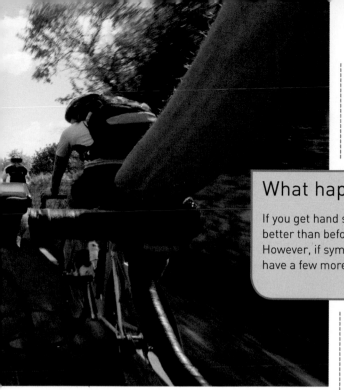

Week 2

You've let things settle down for a week, now's the time to get back on the bike.

What happens if I feel something?

If you get hand symptoms initially, don't worry as they should be better than before – see how they feel once you're fully warmed-up. However, if symptoms progress, stop. Don't push yourself. Rest and have a few more days off before continuing your exercise routine.

Time to start a core excercise routine alongside your other exercises. See the rehab toolkit page 202.

Week 1

MOVING ON

The first week is about keeping symptoms at bay while working on areas of the body that can help support comfort and stability for the upper body while on the bike. These exercises can help reduce the pressure and tension on the ulnar nerve while riding. Think of these exercises as core work specifically for the upper back and neck. Continue these exercises as symptoms ease for the next few weeks

REHAB TOOL KIT EX.	EX. NO.	PAGE
1. Improve your breathing	n/a	159
2. Neck rotation	1.1	163
3. Scapular stabiliser activation	1.6	167
4. The wall angel	1.7	167
5. Deep neck flexor activation	1.4	165
6. Deep neck flexor strengthening	1.5	166
7. Ulnar nerve flossing	2.7	173

Week 5

STILL HAVE PAIN: WHO SHOULD YOU CALL?

If after four weeks you literally cannot shake off the hand symptoms while riding or in the unlikely event you're still getting symptoms off the bike after two weeks, it's time to seek assistance, but who should you call?

PLAN A

PLAN B

16 CONCUSSION

Sixty mile per hour descents, sharp bends, rush hour traffic; it's no surprise cycling enthusiasts succumb to the odd crash. And with any impact crash there is a risk of concussion, a vague catch-all term that can be responsible for a host of symptoms including headache, dizziness, confusion, blurred vision and even slurred speech. But what you might not know is that you don't necessarily have to have banged your head to get it, and that while a one-off concussion is rarely serious, it can significantly affect you both on and off the bike and needs adequate recovery time. Getting to know the danger signs so that you can give your body the time it needs to recover *and* rule out anything more serious is just common sense.

The lowdown

During the first week of every Tour de France there are many high-speed crashes and many of those that crash will leave the race because of their injuries. Following a crash if the rider gets up independently, one of the first things the medical team in the follow car will be looking out for is symptoms of concussion.

A forceful blow to the head or severe whiplash, when the body stops and the head keeps moving before suddenly stopping, can lead to a temporary disturbance of the brain's normal function, this is concussion. Relatively little is known about the intricacies of this injury because it's only been in the last few years that more emphasis has been placed on getting a deeper understanding

of it. Knowledge is now increasing on an almost daily basis and this is because of the high-profile longer-term consequences (such as the early onset of dementia) that are now being associated with concussion as seen in sports people such as retired American footballers and boxers.

What is definitely known is that it causes physical damage to the tissue of the brain, which results in wide-ranging symptoms that can last anything from a few hours up to a few months. What remains largely unknown is exactly what *causes* these symptoms.

Symptom checker

Following a crash where you suspect concussion:
- ✔ Headache
- ✔ Dizziness
- ✔ Feeling nausea or vomiting
- ✔ Loss of balance
- ✔ Feeling confused
- ✔ Unawareness of where you are or what has just happened
- ✔ Ringing in your ears
- ✔ Double or blurred vision
- ✔ Loss of consciousness

If *any* of the above sounds familiar either immediately after, later that day or even the next few days, a concussion should be suspected.

The symptoms may seem vague and general as they cover a lot of symptoms you might expect when you come off a bike anyway. This is because the variety of different presentations of a concussed person are huge, so if you suspect at all that you may be concussed, medical assessment should be sought as a matter of course.

If you have come off your bike and landed heavily and impacted your head on the ground, or had a big whiplash, then the chances are, if it's a high-speed crash, other parts of your body may also be damaged. But for now, let's assume they've been taken care of. Now's the time to find out if you are concussed.

The first thing to do is to check your helmet as it may give you an indication of where and how badly you may have hit your head. Is it cracked, is it completely broken? If you crashed at speed, you'll feel stunned, you may feel slightly nauseous and dizzy and you may feel a bit confused. However, these don't necessarily mean you have a concussion, but if these symptoms continue along with any others, then it's a possibility. There's a lot of crossover between symptoms of concussion and other injuries so this should always be at the back of your mind.

Equally, any of the symptoms of concussion can come on from a few minutes or even hours later while some may take a few days before they develop.

If you feel totally fine, and your bike hasn't been damaged beyond the ability to ride it, you will normally be OK to ride home slowly, but if you suspect a concussion, it's time to call it a day on the bike. Phone a friend or call a cab and get yourself home. **DO NOT RIDE YOUR BIKE HOME.**

The science bit

The skull and brain

- The skull is hard, like a shell and surrounds and protects the brain and other sensory organs such as the eyes, ears and nasal cavities.
- The soft brain is suspended inside the skull, in the cranial cavity and is surrounded by fluid that both nourishes it and protects it against the skull.

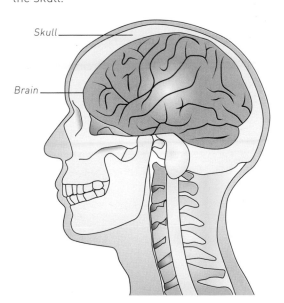

Skull

Brain

Riding with others

Riding with others, see a crash and suspect concussion? It's as important to be able to recognise possible concussion in others as it is to understand you may have it yourself. Any one or more of the following visual clues may indicate concussion. Witness this then call an ambulance:

- Loss of consciousness or responsiveness.
- Lying motionless on the ground or slow to get up.
- Unsteady on their feet/balance problems or falling over.
- Grabbing/clutching of the head.
- Dazed/blank or vacant look.
- Confused/not aware of where they are.
- Neck pain.
- Increasing confusion or irritability.
- Repeated vomiting.
- Seizure or convulsion.
- Weakness or tingling in arms or legs.
- Deteriorating conscious state.
- Severe or increasing headache.
- Unusual behaviour change.
- Double vision.

PROFESSIONAL INSIGHT

Tyler Farrar AMERICAN PRO AND TOUR DE FRANCE, GIRO D'ITALIA AND VUELTA A ESPAÑA STAGE WINNER

■ *'During stage one of the 2012 Tour of Britain, I crashed pretty hard and landed on my head. I was messed up for about a week. Eating was really hard; I had no appetite and would sleep for 16 hours a day. It just felt like my thought process was moving through molasses. I felt slowed down. Over the next two weeks I slowly got better but my attention span wasn't too good and I remember feeling overly emotional. It took me at least a month to feel totally normal again. Luckily it was late in the season, so I hung up my bike for the month which in hindsight was very lucky.*

Even some few weeks after, although I physically felt OK, mentally I wasn't quite right, everything was still slow. It was incredibly frustrating and actually really scary. Because the brain is so unpredictable, nobody will give you a definite answer; it's not like breaking a bone that heals in six weeks. There's no definitive timeline for recovery so you're always waiting for certain symptoms to get better.

My advice for those who have been concussed, is don't rush it, and listen to your doctors as you don't have the judgement to make real calls on what you should be doing and what you can expect. Yes, you want to get back on the bike, but you have to be patient and recover fully.

I saw a neurosurgeon and had to go one week with no music, no television, no reading, no computer and no phone. They want your brain to be as rested as possible. I walked around the house wearing dark sunglasses as I was very light sensitive, which is also a symptom. If you think you have been concussed, go and see a doctor and they will help. Don't think the symptoms will just go away, or that they aren't serious. They are.'

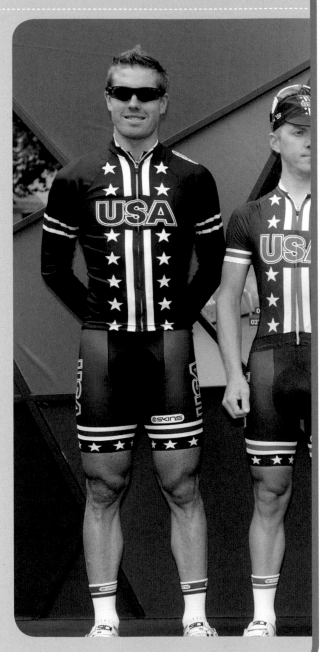

Loss of consciousness

Up until 1986 the criteria for grading sports concussion relied upon having loss of consciousness (LOC) present for a diagnosis to be made. Less than 10 per cent of concussions involve LOC and nowadays you don't have to have lost consciousness to be classed as concussed.

Every four years a group of eminent scientists and medics, the Concussion in Sports Group, meet and create a consensus paper outlining the latest thoughts and recommendations on concussion. For the last three meetings in 2004, 2008 and 2012, the definition of what concussion *is* has changed each time. It's no wonder there are mixed messages and confusion in the public domain on what concussion actually *is* and why it may still be so generally poorly understood when even the definition is still in flux.

Causes of concussion

A helmet may save your life in a fall, but it won't necessarily prevent you from concussion. There are two mechanisms to get concussed, direct and indirect. Direct would be a forceful blow to the head, which is most likely a result of falling off your bike and landing on your head. The second way is by an indirect force to the body that causes a rapid acceleration and deceleration, or 'shaking' of the head. You may recognise this as whiplash.

BELOW Whiplash can cause concussion indirectly

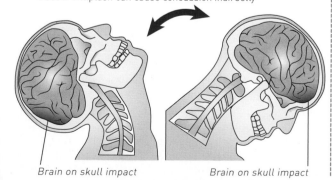

Brain on skull impact   *Brain on skull impact*

The word 'concussion' comes from the Latin verb *concutere* – 'to shake violently', which accurately describes the indirect method of getting concussed.

If you crash and your helmet is badly damaged, you may more readily suspect concussion. However, it's the indirect method for cyclists which is imperative to understand. It's important to note that in a lot of these cases, your helmet may not have a scratch on it at all. A lot of cyclists will think that because they haven't 'hit their head', concussion isn't a concern, but if the fall itself was violent enough, concussion may still be a possibility.

What has happened?

The brain makes up the majority of the central nervous system and governs all function within the body. Concussion is the mildest form of traumatic brain injury and the most common. Concussion occurs when the soft gelatinous brain is 'shaken' inside the hard skull (like a wet sponge in a bucket) and the rotation and bruising that occurs as the brain strikes the skull sets off a cascade of events causing the symptoms of concussion:

- The blood flow, oxygen supply and chemical balance of the brain are all disturbed.
- There's injury to the nerve fibres of the brain as the brain rotates on impact causing them to stretch – some repair, some don't.
- Some of the brain cells, neurons, die.

Let's be clear, when a person is concussed, there *is* damage to the brain and this is responsible for the symptoms experienced, especially over the first 10 days or so. It's estimated that an individual's decisions, cognition and emotions are impaired by as much as 50 per cent when concussed. This change is directly due to physical damage to the brain tissue.

Investigation

As there may be no obvious signs of injury, this makes concussion hard to diagnose, assess and manage even for the most skilled practitioner, let alone for self-diagnosis. There is no one specific test or marker that is relied on for accurate diagnosis. The best advice: if you are *at all* in doubt as whether you're concussed you should see your doctor.

 It is possible to crash, hit your head, damage your helmet and not get concussed. If you have no headache, nausea, vomiting, didn't lose consciousness and have no difficulty breathing, you're probably not concussed and won't need to see your doctor.

Complications of concussion

SECOND IMPACT SYNDROME

On very rare occasions, a second blow to the head, before the first one has had time to heal properly, can have catastrophic consequences. It usually only affects younger people – those under 18 years old – and this phenomena is called 'second impact syndrome' and happens when swelling of the brain occurs and the pressure inside the skull builds quickly.

The skull is hard and so cannot expand to accommodate the swelling; the swelling gets forced downwards out of the opening of the brain stem at the bottom of the skull. Huge pressure on the brainstem occurs and leads to brain damage and death within 2–5 minutes. The chances of sudden impact syndrome are rare. However, it highlights the importance of recognising and understanding concussion the first time so appropriate measures to help recovery are put in place and the risk of follow-up head injury and second impact syndrome are absolutely minimised.

POST-CONCUSSION SYNDROME

Post-concussion syndrome (PCS) is a complication of concussion and is where a variety of the symptoms that were experienced during the initial concussion become prolonged and last longer than 10 days. Symptoms that usually have eased off by this time such as headache and

dizziness can go on for weeks, or even months in some cases. The difficulty with this disorder is that it's not easy to predict or prevent as the risk of it occurring isn't linked to the severity of the initial concussion.

Experts are undecided on how many people who develop concussion will go on to get PCS, and estimates vary widely between 30–90 per cent. Normally symptoms of PCS will occur within the first 7–10 days after getting concussed and resolve within 3–6 months, although 10 per cent of people will still be getting symptoms a year later. Even in 2015, nobody can state what the actual cause of PCS is and there are a couple of theories ranging from chemical imbalance in the brain caused by the initial concussion to it being a possible emotional and psychological response to the initial head injury, described as almost a milder form of post-traumatic stress disorder.

Symptom checker

Symptoms of PCS can include any of the issues of the initial concussion (see page 132) in addition to:
✔ Fatigue
✔ Irritability
✔ Anxiety
✔ Insomnia or disturbed sleep
✔ Loss of concentration and memory
✔ Noise and light sensitivity
✔ Appetite changes
✔ Reduced sex-drive

Chronic traumatic encephalopathy

Evidence is emerging that some people who have been concussed multiple times over the course of their lives – or sporting careers – are at increased risk of developing lasting and even progressive impairment, which limits their ability to function properly. Chronic traumatic encephalopathy (CTE) is a form of neuro-degeneration – breakdown and damage of the nerves of the brain – that is thought to be secondary to repetitive head injury. Previously this condition was known as *dementia pugilistica* because of the association between repetitive head injuries and the early onset of disorders, such as dementia, seen in boxers. It's now known that repetitive blows to the head in any form can lead to impairments and the condition has since been renamed CTE.

Adequate time must be taken to allow healing after concussion as it's now understood there's a cumulative impact from multiple injuries and CTE may well be the end result. Whereas concussion and PCS are temporary brain damage, CTE is a degenerative condition that may come on years or even decades after the 'recovery' of head injury and the impairment is permanent.

Early signs of CTE developing might often be spotted by family or friends and include an increased incidence of the individual being angry, irritable, depressed, lacking in emotion and/or having a shorter fuse. As the disease progresses, movement becomes difficult and may mimic symptoms of Parkinson's disease (Muhammad Ali's personal doctor Ferdie Pacheco mentioned in his book 'Fight Doctor' that Ali 'doesn't have CTE but true Parkinson's disease, brought on by trauma to the head' – although CTE can only be properly diagnosed in a post-mortem when the cells of the brain are studied under a microscope). Speech and eye problems can also develop and the memory can get worse and in some cases dementia can set in.

Treatment

Injury at a glance

Pain scale	Mild to moderate
Time off bike	Minimum 1 week
Call in the professionals?	Yes
Surgery?	No

First thought

You've been diagnosed with concussion or have suspected concussion, but where do you go from here? It's reasonable that you might not have been to see your doctor if symptoms described earlier didn't warrant it. The good news is that as daunting as concussion may seem and as significant an issue it is, the reality is that the actual extent of damage to the brain is normally minimal and the problem will get better without treatment. In the vast majority of cases – almost 90 per cent – symptoms of concussion resolve spontaneously over 7–10 days. However, if there are signs of more serious injury (as mentioned previously), they may need emergency treatment.

 If you suspect concussion, you should not get back on your bike and ride home. Studies have shown that balance deficits last for approximately three days following sports related concussion, which obviously rules out returning to cycling during this period.

First action

Symptoms of concussion can progress and if they do it will usually be within the first 48–72 hours. It's important to remain alert to the possible symptoms of the problem progressing into something more serious. If you have somebody that can stay with you for the first 2–3 days, they can help to monitor you and will be there if things worsen.

If you or someone in your care notices any of the following symptoms, go to the nearest hospital, as they could be signs of a medical emergency:

- Mental confusion
- Drowsiness that goes on for longer than an hour
- Difficulty speaking
- Loss of balance
- Persistent painful headache
- Lack of consciousness
- Fits or seizures
- Repeated vomiting

FIRST AID FOR MILD SYMPTOMS OF CONCUSSION

 Apply ice every 2–4 hours to the head injury to reduce local pain and swelling for 20 minutes at a time.

Over-the-counter medication

 PARACETAMOL ONLY

DO NOT use NSAID type painkillers for FIVE DAYS after suspected concussion. These include aspirin and ibuprofen. These medications increase the risk of bleeding at the site of the injury that can make the situation worse.

See pages 62–63

The next step

The cornerstone to dealing with concussion is complete physical and mental rest over the first 24–48 hours, or until the symptoms have gone. Rest is the best and most appropriate way to allow your brain to recover from concussion. During this time, limiting brain stimulation is important. This means limiting or avoiding the following activities that require thinking or mental concentration:

- Watching TV
- Using your phone including texting
- Bright lights
- Schoolwork/studying/work
- Using the computer or playing video games
- Speaking on the phone
- General physical exertion – no exercise!
- Reading
- Any activity that requires you to 'think'
- Alcohol

Other things that will help:
- Getting appropriate sleep
- Remaining in a lowly lit room when possible

These can be reintroduced as your symptoms start to improve.

 If you are getting a persistent headache 24 hours after complete physical and mental rest, you should see your doctor for assessment.

Headaches

When you get headaches following a concussion they may often feel like tension-type or migraine headaches. The most commonly associated headaches would be tension-type or cervicogenic (neck-related) headaches. These headaches can be associated with a neck injury sustained at the time of concussion. Seeking help from either a chiropractor, osteopath or physiotherapist, can help to reduce neck irritation that may be causing the headache.

Returning to cycling

Regardless of the level of cyclist you are or how fit you may be, when it comes to getting back on the bike after concussion everyone should be managed using the same approach.

You should not return to cycling until you have completely recovered from your symptoms of concussion. Once they have disappeared then it's recommended that exercise, when started, should be introduced in a graduated stepwise approach. This follows a sensible path for you to restart cycling while monitoring your recovery and checking to see if any concussion symptoms return which would be cause to back off. The protocol has been modified and adapted from the latest Concussion in Sports Group Consensus statement to help you structure your return to cycling following concussion:

Five-step return to cycling after concussion guidelines

REHABILITATION STAGE	FUNCTIONAL EXERCISE AT EACH STAGE	OBJECTIVE OF EACH STAGE	LENGTH OF TIME
1. No activity	None – Still experiencing symptoms	Recovery	3–10 days
2. Light aerobic exercise	Gentle walking, swimming or stationary cycling at low/medium intensity. No weights/core training	Increase heart rate	24 hrs +
3. Cycling specific	Stationary cycling with efforts of higher intensity, out of the saddle work	Add movement	24 hrs+
4. Return to the road	Return to road cycling. 'Recovery ride' of medium intensity maximum	Increase cognitive load as return to environment	24 hrs+
5. Normal cycling	Return to cycling as you wish	Restore confidence and reassess skills	24 hrs+

Only proceed to the next stage once you're OK at the current level and experience NO recurrence of your concussion symptoms.

Once you get past stage 1, progression through each further step should usually take 24 hours, so if everything goes well, the shortest time you could approximately get through the full rehabilitation protocol would be one week.

You may not intend to ride your bike on a daily basis, which is fine, but you should not skip a step even if you have 3–4 days before starting each stage. It will take you longer to reach stage 5 and get back out on the road again but ensuring you get through each step in progression is important. If you have no symptoms during rest *and* provocative exercise such as cycling, you're on your way to being recovered from concussion.

If *any* symptoms of your initial concussion come back while you're going through the stepwise programme, then it's important to stop and rest for 24 hours. The next time you ride drop back to the previous stage and if you get no symptoms attempt to move back up to the next stage again.

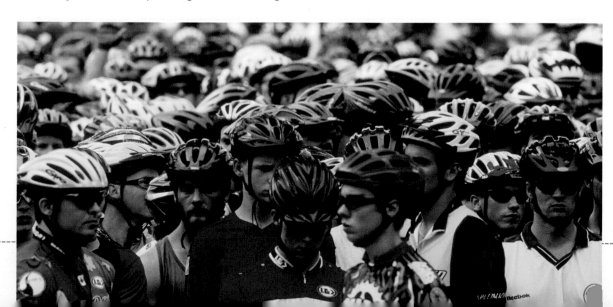

STAGE BY STAGE

Stage 1 Symptoms of concussion will normally have disappeared within 10 days of the initial injury so stage 1 could potentially last as long as this. It's advised you don't get back on your bike the day of concussion and you give your body three days to recover, even if symptoms seemingly disappear in that time, due to the increased possibility of complications of concussion occurring during that time.

Stage 2 After three days you can potentially move on to stage 2 if you no longer have symptoms at rest. The aim is to gently reintroduce the body to mild exercise such as going for a walk. You can even get on the home trainer for a very gentle leg spin.

Stage 3 Here you can begin to increase the effort on the home trainer. You are getting your body used to riding again and doing some mild efforts out of the saddle will help simulate this too.

Stage 4 You can finally get back to cycling on the open road. By cycling on the road you're naturally increasing the mental stress. This means your brain activity is moving up a few notches as you're thinking more about everything from your surroundings, your route, the lights changing, avoiding potholes and much more.

Remember your first ride back should always be an easy recovery ride. The faster and more intense you ride, the faster you have to act and think, putting more stress on the recovering brain. Riding familiar roads will hopefully reduce the chances of coming off the bike and being concussed again.

Stage 5 Now you're back to 'normal'. Continue to build your riding and it will help your confidence return.

Still having symptoms?

If you're experiencing persistent symptoms for longer than 10 days go (back) to your doctor. They will assess you and decide whether you may be developing PCS. While there's no treatment that will speed up your recovery they may be able to help reduce individual symptoms. If you've been diagnosed with PCS, there are some things to consider that can be helpful while you continue to recover:

- **Take your time** – avoid rushing back into things and take things slowly.
- **Sleep** – difficulty sleeping is a common symptom associated with PCS; encouraging good sleep habits (see page 54) can play an important role to optimise your sleep.
- **Stress** – try to limit your stress levels wherever possible.
- **Alcohol** – avoid alcohol as you continue to recover.

Most cases of PCS symptoms resolve within 3–6 months, while 10 per cent of people still have symptoms 12 months later. There's some evidence to suggest that light exercise may be helpful with recovery from PCS. Follow the return to cycling after concussion guidelines and find a stage that causes no progression of your symptoms and you should be OK to ride at that level as you wait for your remaining symptoms to resolve.

MATT SAYS:

'It's one thing to get back to cycling; it's another to get back to your optimal level of performance. I've seen it take from six months to a year following concussion before a cyclist feels they are able to perform at the same level as pre-concussion. It's not as uncommon as it may seem but there's no significant evidence that discusses concussion and returning to performance. It's important not to get too frustrated if your recovery to top form takes longer than you expect and happens a while after you have 'recovered' from your concussion.'

CYCLING NIRVANA

Jack Bauer NEW ZEALAND | 2014 COMMONWEALTH GAMES SILVER MEDALLIST

■ 'I'd never won anything on a road bike. I sold up back home in New Zealand and moved to Europe to try and make it as a pro bike rider.

It was in the middle of a five-month stint I was doing living in Ghent. I was in the heart of cycling's mainland trying to chase my dream. I was still an amateur. In those days I knew little about cycling but I knew some of the names of previous winners of this one particular race.

In the last lap of the race there was a moment the pace lulled with a couple of kilometres to go, as we approached a corner. My teammate, an older Belgian dude, told me to attack if I had the legs. I listened, attacked and had a huge exhilarating feeling as my legs fired up and I was at the front of the race. Prior to this I had won nothing on a road bike. I attacked with 4 km to go and the harder I went the more exhilarated I felt. I felt on a high for the last 4 km and that was my Cycling Nirvana moment. It gave me confidence in my ability to make a telling effort as I'd often thought I couldn't do it.'

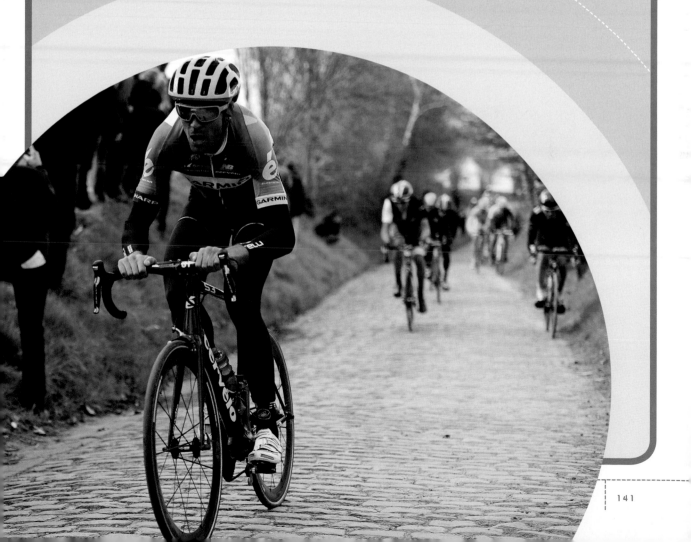

17 *FRACTURES*

Crashing itself is harmless; it's landing that causes the damage. You may not think it, but when you're riding your bike, you're pretty high up and falling could send you crashing down from over six foot if you're thrown up into the air before landing, all while wearing Lycra – which offers virtually no padding at all (you might as well be in your underwear for the protection you get). So if you land with enough force, it's possible to break a bone or two.

From the pro perspective, large crashes, broken bones and the chaotic first week of the Tour de France almost go hand in hand. The sight of a rider getting up slowly from a crash is all too familiar. Who could forget when Bradley Wiggins fell off his bike, succumbing to a collarbone break, 40 km from the finish in Chataeraux of stage seven at the 2011 Tour de France (as image shows). A race he was a favourite to win. Prepare all you like and train as hard as you can. Sometimes, crashes are inevitable.

Breaks

Crashes in cycling tend to see common fractures occur over and over again. And this is all to do with the likelihood of landing on particular parts of the body when you crash. What are you most likely to break?

- The collarbone
- The scaphoid bone of the wrist
- The ribs

These three common cycling fractures have certain features that make them important to understand and recognise. Each of them can impact your cycling and it's important they're properly addressed and given the suitable amount of time to let healing occur before being stressed again on the bike. So let's go through them and explain how they occur and most importantly, how to manage them.

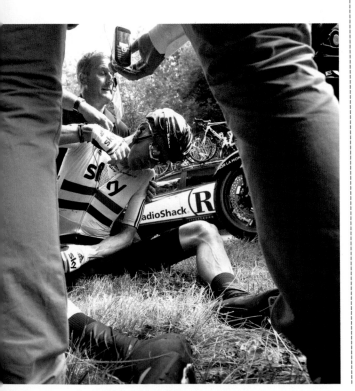

PROFESSIONAL INSIGHT

Alex Howes AMERICAN PRO AND TOUR OF UTAH STAGE WINNER

■ *'Just out of the corner of my eye I saw the strap from the cooler come up. I'll never forget it. We were roughly 150 km into a 260 km "Olympic Race Day Simulation" training ride. A strap attaching a small cooler to the back of the scooter we were motor pacing behind came loose, wrapped itself around my break leaver and, two milliseconds later, I was on the floor. Full sprawl. I remember the adrenaline, the rushing around to get up, get moving, reaching down to put my rear wheel back into my bike after the crash, the light graze as my shoulder brushed my cheek and the casual observation, "My shoulder doesn't normally touch my cheek when I bend forward" ... No Olympics for me. Broken collarbone.*

Broken might actually be the wrong word. Shattered would be a more appropriate word for a bone broken into seven pieces. One plate and 12 screws later I was good as new. According to the surgeon that is. It took 11 focused days of rehab to get back on the open road, three weeks before I could race again and another three months of rehab before I felt fully normal. Rehab consisted mainly of stretching, a few push-ups and light dumbbell (aka a small can of soup) work, focusing on bringing the AC joint back to full mobility. Going on two years now after the accident and I'm still not fully done. I will see rehab version 2.0 after removing the surgical hardware that still prevents me from properly wearing a backpack and gives me pain when sleeping on my side.

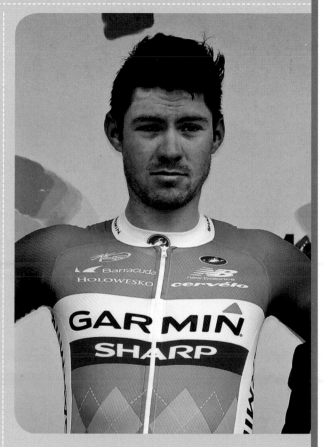

But in all honesty folks, the old, "droopy shoulder" is not a death sentence. Usually surgery can be avoided. A couple weeks rest, some stretching and a glass of milk fixes most of them. Not to mention, a sling is a great conversation-starter at the pub.'

PART 1: COLLARBONE FRACTURE

The collarbone – or clavicle – is the most commonly fractured bone in the body representing approximately 5 per cent of all human fractures. A study in the *International Journal of Sports Medicine* in 2014 summarised that, in sport, cycling was the most common cause of clavicle fracture. Look closely enough at the shoulders of most pro cyclists and you'll see the battle scars that tell the story of a surgically repaired collarbone or two. In fact, you'll be hard pushed to meet a pro cyclist that hasn't broken their collarbone at some point in their career.

The lowdown

The fracture happens when a rider is thrown from their bike and either lands heavily on their shoulder or from the impact through the arm of an outstretched hand that instinctively goes out to

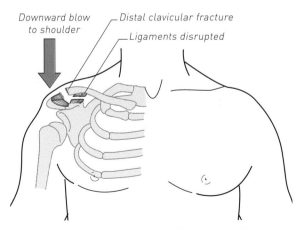

Downward blow to shoulder — *Distal clavicular fracture* — *Ligaments disrupted*

ABOVE Note the dropped shoulder on the fractured side

Symptom checker

Following a crash where you land on the shoulder or an outstretched arm:
- ✔ Extreme pain, tenderness and swelling over the front of the collarbone area usually in the middle.
- ✔ Bruising to the skin over the collarbone.
- ✔ Less commonly, symptoms as above but towards outer third of collarbone.
- ✔ Often a displacement of the bone can be felt.
- ✔ Natural tendency to clutch arm into body.
- ✔ Shoulder may be slumped downwards and forwards as is no longer supported by collarbone.
- ✔ Unable to get back on bike and ride due to obvious pain.
- ✔ 'Tenting' of the skin as the bone pokes through.

break their fall. The collarbone breaks relatively easily as it's one of the weakest bones in the body.

It's not unusual to hear the sound of the bone breaking on impact as it lies so close to the body's surface. The majority – 69–82 per cent – of collarbone fractures occur in the middle third of the bone, which is the weakest point. If you're *really* unlucky you'll separate your shoulder (see page 118–124) at the same time as fracturing your clavicle in a fall when the outer third of the collarbone fractures, although this is rarer.

There are different types of collarbone fracture ranging from a small crack in the bone to a clean break where the clavicle snaps in two like a twig. In some accidents, the bone can break into multiple fragments or even break through the skin creating management challenges. However, in a typical collarbone fracture in the middle third of the bone, the shoulder tends to drop as it's no longer properly supported and the two ends of the fracture move apart. (See diagram opposite).

The science bit

The collarbone

- The collarbone is a relatively short and curved bone yet remains the largest horizontal bone in the body.
- It joins the upper limbs to the trunk by connecting the top of the breastbone to the shoulder girdle on either side.
- It's located directly under the skin at the bottom of the neck where, for most people, it is obviously visible and easy to feel.
- The clavicle is often divided into three sections: the medial end, which is joined to the breastbone; the middle third; and the lateral end, which joins to the scapula at the acromioclavicular (AC) joint.

INVESTIGATION

If you crash and think you have a suspected collarbone fracture, try and keep the arm still, which you'll normally instinctively do, to avoid the two fractured ends moving too much. Unfortunately then, it's off to the hospital you go. An X-ray will be done to confirm if the clavicle has been fractured and then the treatment options will be outlined from there.

Treatment

Injury at a glance

Pain scale	Moderate to severe
Time off bike	2–6 weeks
Call in the professionals?	Yes
Surgery?	Depends

Most collarbone fractures are left to heal naturally while the hospital may provide a simple sling to help support the arm and hold the bones in their normal position. It used to be believed that if you fractured your collarbone, as long as both ends of the clavicle were 'close to one another' then it would heal OK. Well, times and thoughts are changing. With mid-clavicle fractures that most commonly occur it's recognised that there will be displacement of the fractured ends approximately 73 per cent of the time.

The approach taken towards your recovery will be determined by a few factors. The biggest priority is that the fracture heals properly. About two thirds of the time the two ends of the fracture don't fuse together properly. This poor healing response often leads to shortening of the clavicle by on average 1.2 cm. This means after this poor healing response the clavicle on the fractured side will be 1.2 cm shorter than it was pre-fracture.

Shortening of the collarbone up to 1.2 cm isn't really a problem. However, when it gets to 1.4 cm or above, complications can arise such as prolonged pain in the area and into the arm and compromised shoulder function. Simple everyday activities can become difficult and even sleeping on the affected side can be painful. Physiotherapy might help, but it's thought the only real treatment option of choice to prevent long-term issues is surgery to repair the collarbone. This improves shoulder stability by replacing it back to an appropriate length and will normally be done by fixing a plate and screws to bridge the fracture site.

More surgical repairs are done nowadays for collarbone fracture than 15 years ago because there's a much higher incidence of the fracture not healing properly if left than was previously recognised. Now the thought is if it's suspected, it's better to operate initially than treating conservatively and having to potentially do the surgery later anyway.

So you have a confirmed collarbone fracture, but what happens next?

First aid

 Ice over the painful area for 10–20 minutes 2–3 times a day. This can be continued for as long as significant pain persists.

Over-the-counter medication

See pages 62–63

Avoid freeze spray and topical NSAIDs as you risk disturbing the fracture site as you apply them.

First action: help your recovery

Depending on whether you had the operation or not will determine where you begin with your rehabilitation.

NON-OPERATIVE TREATMENT

- Overlapping and shortening of the clavicle will be monitored for the first 3–4 weeks to make sure it doesn't occur as it can lead to significant deformity.
- You'll usually be advised to remain in the sling for 3–4 weeks to help support the collarbone as it heals.
- The aim of treatment is to provide pain relief, which should be continued as indicated as most simple collarbone fractures will usually always heal within 4–6 weeks.
- Avoid heavy lifting with the injured arm for six weeks.
- Focus on good posture and body position – avoid slouching and your shoulders rounding – throughout the duration of using the sling.

Rehab from clavicle fracture

Whether you have the operation or not, your doctor will often refer you for physiotherapy to assist your recovery which is a good idea. If not, the following plan can help your recovery to get you back to cycling in the shortest time.

Weeks 1–6

These exercises focus on reducing stiffness in the shoulder joint while keeping the shoulder muscles working too so once the fracture has healed you're more quickly on the road to recovery. Go through the exercises, starting with the easier exercises, progress through them; however, if any are too painful, skip over them and move on to the next one.

If your collarbone was surgically repaired, it will immediately be more stable. The earlier exercises in this case may be too easy and assuming you can do them with no limitation or pain you can move onwards to find more challenging ones further along. Beware though as you may be instructed not to 'sweat' for the first couple of weeks following surgery to avoid any chance of the wound getting infected.

RECOMMENDATIONS

REHAB TOOL KIT EX.	EX. NO.	PAGE
1. Isometric shoulder activatiom	2.3	170
2. The shoulder swing	2.2	169
3. Passive shoulder movement	2.4	171
4. Tennis ball grip	2.8	174
5. Active shoulder range of motion	2.5	172
6. Scapular stabiliser activation	1.6	167
7. One-sided scapular stabiliser	1.8	168
8. Dynamic shoulder strengthening	2.6	172
9. Pectoral muscle tennis ball release	3.8	179

BACK ON BIKE

As the fracture becomes more stable, pain will be the guide to when you can get back on to your bike.

Typically your doctor or physio will advise you when you can return to cycling. If you still have significant pain or your doctor hasn't signed you off to exercise then you should wait a little

longer. The exercises you've been doing up to now mean that if everything has gone well, now's the earliest you should attempt to get back on your bike.

Your first few rides should be on the home trainer and you can possibly get back to cycling sooner, even if your arm is in a sling, but again, let pain be your guide.

Avoid using the drops initially as the increased weight through your upper body could irritate the shoulder.

Secondary issues

A crash that causes clavicle fracture can also aggravate the soft tissue and muscles around the shoulder. If you think these are slowing your recovery, seek help from a physiotherapist to reduce these problems. Give other areas of the body affected in the crash the attention they require rather than just focusing on the collarbone as you don't want another issue prolonging your eventual return to cycling.

STILL HAVE PAIN – WHO SHOULD YOU CALL?

When you get back to riding and you can't shift the discomfort or you're still experiencing pain and irritation from the shoulder, it's time to find out why you are still suffering.

PLAN A

PLAN B

 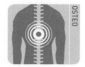

PART 2:
RIB FRACTURES

Rib fractures are common in cycling; in fact they're second only to collarbone fractures. The ribs get fractured usually following a crash when you land on the side of your torso or when you go over the handlebars with enough rotation to land on your back – both scenarios could result in one or multiple ribs being fractured depending on the force and angle of impact. Ribs usually fracture at either the point of impact, or at the angle of the ribs at the back and side of the flank where they are at their weakest point.

The lowdown

When ribs break, the muscles and soft tissue between them normally keep the ribs in place. In big enough impacts, however, the fractures can become displaced causing more damage as the end of the rib can puncture a lung causing either air or blood to seep into the space between the lung and the chest. This significantly interferes with breathing. It's not uncommon to get winded from the impact when ribs fracture but suspicion of complications arise when breathing difficulty persists or comes on a few hours after a crash where a rib fracture is suspected.

Of the 12 pairs of ribs, the most commonly fractured are the fifth to tenth which are found at the mid to lower end of the ribcage. Fracture of the upper four ribs is less common as they're protected to an extent by the shoulder girdle. Additionally, ribs 11 and 12 fracture less frequently as they're classed as 'floating' ribs because they're not attached to the breastbone at the front of the chest, which means they can absorb more impact before breaking.

PROFESSIONAL INSIGHT

Nathan Haas AUSTRALIAN PRO AND TWO-TIME JAPAN CUP WINNER

■ *'I was preparing for an upcoming race and out on my bike. Knowing I was through a hard part of the circuit, I was relaxing and ended up crashing on an easy section. As I was turning a corner I got my balance all wrong, my chest fell on to my handlebar and stem and I fell flat on to my face. I was really badly winded, that feeling where you're a bit scared because you're fighting for your breath.*

As I caught my breath and gathered my thoughts I realised something was wrong but it wasn't so bad that I needed to rush off to hospital. I sat there for about two minutes trying to compose myself and continue to get my breath. As I did I noticed a really deep ache over the front and side of my chest. At the time I thought I'd just bruised myself. It was painful but you're still stinging a bit from the crash. I was only 15 minutes from home so I rolled back with a friend who helped clean up the wounds.

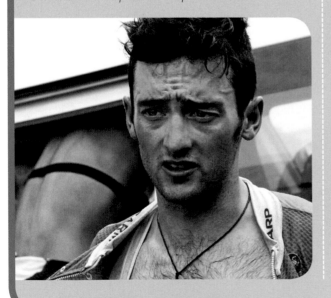

I thought nothing of it but that night I couldn't sleep on my chest and had to sleep on my back. Over the next two days I became strongly aware of an acute hot point on the rib, like a laser-sharp focal pain. On the third day I was still in agony and went to see my doctor. He said there was no point doing a scan and diagnosed a suspected rib fracture. He told me to take two weeks off any sport and told me to take paracetamol and ibuprofen for the pain.

The pain wasn't really bad until I either accidently knocked myself or took a deep breath. At any point of the day I knew it was there, you couldn't really escape it. After two weeks, the pain had almost entirely gone until I was cycling and my diaphragm was expanding as I was breathing more deeply, then I'd notice a twinge.

The problem was once the pain had gone you'd forget about it and then on certain movements it would catch you and I'd get a sharp dagger pain then an ache for two hours after. The hardest point was knowing when to get back into exercise and at what intensity as I'd still feel some pain on certain movements after four weeks. It's a frustrating injury because it's always with you. It takes longer than you might expect to feel really good again.

The advice I'd give is don't get ahead of yourself: because so many things are painless, you'll do something over the top and it's agony and you feel like you've damaged it again. For the first 2–3 weeks, don't mess around with it. Even though it's not that serious, it's far more annoying than you initially give it credit. On the flip side don't be scared for it to hurt a little as you get back into exercising otherwise you'll be sitting around for weeks. Man, it's an annoying injury.'

The science bit

The ribs

- The ribcage is made up of 12 pairs of ribs that wrap around the torso and protect the internal organs found there mainly the heart and lungs.
- The ribcage expands and retracts in normal breathing.
- Ribs 11 and 12 are also known as 'floating ribs' because they have no connection at the front as they're not attached to the breastbone.
- The ribcage is separated from the abdomen below by the diaphragm that controls breathing.

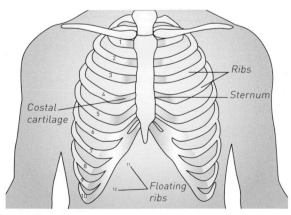

ABOVE The ribcage

Treatment

Injury at a glance

Pain scale	Moderate to severe
Time off bike	2–4 weeks
Call in the professionals?	No
Surgery?	No

Nearly all rib fractures are left to heal naturally and will do so without complications. The biggest issue is pain management during the recovery period. Sometimes you can feel the location of the fracture through the skin – and it will be painful – especially as it starts to heal as a small bony callous can form at the fracture site, which is normal.

The important thing to know is that the fracture can be extremely painful for two or even three weeks, with continued mild discomfort for up to 6–8 weeks. Any movement that causes irritation of the fracture can be excruciating, making everyday activities such as sleeping or getting out of bed difficult and uncomfortable, so be careful. Knowing what to expect can help put your mind to rest so you're not worrying about the pain if it's still bad a couple of weeks later.

Weeks 1–2

Rest from exercise and avoid any activity that produces torsion in the body (twisting) or lifting anything heavy. Usually this will mean two weeks off any exercise.

You shouldn't need to see your doctor unless you have increasing difficulty breathing. If you're still getting a lot of pain on certain movements at the end of the second week it's likely it was a fracture, whereas if the pain has almost disappeared by this time you had probably just badly bruised the rib.

FIRST AID

 Ice over the painful area for 10–20 minutes 2–3 times a day. This can be continued for as long as significant pain persists.

Over-the-counter medication

 See your doctor for stronger pain medication if needed.

See pages 62–63

Week 3

 Start a core exercise programme, pain permitting. See page 202.

Week 4

 No two rib fractures will be the same but there are common threads and after 2–3 weeks you'll normally be OK to start riding again, pain permitting.

By the third week the rib will be beginning to heal and your symptoms will begin to ease as well. If you can give it another week or two of rest from cycling, your pain should be even less giving you more confidence and comfort to ride later.

Make the first few rides easier by using the home trainer.

Kinesio tape?

 A simple way to offer some protection and support for the damaged rib when you get back on the bike. Depending on the location of the fracture you may be able to apply it yourself, or you may need help. You'll be surprised how much support you will get from just two pieces of tape. See the rehab toolkit page 179.

Week 9

STILL HAVE PAIN – WHO SHOULD YOU CALL?

After eight weeks if you are still getting discomfort, it may be due to secondary reasons such as local soft tissue damage that occurred in the crash. If you can't shift the pain in or around the area, it's time to seek help, but from who?

PLAN A

PLAN B

 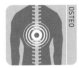

PART 3:
SCAPHOID FRACTURE

The scaphoid is the most commonly fractured carpal bone, one of the eight small bones that make up the wrist, accounting for 70 per cent of carpal fractures. It normally occurs when cycling if you fall from your bike on to an outstretched hand. If the impact is forceful enough, there'll be enough stress put on the scaphoid causing it to fracture. When you fracture your scaphoid it might not be obvious at first.

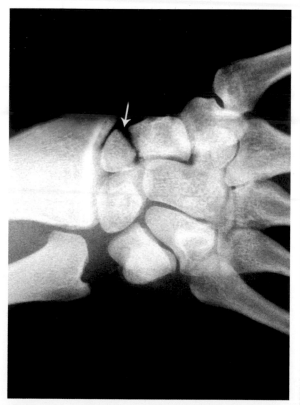

ABOVE Scaphoid fractures are extremely common

Under normal circumstances, a deep dull ache in the wrist at the base of the thumb will be felt which gets worse when gripping or squeezing the hand and is accompanied by swelling in this area. This area is known as the 'anatomical snuffbox.'

This area can be tender when pressure is applied on it *without* scaphoid fracture, as the nerve that runs through the anatomical snuffbox can be irritated. It's far better to err on the side of caution whenever a scaphoid fracture is suspected so it's best to go to hospital where doctors can X-ray or scan you if they suspect it too.

The lowdown

Unless the wrist is deformed, which it might not be, scaphoid fracture may not be suspected; and in some cases, the pain might not be strong enough to suspect a fracture and it can easily get misdiagnosed as a sprain. Any situation where wrist pain persists for longer than a day after a crash on to an outstretched arm, a high level of suspicion of a scaphoid fracture should remain due to the poor outcome and complications of missing it and having a fracture that doesn't heal properly.

The biggest problem with this fracture not healing properly is 'avascular necrosis' (AVN). This happens when the fracture goes right through the scaphoid bone and the pieces don't fuse properly. Now, one of the fractured pieces of bone stops getting proper blood supply and it dies. It's estimated this happens in between 13 to 50 per cent of all scaphoid fractures. When AVN occurs it leads to a longer, drawn out recovery with increased long-term complications such as prolonged aches and pain in the wrist, decreased grip strength, reduced wrist movement and development of arthritis in the wrist.

Attempts are always made to avoid AVN whenever possible and that is why scaphoid injuries are treated with a high level of suspicion until a fracture is ruled out. If scaphoid fracture is confirmed, you can almost guarantee you'll be off your bike outside for at least two months.

PROFESSIONAL INSIGHT

Simon Clarke AUSTRALIAN PRO AND 2012 VUELTA A ESPAÑA MOUNTAIN JERSEY WINNER

■ 'I broke my left scaphoid in the 2011 Paris-Roubaix. It was about halfway through the race and I was coming back past the team cars to the bunch when the Lampre team car passed me on the left and then I came around the next corner and he was stopped, blocking the whole road, and I went straight into the back of the car at about 55 km/h.

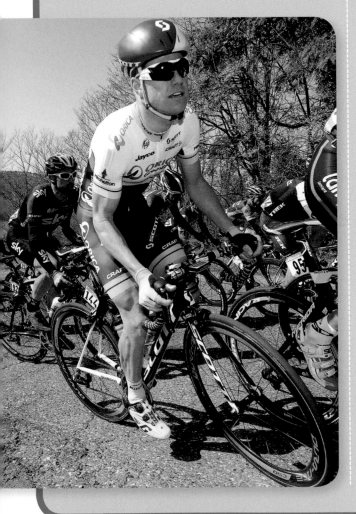

I hit my right knee and my head really hard on the back of the car so they were my first major worries but apart from some pain nothing was too serious. As I got back to the team bus, the doctor checked me and said everything looked fine. I flew home that night and the next day I got on the ergo to test my knee which was quite sore, but didn't prove too bad. It wasn't until that afternoon when I went down to the Aussie centre in Varese to see the physio that I realised that my left wrist was a little sore. No more pain than a slight sprain feeling.

The physio had a look at it and said it definitely needed to be scanned to check everything was OK. He organised for me the next morning to go into a private hospital in Milan. By early afternoon I had the results, which said the scaphoid was broken, basically in half (horizontally).

The specialist explained that we could either just put it in a cast or otherwise do a little operation that would involve inserting a 3mm titanium screw into the scaphoid to pull it together. He recommended the operation as it would mean a better binding of the break and also ensure that the blood supply throughout the bone wouldn't be affected.

On that same evening (two days after the crash), I had the operation and everything went fine. Post op. they made me two casts and four days later, I started riding on the ergo. Every morning I went and saw my physio to work on wrist mobility and after eight days on the ergo I started riding on the road, still with the riding cast. I think I rode on the road for about two weeks with the cast before taking it off.'

The science bit

The Scaphoid bone

- The scaphoid bone is one of the eight small carpal bones in the wrist. It is boat-shaped and the size of a medium-sized cashew.
- It sits between the hand and the forearm on the thumb side of the wrist.
- Its shape and how it joins with other bones see it play an important role in allowing movement of the wrist.
- The scaphoid can be felt at the base of the thumb in the 'anatomical snuffbox', which can be found between the two tendons that pop up when the thumb is extended against resistance or the hand is put into the 'hitchhikers' position.

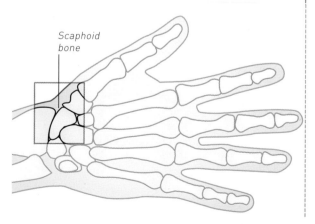

Scaphoid bone

Investigation

Suspect scaphoid fracture and it's important to seek medical opinion and normally X-rays will be done. Sometimes this fracture doesn't show up immediately on X-ray. If X-rays come back normal, a fracture cannot be ruled out. An MRI scan might then be done to detect a fracture. However, usually the X-rays would be repeated two weeks later and, by this time, absorption of the bone around the fracture site will have started and the fracture will be visible on X-ray if present.

Treatment

Injury at a glance

Pain scale	Mild to severe
Time off bike	8 weeks minimum
Call in the professionals?	Yes
Surgery?	Yes

If a scaphoid fracture is confirmed, you'll normally come under the care of a surgeon. If initial X-rays are negative but on examination a fracture was still suspected, then the wrist will usually be cast for two weeks until follow-up X-rays are performed. If two weeks later a scaphoid fracture is confirmed, it will be treated accordingly.

Depending on the nature of the fracture your doctor will make a decision on management. If the fracture is classed as being 'stable' (meaning the two ends of the bone are less than 1 mm apart from each other), the fracture *might* be cast for a further 10 weeks. Even with appropriate casting, up to one-third of these fractures still don't heal properly. This will almost certainly lead to arthritis between the two fragments and AVN in up to 50 per cent of cases, causing prolonged pain and stiffness of the wrist, so surgery is often recommended.

Without surgery this fracture doesn't always heal well and can take up to six months for the bone to heal properly, and if it fails to, it will lead to surgery anyway. So nowadays even 'stable' scaphoid fractures will often be surgically repaired.

Unstable fractures – when there's a gap greater than 1 mm between the two fractured pieces – requires immediate surgery. A screw will usually be placed into the bone to hold it together and encourage healing. The bottom line is, there's no quick fix for a scaphoid fracture. Even if you go down the surgical route, it will still normally result in the wrist being cast for 6–8 weeks *after* surgery.

Home Trainer

 The saving grace is that as long as you're stable and comfortable riding with one arm, you can put the injured hand in a sling and continue on the home trainer when you want. This will at least mean you're less likely to lose as much fitness as if you took 2–3 months off the bike completely. OK, you won't be able to go flat out on the bike with one arm, but it's better than nothing, right?

Week 1
THE NEXT STEP – AFTER CAST REMOVAL
This is when your rehab can begin. Your surgeon will normally have organised follow-up physiotherapy for you to help your recovery.

When the cast comes off you will have lost some muscle tone and strength in and around the wrist. This will need to be improved before you start using both hands comfortably on the bars again. The following exercises will help move you in the right direction and are a guideline.

REHAB TOOL KIT EX.	EX. NO.	PAGE
1. Wrist mobility	2.9	174
2. Tennis ball grip	2.8	174

Week 3
Now's the time to start your riding if you haven't as yet. Try to use both hands on the bars on the home trainer to begin with before moving out on to the road.

Run through your wrist mobility exercises before you ride.

Week 7
STILL HAVE PAIN – WHO SHOULD YOU CALL?
Six weeks from having removed your cast, if you're still getting prominent discomfort in the wrist that's not markedly improving, then it's a good idea to follow up to make sure everything is healing normally as it's now been at least three months since you fractured your wrist. The best option at this stage is to return to see either your surgeon or physio; they will have been following your care from the start and will be best placed to advise you.

PLAN A

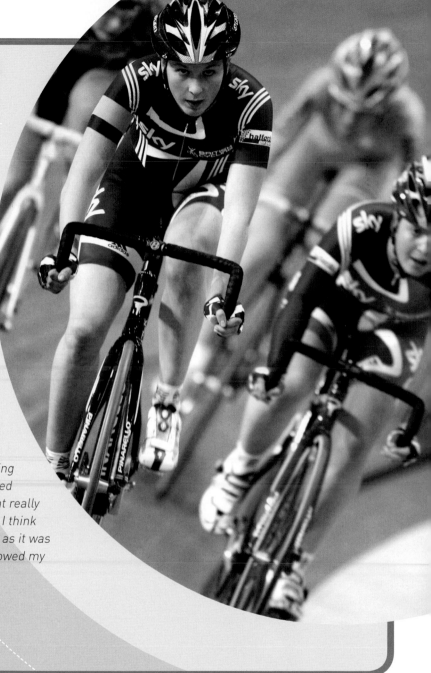

CYCLING NIRVANA

Lucy Martin

GREAT BRITAIN | 2012 TEAM GB OLYMPIAN

■ 'One of my memorable moments in cycling was when I was a junior and won the British national championships. I always just remember the final 500 m, which was up a short climb. I had been so nervous the whole race and felt like everyone else was better than me. Then, as we started up this climb and girls started to sprint, I was going backwards and thought "that's it race over". But then, it really was one of those "no chain" moments: something in my head must have changed and I suddenly was head down, no feeling and just passing all the others until I crossed the line first. I was elated, delighted and couldn't believe it. Complete Cycling Nirvana. Off the back of it I was selected on to the British U23 academy and that really was the proper start of my pro career. I think it's also a memorable moment for me as it was one of the few races that I actually allowed my mum to come and watch.'

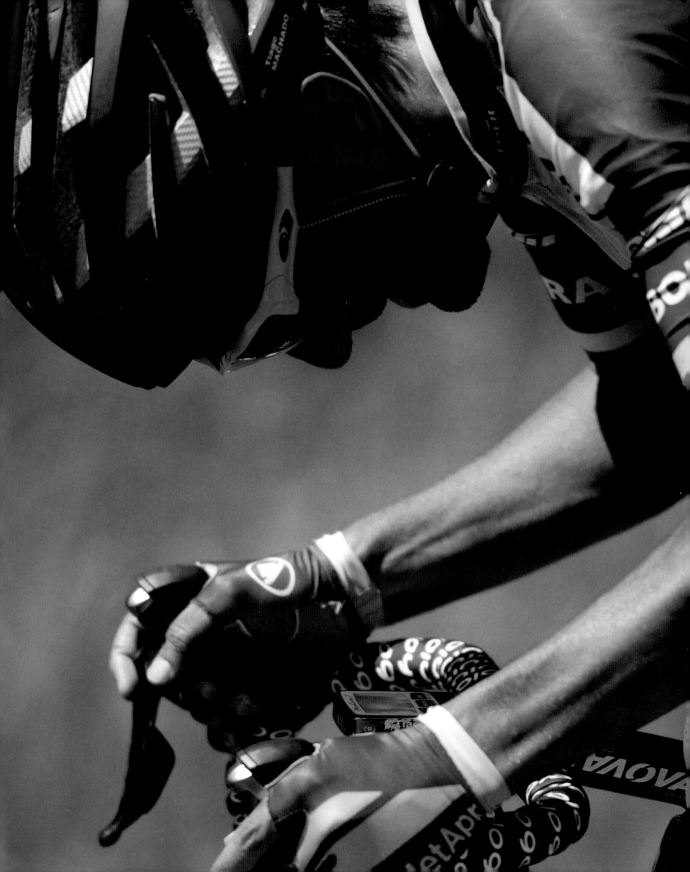

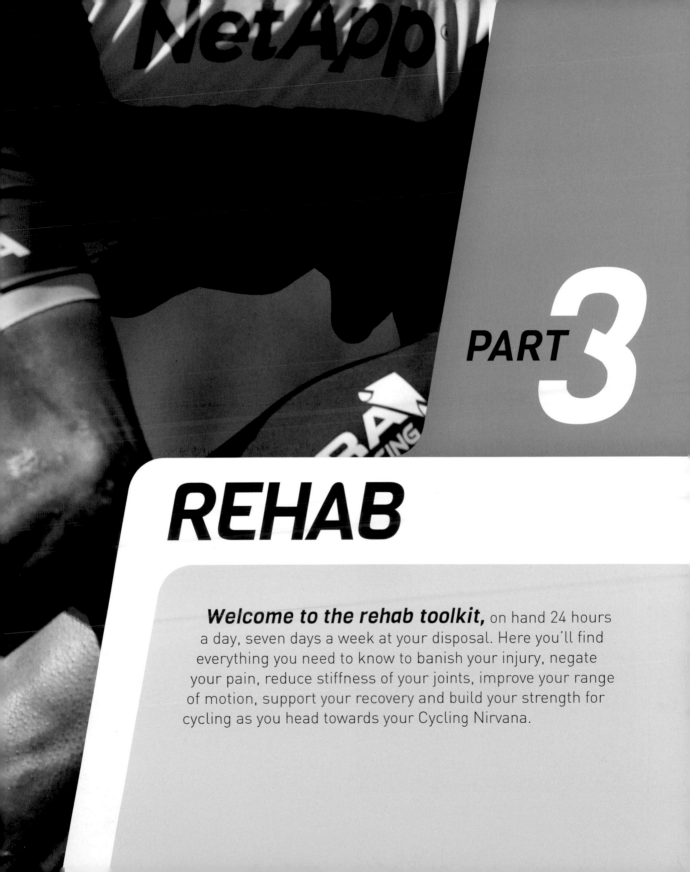

REHAB

Welcome to the rehab toolkit, on hand 24 hours a day, seven days a week at your disposal. Here you'll find everything you need to know to banish your injury, negate your pain, reduce stiffness of your joints, improve your range of motion, support your recovery and build your strength for cycling as you head towards your Cycling Nirvana.

18 THE REHAB TOOLKIT

Everything in the rehab toolkit has been specifically chosen for its ability to optimally *get the job done*, whether it be to strengthen a specific muscle group or help support a joint while riding. The exercises we recommend have nothing to do with increasing muscle bulk, and everything to do with improving the muscle function, and

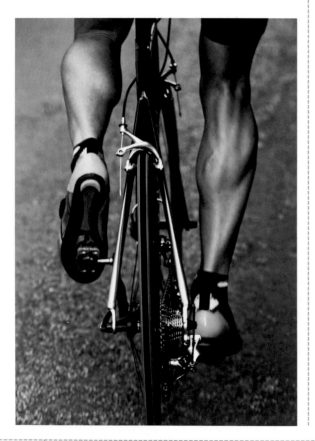

are delivered in a simplified way divided into regions of the body. The exercises presented are deliberately low-tech: all you need is some floor space, time and some application, so there's really nothing stopping you. Our aim is to get you robust enough to enjoy your cycling pain free and far from the worry of overuse injury being around the corner.

As you cast your eye through the exercises you'll notice that every part of the body is covered. Despite only using your legs to pedal, you actually use your whole body to support your riding, and injury isn't restricted to the lower half, far from it. See the rehab toolkit as the building blocks you need to build specific routines to get your injury resolved.

You can read about each area of the body and work through what you think your problem areas are, but we've made it far simpler than that. In the injury section, we recommended the specific exercises that are relevant with the exercise number for ease of reference. So you'll have no problem finding them so you can crack on with them and start to put that injury behind you.

At the end of the rehab toolkit you'll see we've chosen specific exercises we think are most suitable as a warm-up, a streamlined version for when time is limited, as well as selecting specific exercises we think can best help you warm down and recover after your ride. Not only that, we've designed a core exercise programme, with progressive exercises that you can increase in difficulty once you've mastered the initial routine. It's all here, laid out for you.

The 3 golden rules of exercise

Before we get started on the exercises, it's important we inform you of the three golden rules when doing any of the exercises in the rehab toolkit. These three principles are the cornerstone to getting the most out of your exercises and yet are commonly overlooked. Take the time to understand and apply these rules and it will help you make every exercise have a dual purpose, so that some of your deeper core muscles get an additional workout. This is important for building robustness and these rules are even more important to apply when you're returning from an overuse injury compared to a traumatic one. The three golden rules are:

1 Breathe properly
2 Remember to brace
3 Keep your lower back straight

Golden rule no 1: breathe properly

Breathing correctly may seem simple, yet few people manage it, to the detriment of the ability to activate your core muscles. The diaphragm has a double role, firstly in breathing and secondly for posture – where appropriate function helps support trunk core stability. Normal breathing is the cornerstone to spinal stability but is often overlooked.

Faulty breathing needs to be restored, allowing the diaphragm to properly assist in stabilising the core first, before *any* other movements or exercises are started. Your goal is to move from being a 'chest breather' – as most people are – to a 'belly breather', which will mean appropriate use of the diaphragm throughout breathing.

ARE YOU A CHEST BREATHER?
Lie on the floor with your knees lifted and your feet flat on the floor, then place one hand on your stomach and one on your chest before taking a deep breath in. If you feel your chest expand as much or more than your stomach, you're a chest breather and have less than an optimal breathing pattern.

IMPROVE YOUR BREATHING
- Lie on the floor, hips and knees bent, feet flat on the floor.
- Place one hand on the stomach and one on the chest.
- As you inhale focus on moving your stomach outwards while your chest remains still.
- Focus on long and slow breaths building up from normal breathing.
- After a few breaths, aim for a 2–3 second inhalation phase and a longer 4–6 second exhalation phase (6–8 breaths a minute). **(Reps – 10–20 breaths, 1–2 times a day.)**

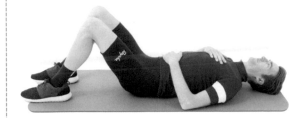

MATT SAYS:

'This exercise will help you draw breath in from your diaphragm while trying not to expand your ribs as you inhale. This is normal breathing. You may feel light-headed as you begin; if this happens take shorter normal breaths to start with before increasing their duration. Once you've nailed it lying down, breathing training, like any new motor skill, is best repeated throughout the day while in different positions, at the desk or when you're back on the bike, for example – this will help commit this new movement pattern into your brain's hard wiring making it automatic.'

Golden rule no 2: lumbar spine bracing

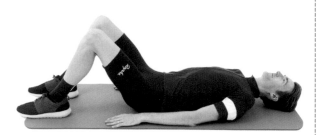

Activating all three layers of the abdominal wall when bracing enhances the stability offered to the lumbar spine and lower back throughout any other exercise. Bracing improves the ability to withstand load and stresses placed on the lumbar spine in everyday activity as well as withstanding sudden unexpected load.

- Lie on the floor with hips and knees bent, feet flat on the floor.
- Tense the muscles 360 degrees around the abdomen and lower lumbar spine while continuing to breathe normally.
- Muscles should be tensed gently between 10–20 per cent of your maximum (it should feel like a gentle tightening of the core).
- Hold this contraction for 30 seconds. **(Reps – repeat 3 times.)**

MATT SAYS:

'Once you've mastered this exercise in this position, repeat on all fours ensuring you keep the back straight. A key to learning this exercise is to be able to do it during everyday activities so when you've got it nailed, try it sitting at your desk, in bed, or while driving or cycling.'

Golden rule no 3: a neutral lumbar spine

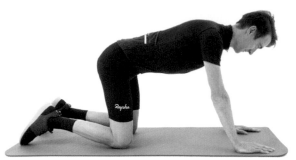

In simple terms this means keeping your back 'straight', in particular the lower back. This is the cornerstone of maintaining 'good posture'. By keeping the lumbar spine in a neutral position you provide a more stable platform for the rest of the body to be supported.

The hips and gluteal muscles of the buttock are far stronger than the lumbar spine's small joints and muscles so should bear the brunt of the weight of the upper body, and keeping the lumber spine in neutral helps support this. As soon as you move away from a neutral position, for example, into flexion – leaning forwards – increased stress is put through the discs of the lower back making this area vulnerable to injury (for more info on anatomy of the lower back see page 80).

Practising 'finding' a neutral lumbar spine will help you to recognise the position so you can more readily adopt it in both the exercises in everyday life. Once you can maintain a neutral lumbar spine while cycling it will also help to reduce tension and mild discomfort in the lower back that you may experience when you ride. Finding a neutral lumbar spine:

- Adopt the all fours position, with your hands directly underneath your shoulders, knees beneath your hips and arms and legs shoulder-width apart.
- Spend a few seconds practising your breathing and bracing in this position.
- Keeping your upper body stable, rock your pelvis as far forwards as you can, then as

far back as you can, and then find a position halfway between the two – this will be a neutral lumbar spine position.

Practise finding a neutral lumbar spine in other positions such as lying on your back (knees lifted and feet flat) or sitting at your desk.

Applying the three golden rules

The three golden rules are relatively easy to keep, but making them a habit and adopting them when you perform any other exercise is the harder aspect to master. So practise throughout the day, even when you're not doing the exercises. Once you can consistently apply them while performing other exercises, you'll not only enhance the benefit of the exercises but you'll also increase the protection of your lumbar spine and lower back while doing them too. Once you have *really* mastered them, you'll be able to apply the rules automatically, without thinking, in everyday life, including your cycling. And when you can, it will provide the perfect foundation for the improving robustness of your body.

BELOW It's important to remember the three golden rules

Exercise guidance

- All the exercises should ideally be done five days a week unless otherwise stated.
- Remember the three golden rules when you're going through each of the exercises, we can't stress that enough.
- Allocate enough time to go through your recommended exercises methodically, remembering that good form is essential throughout.
- As soon as you lose form during any exercise that exercise is finished for the day; stop and come back to it as you repeat the exercises the next time.
- If you get any pain related to an injury as you perform the exercises, avoid that exercise for the day and move on to the next one unless otherwise stated.
- If you don't have time to do a complete routine that's recommended, pick up where you left off the next time you perform the routine, e.g. performing three or four exercises of the core exercise routine at each session, this way you still get the complete cycle.

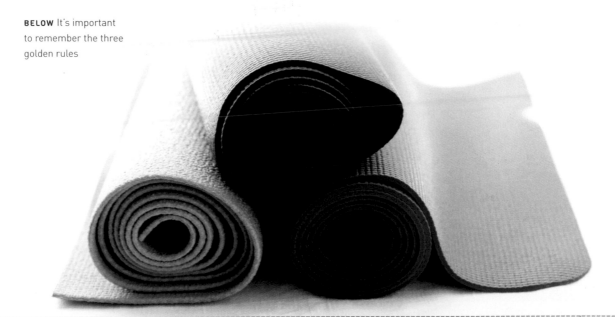

The rehab toolkit contents

1 Head, neck and upper back

1.1 NECK ROTATION

This exercise improves the function and mobility of the cervical spine.

- Sit upright and make your neck tall, gently tuck in your chin.
- Slowly turn your head as far as you can (without pain) to the left and hold it there for a count of 3 seconds.

- Slowly return your head to the midline and repeat the procedure to the right and then returning to the midline. This is 1 repetition.
- As you turn your head, keep your chin tucked in. At the end of the rotation, your eye line should be on your shoulder. This prevents you moving the neck backwards into extension at the same time as rotating it – a common mistake.
(Reps – repeat every couple of hours).

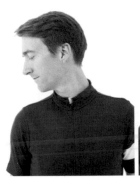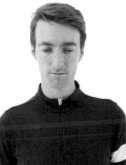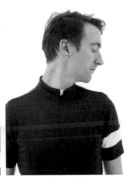

LEFT This is a great exercise to do while sat at the desk to relieve tension.

MATT SAYS:

'I always recommend avoiding side bending (lateral flexion) of the neck. For some reason it's often advised for neck discomfort and is recommended in many exercise classes. Yes, the neck can laterally flex, but it's not really designed for that motion.

Side bending can aggravate already irritated joints, making neck pain worse. When you rotate your head, there's a slight amount of natural lateral flexion that occurs, and this "coupled motion" is enough to improve general neck mobility. Worse, is when people "crack" their own necks in an attempt to self-manipulate. This "cavitation" occurs when gasses dissolved in the fluid of the joint get released when there's a rapid change in pressure inside the joint. This is to be avoided: it might feel good in the short term, but the more you do it, the more you will feel like you need to. Also, it will often be the same joint that "cracks" but it may well not be that joint that's causing discomfort. You don't want to create more of a problem by cracking your own neck so avoid it altogether.'

1.2 UPPER BACK MOBILITY

The thoracic spine is an under-appreciated region of the spine. This exercise helps mobilise this often stiff and restricted area of the body. Modern lifestyles mean this area is under continued stress – dysfunction and immobility in this area can significantly contribute to discomfort on the bike, making it imperative to increase mobility in this area.

- Lie on your left side, head resting on a cushion, with your right knee bent and touching the floor, left leg straight and arms stretched out in front of you with your palms together. Trap the foot of your top leg underneath the bottom outstretched leg. (This keeps your pelvis straight throughout the exercise ensuring the movement comes from the upper back.)
- Keeping the left hand and right knee touching the floor, slowly move your right hand away in an arc up and round until the back of your right palm is as close as possible to the floor on the opposite side while maintaining the right knee contact on the floor. This should take between 3–5 seconds.
- Slowly rotate your head so your eye-line follows the moving arm.
- Once rotated as far as you can, hold this pose for 2 seconds before slowly returning to the starting position. This is one repetition.

Repeat 10 times on each side.

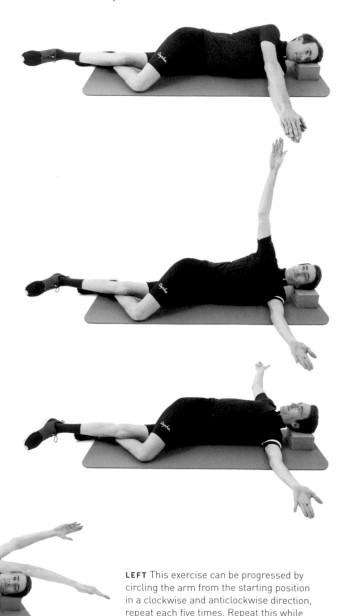

LEFT This exercise can be progressed by circling the arm from the starting position in a clockwise and anticlockwise direction, repeat each five times. Repeat this while lying on the other side.

1.3 NECK STRETCH (LEVATOR SCAPULAE MUSCLE)

Gently stretching the muscles at the back of the neck as they join the upper back can help to reduce tension in the neck and relieve symptoms. This stretch will usually feel quite sore in the early stages of neck pain but will soon become easier.

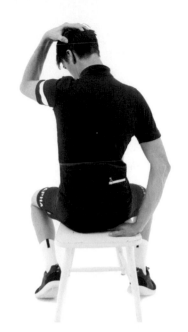

- Sit upright with your shoulders back and make your neck long.
- Place your right hand underneath your right buttock, with the palm faced down.
- Turn your head 45 degrees to the left, and drop your head forwards.
- Add to the stretch by gently pulling your head further forwards and hold this for 10 seconds. (You should feel the stretch on the right side of your neck as it joins the shoulder/ upper back region).
Reps – Repeat on both sides 3 times.

1.4 DEEP NECK FLEXOR ACTIVATION (CHIN RETRACTIONS)

This is a principal exercise to wake up the 'core' muscles that control the neck, which often become weakened through poor posture or injury.

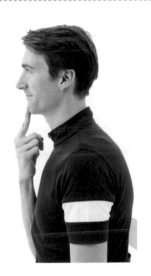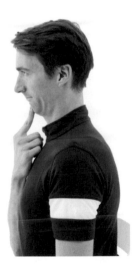

- Sit up with your head straight and make your neck long.
- Gently draw the chin backwards and drop it ever so slightly (imagine you are gently trying to hold a grapefruit under the chin without squashing it while there is a helium balloon lifting the back of your head).
- Hold this position for 10 seconds.
Reps – Repeat 3 times.

MATT SAYS:

'This is a subtle exercise, you shouldn't be either jamming your chin backwards or nodding it too hard. Once you think you are in the right position, try and swallow. If it's more difficult to do so, then you're activating your deep neck flexor muscles. This is a great exercise to help reduce the forward head position (anterior head carriage), which is also associated with increased strain on the neck.'

1.5 DEEP NECK FLEXOR STRENGTHENING (HEAD LIFT)

A progression of the previous exercise that more deeply stimulates and improves endurance strength of the deep neck flexor muscles, which is so often weak in neck pain sufferers.

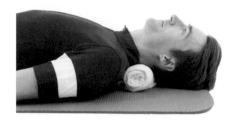

- Lie on your back and place a rolled-up towel underneath your neck.
- Make your neck long and relax your shoulders.
- Gently drop your chin and slightly nod, gently pulling your head into the rolled-up pillow at the same time as making your neck 'longer' – this engages the deep neck flexor muscles.
- Lift your head off the pillow about an inch, remembering to keep your chin tucked in (just enough so your head is no longer supported on the pillow).
- Hold this position for 30 seconds
  Reps: Repeat up to 3 times.

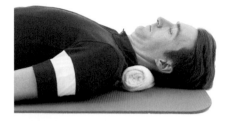

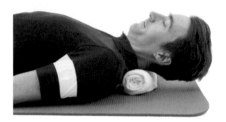

When you lift your head up, look down towards your toes, which will naturally encourage you to keep your chin tucked in. Avoid sticking your chin out as this puts more stress on the cervical spine so is more likely to irritate the injury.

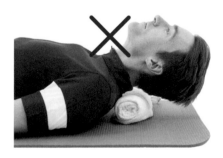

MATT SAYS:

'This is not an easy exercise. The first few times you do it you will probably find it difficult to reach 30 seconds once, let alone 3 times. Don't worry, only do it for as long as you can and work to build it up to 3 reps of 30 seconds. Your head may shake quite violently as you attempt to hold your head in position to begin with; this is normal and typically a sign that weakness in these muscles exist that need to be worked on – so stick with it.'

1.6 SCAPULAR STABILISER ACTIVATION

This exercise helps engage the muscles between the shoulder blades that are important for upper body and shoulder stability, especially on the bike. By getting these muscles switched on, it reflexively helps reduce the tension and tightness in the upper traps (shoulder) muscles, reducing the chances of this tightness influencing your injury.

- Lie on your back, knees raised and feet flat on the floor, arms by your side.
- Slowly draw your shoulders downwards and backwards and gently squeeze the muscles between your shoulder blades while continuing to breathe normally.
- Hold this position for 30 seconds then relax. This is one repetition.
Reps – Repeat 3 times.

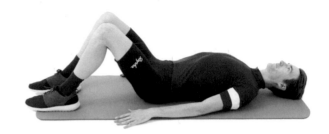

1.7 THE WALL ANGEL

An excellent approach to help improve muscle imbalance in the upper body, as well as helping with upper back pain and neck pain, in particular the shoulders. This exercise involves movement and more deeply engages the muscles. The wall angel also helps switch on the lower scapula stabiliser muscles, which are important to help improve cervical spine stability.

- Stand leaning against a wall with your feet slightly wider than shoulder-width apart.
- Ensure your pelvis, upper back and the back of your head are all touching the wall and bring your arms out and back with your hands above your head and elbows touching the wall.
- Slowly lower your elbows, sliding them down against the wall over the count of 3 seconds as low as you can – as you do so gently squeeze the muscles between your shoulder blades.
- Hold the lowered position for a count of 3 seconds before returning to the starting position and repeat 10 times.
Reps – Build up to repeat this exercise 3 times.

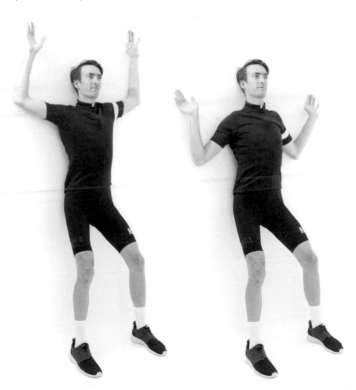

1.8 ONE-SIDED SCAPULAR STABILISERS

This exercise more deeply engages the lower scapular stabilisers, allows the injured side to be more specifically worked on and will help shoulder mobility.

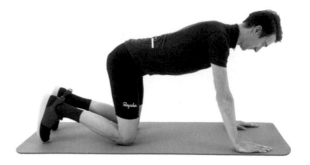

- Begin in an all-fours position, with your hands and knees shoulder-width apart, knees underneath your hips, and hands underneath your shoulders.
- Gently squeeze between the shoulder blades, and take the arm of the injured shoulder out to the side of the body until the arm is horizontal to the body with the palm facing the floor, over the count of 3.
- Hold for the count of 2 and return to the starting position. Repeat 10 times.
  Reps – repeat 3 times.

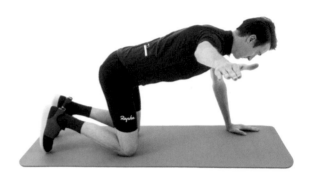

1.9 UPPER BACK TENNIS BALL RELEASE

Hours spent on the saddle can mean the upper back can get tight as the muscles are engaged to support the head. Working through them with self-massage can improve comfort on the bike.

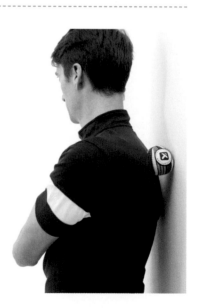

- Place the ball between your back and a hard surface such as a wall.
- Roll the ball around until you find the tender spot that has been bothering you.
- Spend 10–15 seconds slightly moving the body and rolling the ball over and around the tight muscle.
  Reps – find 3–4 tender areas, though there may be less.

MATT SAYS:

'Moving your arm across your chest exposes deeper upper back muscles where your tightness might be coming from.'

2 Shoulders and arms

2.1 THE SHOULDER ROLL

Rolling the shoulders will improve general mobility in the shoulder girdle and upper back regions. Both are areas that can get tight and restricted through cycling. This is a great exercise to do while sat at the desk to relieve tension, repeated every couple of hours.

- Sitting upright, make your neck tall, roll your shoulders from down and forwards to up and backwards in a circle.
  Reps – repeat 3 times.

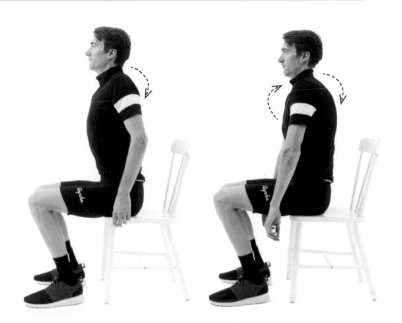

2.2 THE SHOULDER SWING

This exercise will help to reduce stiffness in the shoulder joint itself while limiting the load on the joint.

- Standing and supporting your body with your good arm, lean over and let the injured arm hang freely.
- Gently let your arm swing forwards and backwards like a pendulum for 1 minute then stop.
- Gently move the arm in small circles swinging like a pendulum in clockwise circles for 1 minute.
- Stop and perform the same exercise counter clockwise for one minute – 1 repetition.
  Reps – repeat twice.

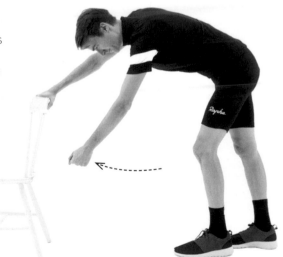

Once this gets easier, you can hold a small weight in the arm. Place a bag of sugar in a carrier bag or something like this to slightly increase the pendulum action. It will feel surprisingly comfortable to do this.

2.3 ISOMETRIC SHOULDER ACTIVATION

Isometric exercises contract the muscles without any movement of the joint. This allows muscle function to be retained or slight strength to be improved with minimal risk to stress on an injured area.

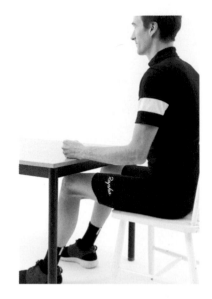

Triceps: Gently engages the muscle at the back of the arm responsible for extension.

- Rest your injured arm on a tabletop with your elbow at 90 degrees and make a fist.
- Press the fist and forearm down into the tabletop. Your triceps muscle will contract but your arm will not move. (Begin gently and, as you feel more comfortable, you can slightly increase the pressure).
- Hold this for 10 seconds.
  Reps – repeat 3 times.

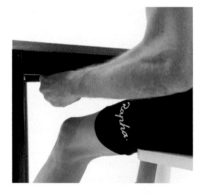

Biceps: Gently engages the muscle at the front of the arm responsible for flexion.

- Make a fist and place your injured arm under a tabletop with your elbow at 90 degrees.
- Press the fist and forearm up into the underside of the tabletop. Your bicep muscle will contract but your arm will not move. (Begin gently and as you feel more comfortable you can slightly increase the pressure).
- Hold this for 10 seconds.
  Reps – repeat 3 times.

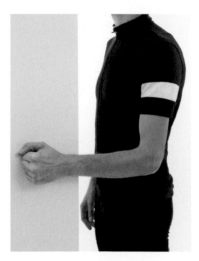

Rotator cuff – internal rotators: This exercise gently engages the muscles responsible for shoulder rotation.

- Standing in a doorway, arms down by your side, bend your elbow to 90 degrees, make a fist and place the inside of your forearm against the inside of the door frame.
- Press your forearm into the door frame.
- Your arm will not move but the internal rotator muscles of your shoulder will contract.
- Hold this for ten seconds.
  Reps – repeat 3 times.

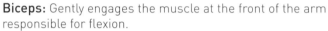

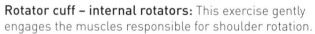

Rotator cuff – external rotators: Gently engages the muscles responsible for shoulder rotation.

- Same procedure as internal rotators except this time place the outside of your elbow against the door frame and reverse the movement, and press the outside of the forearm against the door frame as if you are attempting to move your forearm away from the body. **Reps – repeat three times.**

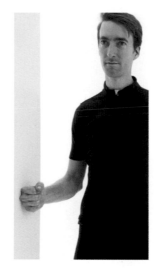

Deltoid: Gently engages the muscles of the shoulder responsible for abduction.

- Stand against a wall or door frame with the elbow bent to 90 degress.
- Gently press the outside of the elbow against the wall.
- Your arm will not move but the deltoid muscle of your shoulder will contract.
- Hold this for ten seconds. **Reps – repeat three times.**

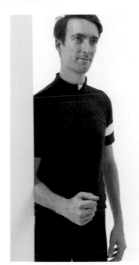

2.4 PASSIVE SHOULDER MOVEMENT

Gently increases shoulder range of motion without having to use the muscles of the damaged shoulder to move it.

- Can be done standing or lying down.
- Begin with your hands straight in front of your abdomen and hold the injured hand of your bad arm with the other one.
- Let your injured shoulder relax as best you can, while you lift the arm with the other hand.
- Lift the arm to 90 degrees and then back down again – 1 repetition. **Reps – repeat 10 times.**

As your arm becomes more mobile you can lift it slightly higher, only as far as is comfortable.

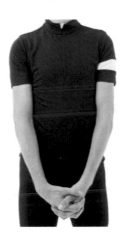

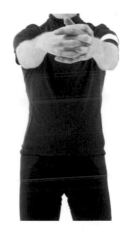

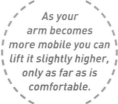

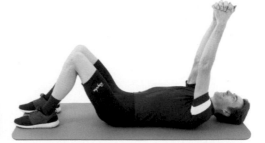

2.5 ACTIVE SHOULDER RANGE OF MOTION

Improving the active range of motion of your shoulder begins to use the shoulder in a more normal capacity.

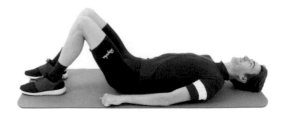

- Lying on your back, hands down by your side.
- Slowly lift the arm upwards until it is perpendicular to the floor.
- While gently squeezing between your shoulder blades, slowly take your arm backwards over your head as far as is comfortable, and then lower, returning to the starting position.
  Reps – repeat 10 times

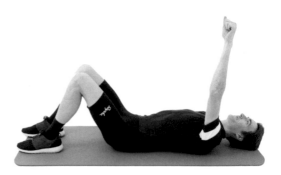

MATT SAYS:

'After a collarbone fracture only bring your arm to 90 degrees in each direction until four weeks have passed or until you feel totally comfortable doing so. After this begin to progress the range of motion further while remembering to stay within your comfort zone.'

2.6 DYNAMIC SHOULDER STRENGTHENING

Rotators: Improves general strength in the rotator cuff muscles, the key shoulder stabilising muscles.

- Side lying with the injured shoulder on the upwards side.
- Place a rolled up towel between the elbow and the side of the body and bend the elbow to 90 degrees.
- Hold a 1 kg weight in your hand (you can use a water bottle or tin of food if no weight available).
- Begin with the weight lowered almost on to the floor.

- Gently squeeze between your shoulder blades and lift the weight upwards in an arc over the count of 3, keeping the towel pinned against your side.
- As you rotate your forearm backwards keep the shoulder still, making sure the only movement in the body is coming from the arm.
- Lower the arm down to the starting position and repeat 10 times.
  Reps – repeat 3 times.

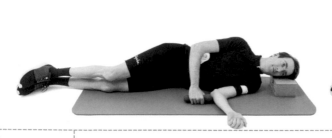

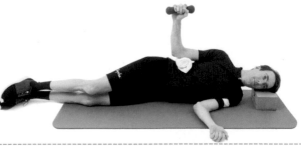

Extensors: Works the lower scapular stabilisers as well as the shoulder extensor muscles, both used to help upper body stability on the bike.

- Lie on your front with the injured arm down by your side.
- Place a 1 kg weight in your hand, facing upwards (you can use a water bottle or tin of food if no weight available).
- Gently squeeze between the shoulder blades and extend your arm lifting the weight backwards as far as comfortable, count to 3 seconds before lowering. **Reps – repeat 3 times.**

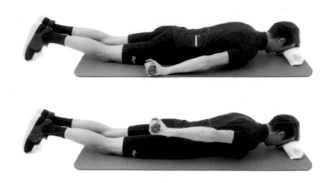

2.7 ULNAR NERVE FLOSSING

This simple yet strange looking dynamic set of exercises can help to reduce snagging of the glide and ulnar nerve as it passes from the neck down the arm and into the hand through the wrist. Improving the slide on the nerve can help relieve discomfort and symptoms by releasing tension on this nerve. These exercises must be done gently and with care; back off if symptoms are made at all worse.

EXERCISE ONE

- Begin with your elbow bent and your palm in front of your face with your head straight.
- Extend the elbow out in front of you keeping it horizontal to the floor and slowly extend your wrist until your palm is facing away from you and your fingers point to the floor.
- With the other hand gently pull your 4th and 5th fingers further into extension. Drop your head into flexion and hold for 3 seconds.
- Let go and return to starting position.
- The exercise should be done in one fluid movement **Reps – repeat 10 times.**

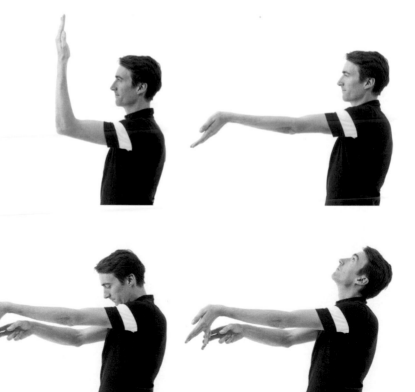

EXERCISE TWO

- Repeat the exercise exactly the same as the first one, but take the head back into extension rather than flexion this time.

EXERCISE THREE

- Make the 'OK' sign with your thumb and first finger, extend the other three fingers and hold your elbow out to the side.
- Over 3 seconds rotate your hand towards you so your 3 fingers point towards the floor, this builds tension in the nerve.
- Bring your hand towards your face so you are looking through the 'O' between your finger and thumb as your fingers remain pointing downwards and hold this position for 3 seconds.
- Let go and return to starting position.
- All exercises should be done in one fluid movement. **Reps – repeat 10 times.**

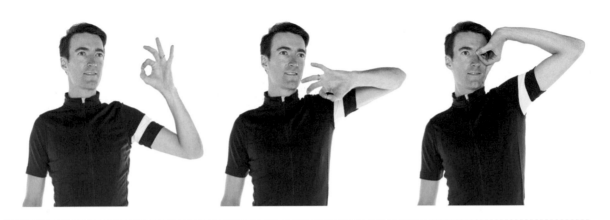

2.8 TENNIS BALL GRIP

An easy exercise to perform that will engage the muscles of the hand. Improving grip strength can help improve upper body stability on the bike after a hand or wrist injury.

- Hold a tennis ball in your outstretched hand and grip as hard as you can for 10 seconds. **Reps – multiple times throughout the day.**

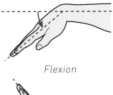

2.9 WRIST MOBILITY

Improving range of motion will help reduce stiffness in the joints following wrist injury.

- Take the wrist actively through all the different ranges of motion and hold the end range of motion for 10 seconds. **Reps – repeat 3 times.**

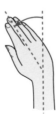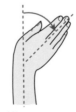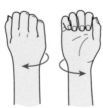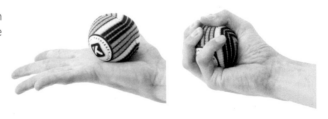

Radial deviation   Ulnar deviation   Pronation   Supination   Flexion   Extension

2.10 KINESIO TAPE FOR THE ACROMIOCLAVICULAR JOINT

A useful tape application following separation of the shoulder (see pages 118–124). Can be used for the first few weeks after injuring the acromioclavicular (AC) joint as it will provide support to the damaged ligaments at the same time as allowing the shoulder joint itself to move freely, unlike a sling. This application can help support the joint from the stress of riding. You'll need to get someone else to apply this tape for you.

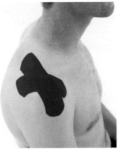
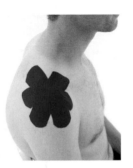
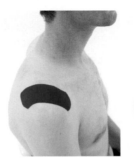

- Cut three pieces of tape approximately 15–20 cm in length.
- Tear the middle of the tape and apply like a Band-Aid, keeping the AC joint right in the centre.
- Applying full stretch on the middle 5 cm or so, stick the tape over the AC joint while letting the ends stick down with no tension.
- Apply the second piece of tape on top of the first, slightly rotated to allow the ends to stick down on the skin.
- Apply the third piece of tape, offset slightly again.

> **MATT SAYS:**
>
> 'An application I consistently use for cyclists off the bike as well as on it because AC joint injury is one you carry around with you and notice all the time even when you are not riding. This tape provides that little bit of extra support to help ease symptoms during recovery.'

3 Torso

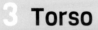

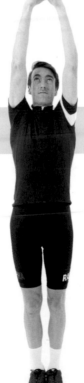

3.1 THE STAND TALL AND REACH STRETCH

Will help decompress and reduce tension in the spine, which can help symmetry when you ride.

- Knees and feet together and arms straight up overhead.
- Gently squeeze the knees together at the same time as reaching both arms upwards as high as you can.
- From this position, gently alternate stretching the left arm upwards for 2 seconds and then the right arm. Repeat 10 times.
  Reps – repeat 3 times.

3.2 THE PRESS-UP

When done correctly this classic exercise will help strengthen your chest and arms, and will help stabilise your bike handling. Increasing muscle bulk isn't required for cycling but this dynamic exercise will build strength not bulk when performed as suggested.

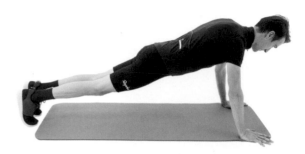

- Start on your front, up on your hands with your arms a little wider than shoulder-width apart and your toes dug into the ground about shoulder-width apart.
- Begin in a straight plank like position with your chin gently tucked in.
- Maintaining a straight torso, lower your body towards the floor keeping your elbows tucked in close to your body over the count of three seconds until your elbows are at 45 degrees at the bottom of the push-up position.
- Making sure your body doesn't sag as you reach the bottom and maintaining a straight spine, push your body back upwards to the starting position over the duration of one second.
  Reps – repeat 10 times (build up to 3 sets).

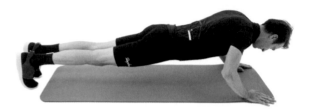

Don't rush this exercise just because of its familiarity. If you don't have the upper body strength to do the above full press-up, doing the same procedure on your knees will be easier to perform and have the same desired effect.

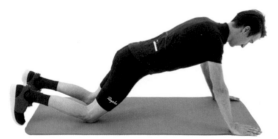

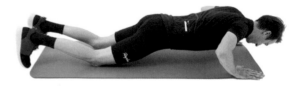

3.3 THE PLANK

This isometric hold will engage the deep core muscles for stability, improving their strength.

- On elbows and toes, maintain a straight and long spine.
- Elbows should be directly underneath the shoulder and chin should be slightly tucked in (eyes looking towards the floor to maintain neutral cervical spine). Hold for 1 minute.
  Reps – repeat 3 times.

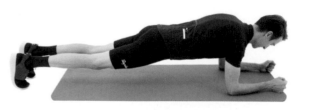

3.4 THE SIDE PLANK

This isometric hold will call on the deep core muscles, especially the lateral oblique muscles – the muscles at the side of the torso. Building strength in this area is important for helping stabilise the side walls of the abdomen.

MATT SAYS:

'If this is too hard to hold for one minute to begin with, do the same exercise resting on your knees (see second image) rather than your feet. This will be easier to do and you can build up to doing the exercise on the feet from there.'

- Lie on your side on your elbow with your feet outstretched, one on top of the other.
- The elbow on the floor should be directly underneath the shoulder to minimise tension in the shoulder.
- Gently tuck in the chin and keep your head in a straight line with your body.
- Raise up into side plank position, maintaining the straight line. Hold position for 1 minute. **Reps – repeat 3 times.**

BELOW The right-hand image shows an adaptation requiring less upper body strength

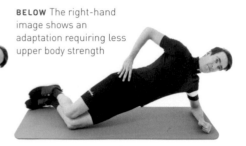

3.5 THE PLANK TO SIDE PLANK

This exercise takes the plank and the side plank to the next level as you advance your core work, requiring increased strength of the deep abdominal core muscles while the dynamic nature of the exercise requires good core muscle activation during transfer of weight between moving positions.

MATT SAYS:

'A natural progression is to hold the position for longer and to increase the number of reps.'

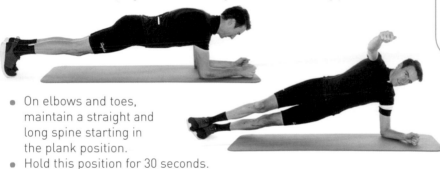

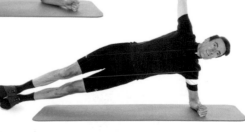

- On elbows and toes, maintain a straight and long spine starting in the plank position.
- Hold this position for 30 seconds.
- From the front plank position, shift the weight on to your left elbow and turn your body, moving into the side plank position. Hold this position for 30 seconds.
- Maintaining good core activation, return to the plank position for 30 seconds.
- Shift the weight on to the left elbow and into the side plank position on your left side. Hold this position for 30 seconds.
- Slowly return to the plank position and finish off here for 30 seconds to a minute.
- Should be a seamless movement between positions while maintaining the long straight plank position throughout.
Reps – repeat twice (each rep is 2.30 min).

3.6 THE FOUNDATION EIGHT POINT PLANK

This exercise ramps up the difficulty of the plank to epic proportions, building more deeply on to abdominal core strength. This isometric hold looks and sounds easy, but it's far from it.

- Start in a prone position, face down, chin slightly tucked in.
- Using your fingertips (with your hand in a position as if you were taking a snooker or pool shot), elbows, knees and toes (eight points), lift your torso off the floor.
- Try and draw your elbows towards your knees and vice versa – further engaging the abdominal muscles.
- Hold this position for 1 minute before lowering the body.
Reps – repeat twice.

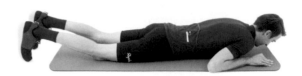
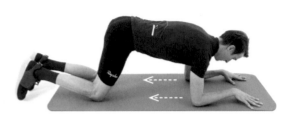

3.7 ABDOMINAL CURL DOWNS

This 'reverse sit-up' routine increases the load through the torso, building strength in the abdominal muscle wall that supports the core. This is an excellent way to increase abdominal strength without compromising the lower back as can happen in a regular sit-up exercise.

- Start in a sitting up position with the knees bent and the feet flat on the floor and arms reached out in front of you and your chin tucked in.
- Slowly uncurl your spine down backwards over the count of 3 seconds, imagining you are releasing your spine one segment at a time while keeping your arms reached out in front of you and your feet on the floor.
- Just before your shoulders reach the floor, try and resist collapsing and your feet lifting.
- Curl down backwards until you feel your shoulder blades reach the floor. Return to the starting position using your arms to sit upwards, pushing off the floor, this is 1 repetition.
Reps – 10 (build up to 3 sets).

Progression – once you have mastered this exercise, make it harder. As your shoulders reach the floor, reverse the procedure by slowly sitting back upright using your abdominal muscles, keeping your arms out in front of you with your heels remaining on the floor.

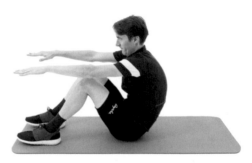
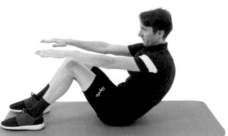
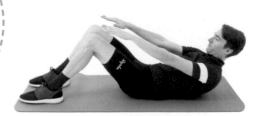

'It's easy to want to hold the feet against the wall if they have a tendency to lift off the ground but avoid this as you'll just start to work the psoas muscle (hip flexor), rather than the deep muscles of the abdominal wall that you're trying to engage so you won't get the same benefit.'

You can progress this exercise even further by crossing your arms in front of your chest rather than reaching out in front of you. If you find yourself getting to a level that is difficult to move beyond, stay at the level you're able to do with good form rather moving on and having bad technique at the next level.'

3.8 PECTORAL MUSCLE TENNIS BALL RELEASE

Hours spent on the saddle, holding on to the handlebars, can result in extremely tight pectoral muscles. The pectoral muscles often get tight following certain injuries such as collarbone fracture due to either ongoing sling use or the naturally protective posture commonly held in the first few weeks after the injury. Massaging the muscles will make the chest wall feel more open and may help prevent slouching.

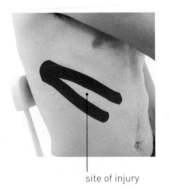

- Place the ball over the pec muscle applying gentle pressure with a reinforced hand.
- Roll the ball around until you find a tender spot and spend 10–15 seconds rolling the ball over and around the tight muscle area. **Reps – Find 3–4 tender areas, there may be less.**

3.9 KINESIO TAPE FOR SUSPECTED RIB FRACTURE

- Cut two pieces of tape approximately 20 cm each and split down the middle of each piece, two-thirds of the way to create a 'Y' shape.
- Keep the site of injury in the centre of your intended tape location.
- Place the first piece of tape down at the single end while pulling each ends of the 'Y' to stretch them slightly before placing them down.
- Apply the second piece of tape at a 90-degree angle to the first piece in the same way.

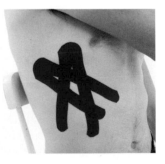

site of injury

4 Whole body

4.1 THE LOW LUNGE

This exercise will deeply engage the glute muscles, which are imperative for cycling as well as help loosen and lengthen the psoas muscles and mobilise the shoulders.

- Slowly take a lunge step forwards, reach your arms straight above you and lower your body until the back knee almost touches the floor.
- Hold for 1 second.
- Squeeze the glute as you stand upwards, bringing your rear foot forwards and lower your arms to the starting position.
- Repeat on the opposite side.
Reps – repeat 10 times.

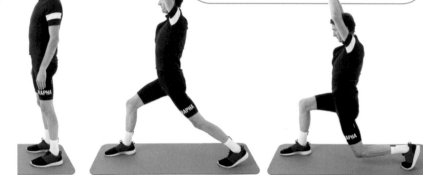

MATT SAYS:

'As you take the lunge step forwards, make sure the front knee comes no further forwards than the ankle to avoid putting too much stress through the knee.'

4.2 THE FOUNDATION LUNGE

This will help stretch and lengthen the hip flexors. It will also help decompress the spine as well as aiding shoulder mobility.

- Take a lunge step forwards, keeping the knee from travelling further forwards than the ankle.
- Square the body up so your hips are pointing forwards (as they will be slightly twisted from stepping forwards).
- Reach both arms over your head straight upwards.
- Raise up on tiptoes on your back foot as you squeeze that buttock and reach your hands even further upwards, and hold for 2 seconds before lowering the foot to the starting position.
Reps – repeat 10 times.

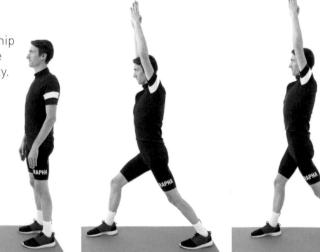

MATT SAYS:

'You should step forwards enough that about 30per cent of your energy is being used to maintain balance, and make sure both feet are pointing forwards to engage the correct muscles.'

4.3 THE HAND WALK

This will dynamically loosen the calf and hamstring muscles as well as deeply activating the core muscles. It will also improve ankle range of motion (dorsiflexion), and also helps to engage the upper body muscles that are important for bike stability.

- From standing, slowly fold forwards not allowing your legs to bend and keeping lumbar spine straight until your hands softly meet the floor in front of you.
- Walk your hands outwards as far as they can go while keeping your legs and spine straight and your feet in the same position.
- Take small steps walking your feet forwards to meet your hands.
  Reps – repeat 5 times.

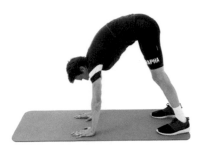 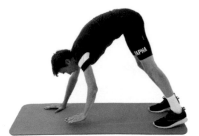 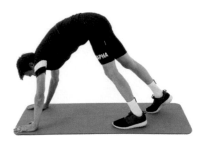

4.4 THE SQUAT

Every cyclist knows (or should know) about the squat. This simple whole body exercise engages and can strengthen many of the muscles used for cycling.

- With feet slightly wider than shoulder width, keep your lumbar spine straight, and your weight shifted back on to the heels.
- Push the bum backwards and reach hands forwards as you slowly lower your body into a squat position (no need to lower the legs past horizontal).
- As you squat, don't let your knees come further forwards than your toes to avoid stressing the knee too much. Keeping the weight back on your heels will help this.
- Take 3 seconds to lower yourself into the squat and 1 second to stand back up.
- Squeeze your buttocks as you stand up from the squat.
  Reps – repeat 10 times.

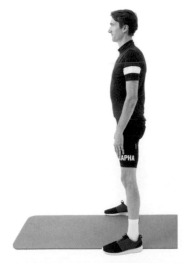 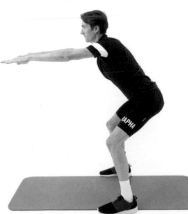 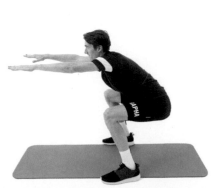

5 Lower back and hips

5.1 LUMBAR SPINE MOVEMENT
Loosens tension in the lower back.

- Lie on your back, knees bent, feet flat on the floor, hands by your sides.
- Gently let your knees rock from side to side. **Reps – 1 minute.**

MATT SAYS:

'This can be done with arms outstretched to the side too, opening up the chest wall. If your whole lower back is coming off the floor as you rock from side to side, you're going too far.'

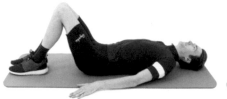 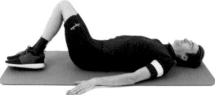 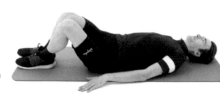

5.2 THE CAT AND CAMEL
An effective exercise for loosening the spine and reducing tension in the lower back.

- Go on all fours, making sure the knees are directly under the hips and hands are directly under the shoulders. Hands and legs shoulder-width apart.
- As you inhale, raise your chest to the ceiling, arching your back. Let your head drop and rock your pelvis backwards while keeping your arms and legs still.
- As you exhale, lower your abdomen towards the floor, let your head slightly tilt backwards, and rock your pelvis forwards, while keeping your arms and legs still. **Reps – one minute.**

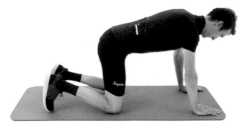
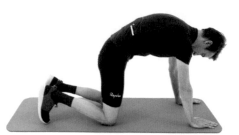
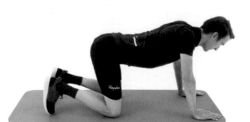

MATT SAYS:

'A common mistake is for the movement to come from the hips or shoulders, not the spine. The arms and legs should remain still. Practising in front of a mirror initially can help you to maintain good form.'

5.3 THE CHILD'S POSE

A similar exercise to the cat and camel, but by changing the action slightly, it will gently stretch the lower back muscles and joints, reducing tension as well as loosening the hip, knee and ankle joints by taking the joints through their range of motion.

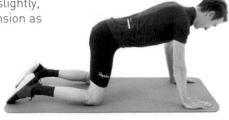

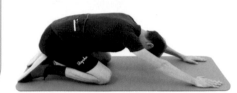

- Start on all fours, knees hip-width apart and hands shoulder-width apart. Keep your back straight and head pointed out.
- Tilt your pelvis backwards, lowering your body and shift back on to your haunches as your reach your hands forwards out in front of you.
Reps – 30 seconds.

> **MATT SAYS:**
>
> *'If you have knee issues, this can be painful, so only go as low as you are able, don't try and force it.'*

5.4 THE KNEES TO CHEST HUG

This will gently stretch the lumbar and gluteal muscles helping to relax the lower back.

- Start laying on the floor with your back flat.
- Draw your knees up to your chest as high as you can and hold them there.
- Hold from behind the knees rather than pulling on the knees themselves to avoid stressing the knee joints straight after cycling.
Reps – 30 second hold.

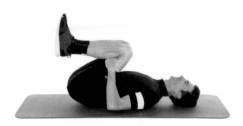

5.5 THE SPHINX

An antidote to extended time spent on the bike in the flexed position. Stretching the hip flexors will help reduce tension in these muscles, which often get overworked, becoming shortened and tight from cycling. Lengthening the neck and gently tucking in the chin engages the deep neck flexors, working on the muscles considered the 'core' ones that stabilise the neck.

- Begin flat on your stomach.
- Prop yourself up on to your elbows keeping your chin gently tucked in.
- From this position gently push your tummy into the floor as you gently put pressure through your elbows arching your back slightly backwards further into extension.
- Hold this position for 10 seconds.
Reps – repeat 3 times.

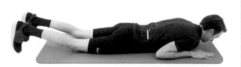

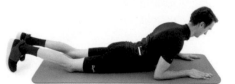

> **MATT SAYS:**
>
> *'You should gently feel this stretching your hip flexors and maybe some mild tightness in the lower back. It's important not to extend too far as you can cause irritation to the lower back. Getting the balance between gently stretching the hip flexors and not aggravating the back is key. Less is more to begin with.'*

5.6 THE CLAM SHELL

Designed to engage, activate and gently strengthen the gluteus medius muscle, one of the stabilisers of the hip and pelvis.

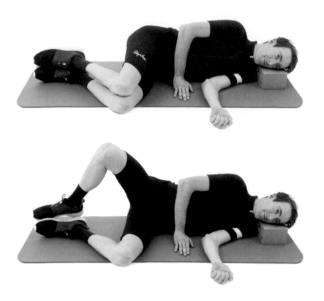

- Lie on your left side with your hips slightly flexed, your knees bent and your legs on top of one another.
- Keeping the heels together, over the count of 2 seconds, slowly raise your right knee up as high as you can, making sure your pelvis stays still. (The only motion comes from the hip joint not the lower back).
- Lower the knee to the starting position over the count of 2 seconds and repeat 10 times.
**Reps – build up to 3 times
(and don't forget to do the other leg too).**

MATT SAYS:

'It's a good idea to maintain muscle balance, so do the exercise on both sides even if you're only injured on one side. You'll often find it more difficult to perform the exercise on the injured side. Form is really important with this exercise. As you lift your knee, your pelvis should always remain solid; when it starts to move, you've lost isolation of the muscle you're trying to target.'

5.7 THE SITTING GLUTEAL STRETCH

During cycling the gluteal muscles often become overworked and tight. This stretch will help relieve tightness and tension in these muscles as well as relieve lower back rotary stiffness.

MATT SAYS:

'The depth of the stretch can be increased by adding slightly more rotation to the spine.'

- Bring the knee towards the chest and cross the foot to the other side of the outstretched leg.
- Draw the knee closer to the chest with the opposite hand at the same time as you rotate the body towards the leg being stretched, ensuring the back stays upright.
- Use the other hand to stabilise yourself or to pull the leg in closer for a deeper stretch.
- Hold this position for 20 seconds.
- Repeat on the other leg.
Reps – repeat twice.

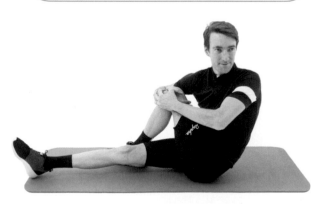

5.8 THE MOVING KNEE HUG

Dynamically stretches and prepares the gluteal muscles for cycling.

- Maintaining a straight back, lean forwards, grab your leg just below the knee and lift it upwards towards your chest.
- As you lift one knee, contract the glute of the other leg and stand tall up on to your tiptoes.
- Hold for 1–2 seconds.
- Lower the leg and repeat on the other side.
  Reps – repeat 10 times.

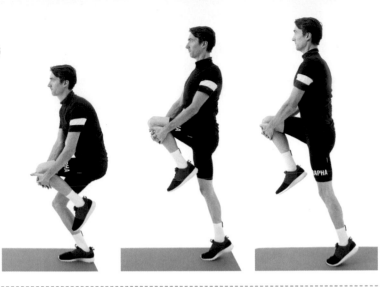

5.9 THE MOVING LEG CRADLE

Dynamically stretches muscles you'll need for stability while cycling – specifically your gluteus medius and piriformis.

- Exactly the same routine as Ex 5.8 except this time you cradle the leg (as shown in the picture).
- Maintaining a straight back, lean forwards and lift one leg up so it's cradled.
- While cradling the leg, stand up tall while gently pulling the cradled leg upwards.
- Hold for 1–2 seconds.
- Release the leg and repeat with the other leg.
  Reps – repeat 10 times.

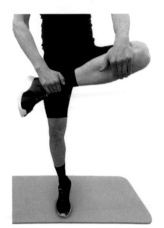

> **MATT SAYS:**
>
> *'As you stand tall, go up on to the tiptoes of the standing leg to get a deeper stretch and engage the calf muscles at the same time.'*

5.10 THE BRIDGE

Engages and gently strengthens the large gluteal muscles (and hamstrings), and will also loosen and lengthen the psoas muscle, a key muscle used in cycling. Encouraging strength in the glutes helps work on some of the major stabilisers of the lower back and pelvis when riding.

> **MATT SAYS:**
>
> *'A common mistake is not lifting up high enough, so practise in front of a mirror.'*

- Lie flat on the floor, with your knees raised and hands by your side.
- Engage your glutes and lift your bum off the floor until your abdomen and thighs are in a straight line.
- Hold for a count of 2 seconds and then lower down, returning to a starting position.
  Reps – repeat 10 times.

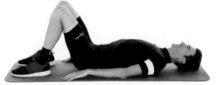
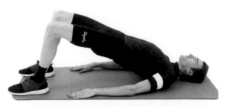

5.11 THE SINGLE LEG BRIDGE

This advanced exercise will engage the large gluteal muscles (and hamstrings) more deeply than the bridge, enhancing strength in these muscles and the lumbar rotator muscles as you attempt to hold the pelvis stable. Doing the exercise on one leg at a time more realistically functionally mimics how the muscles are used while cycling.

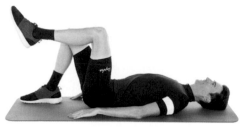

- Lie flat on the floor, with your knees raised and hands by your side.
- Lift the left foot off the floor.
- Engage the right gluteus muscle and lift your bum off the floor until your abdomen and thigh are in a straight line.
- Make sure you keep the hips level as you lift up the pelvis.
- Hold for a count of 2 seconds and then lower down, returning to a starting position and then repeat.
Reps – repeat 10 times, holding for 2 seconds (then repeat on the other side).

MATT SAYS:

'Make sure you lift high enough and don't let the opposite hip drop. You should feel a deep activation of the glutes, lower back and hamstrings (on the active side).'

5.12 THE MARCHING BRIDGE

Will build strength into the lower abdomen, lower back and gluteal muscles, as well as engaging the lumbar rotator muscles that help with rotary stability on the bike. Not an easy exercise to do well. You should feel deep activation within your glutes, hamstrings, lower back and abdominal muscles.

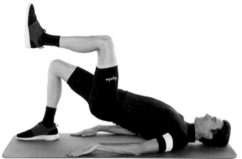

- Lie flat on the floor, with knees raised and hands by your side.
- Engage your glutes and lift your bum off the floor until abdomen and thighs are in a straight line in the bridge position.
- Maintaining this starting position, slowly raise the right foot off the ground bringing the knee up to 90 degrees while maintaining level hips.
- Slowly lower the right leg to return to the bridge position.
- From this position, shift the weight to the other side and repeat the movement with the left leg. One repetition.
Reps – 10 repeated twice.

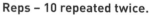

5.13 THE FOUNDER

Engages the muscles of the posterior chain – calf muscles, hamstrings, glutes, lower back and shoulder blade stabilisers. By working them in a chain, the muscles will be working in groups as they do when you ride. This exercise will also stretch and lengthen the muscles as they're engaged allowing both better stability and increased comfort both on and off the bike.

- Standing with legs slightly wider than shoulder and knees unlocked (but not bent), rock back so the weight is on your heels.
- Keeping your chest high and lumbar spine straight, gently pull the buttocks backwards (hinging at the hip).
- Take your hands down by your sides, opening the chest wall, and direct them down and backwards behind your hips while engaging the muscles between your shoulder blades. Hold for 10 seconds.
- Gently push your bum further backwards, feeling the tension in your hamstrings, glutes and lower back while slowly bringing your hands forwards above your head.
- Gently press your hands together as you stretch your hands upwards and forwards away from your body while trying to move your bum further back – pushing your hands and bum as far apart from each other as you can. Hold for 10 seconds.
- Maintain your body position and move your hands back down behind you and repeat.
Reps – repeat 3 times.

MATT SAYS:

'Point the toes straight forwards parallel to each other rather than slightly outwards and you'll better engage the glute medius muscle. Make sure the hinge happens at the hip and you don't fold at the lower back. Keeping the chest high and chin tucked in will help this. This is a great antidote to long periods spent sitting.'

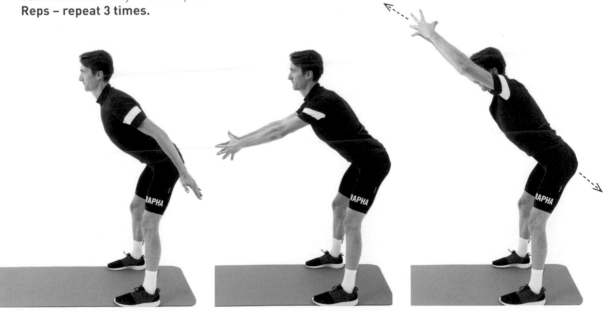

5.14 THE FOUNDATION WOODPECKER

This will deeply stretch the gluteal muscles, relieving tension. This exercise will also help stretch and lengthen the muscles of the posterior chain, which can tighten through cycling.

- Take a lunge step forwards, keeping the knee from travelling further forwards than the ankle. (The back heel may come off the floor).
- Square the body up so your hips are pointing forwards (as they will be slightly twisted from stepping forwards). (a)
- Maintaining a completely still lower body, lean forwards, hinging at the hips.
- Reach your hands forwards, as you gently push your hips backwards and the heel of the forward foot gently pushes into the floor. (b)
- Hold this for 10 seconds before bringing your body back upright to the starting position. **Reps – repeat 3 times.**

MATT SAYS:

'Make the exercise harder by gently drawing the feet together on the floor once you've taken the step forwards (without actually moving your feet) before you hinge the hip to additionally engage the adductor muscles when you do the exercise.'

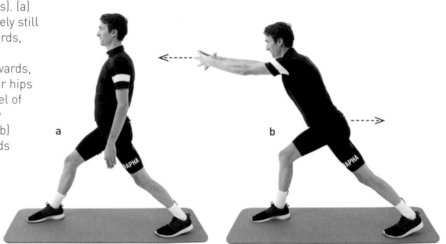

a   b

5.15 THE FOUNDATION WOODPECKER WITH ROTATION

Strongly engages the deepest fibres of the large gluteus muscles and gets them working while in a lengthened position mimicking how they're used when cycling. At the same time, the hamstrings and other posterior chain muscles are engaged, while the stabilisers of the hip and lower back and the rotator muscles of the lumbar spine are all engaged helping to build strength for these muscles, which that are other key for cycling.

- Start from position b of exercise 5.14.
- Slowly rotate your upper body 45 degrees to the right while keeping a still lower body and your arms stretched out in front of you – taking about 3 seconds to get there.
- Engage your right glute muscle as you rotate your body back towards the midline, before repeating the rotation to the left. **Reps – 10, then repeat the exercise with the left leg forwards.**

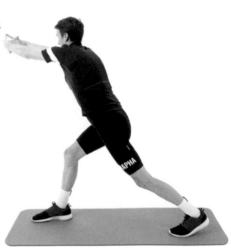

5.16 THE BIRD DOG

This is recommended for general back tightness and will encourage balance, proprioception (spatial awareness) and coordination before you ride. It will also start to engage the gluteal and hamstrings muscles and work the core muscles more deeply as well as helping improve shoulder mobility

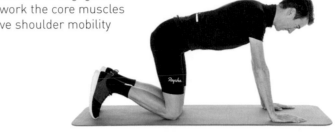

- Start in an all-fours position similar to the cat and camel.
- Maintaining a straight spine, reach forwards with one arm as far as you can while at the same time extending the opposite leg backwards as far as you can.
- Each extension should take 3 seconds to get into position and be held for 2–3 seconds.
- Return to starting position and repeat with opposite arm and leg.
  Reps – repeat 10 times.

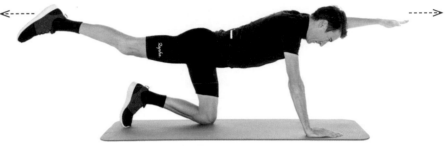

MATT SAYS:

'It's a difficult exercise to master and doing it in front of a mirror to begin with can help encourage stability throughout the exercise.'

5.17 THE HARD BIRD DOG

Building on the bird dog this exercise is slightly harder and places more demands on balance. It helps to improve both strength and stability that will help you on the bike.

- The same exercise as the bird dog but rather than returning to all-fours position between each extension, draw the elbow of the extended arm in to touch the opposite knee that was extended before repeating the extension on the same side.
- Repeat 10 times, with the left arm and right leg before returning to all-fours position and repeating on the other side. One repetition.
  Reps – repeat twice. Progress by holding the extension for 10 seconds.

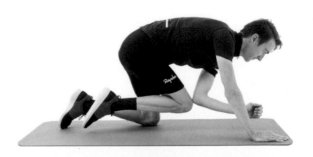

5.18 THE FOUNDATION BACK EXTENSIONS

Strengthens the back extensor muscles that are continuously used to maintain cycling position, supporting you for lengthy spells on the bike.

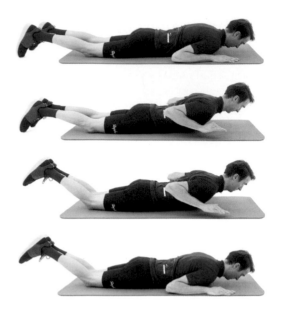

- Start flat on your stomach arms reached out in front of you keeping your chin gently tucked in so you're looking at the floor a couple of inches in front of you (not extending your neck).
- Pull your elbows and forearms back into your side raising them off the ground, engaging your shoulder blades and keeping these muscles contracted hard throughout the exercise.
- Hold this extended position for 30 seconds. **Reps – 2–3 times.**

MATT SAYS:

'A common mistake is extending the neck as you do the exercise to try and increase back extension. Keep the neck straight and in a neutral position, avoiding extension so you're less likely to strain it. This exercise can be progressed; at the same time as extending your back off the floor, press your knees and feet firmly together and bend the knee until your feet are just off the ground. Continue to press your knees and feet together firmly throughout the duration of the exercise.'

5.19 THE GLUTES AND PIRIFORMIS FOAM ROLL

These muscles do a lot of work when cycling, so it's important they are functioning optimally. This foam roll will improve comfort when riding and can be used for recovery too to relieve tension.

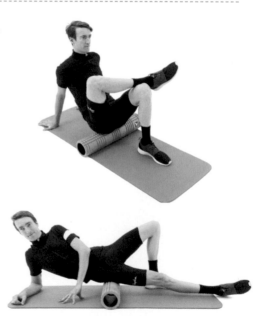

- Place one leg over the other and 'sit' on the roller, supporting your weight with your arms (it's the glute of the crossed leg that will be worked on).
- Roll your buttock forwards and backwards on the roller scanning for any areas of tenderness.
- When you have a tender spot, stop on top of it for ten seconds or until pain has reduced by about 75 per cent.
- Roll backwards and forwards a few centimetres over the tender spot to work and break up the focal tight muscle.
- Change positions on the roller (see second picture) to get the outside of the muscle ensuring the whole glute is scanned and rolled where necessary. **Reps – do for 5 minutes.**

5.20 THE TENSOR FASCIA LATAE FOAM ROLL

These muscles can become extremely tight when out riding, as they're constantly used during the pedalling action. This is often a sore, tender area, but when rolled out, will provide immediate relief.

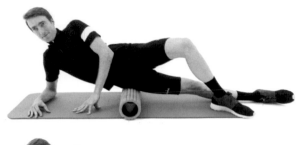

- In a side plank position, place the roller to the outside and just below your 'hip bone'.
- Roll slightly up and down – approx 10–15 cm – and locate a tender spot.
- When you have a tender spot, stop on top of it for 10 seconds or until the pain has reduced by about 75 per cent.
- Roll over the tender spot a few centimetres in each direction to work through the tight muscle.
- Change positions on the roller rolling forwards (see second picture) to make sure the whole TFL is scanned and rolled where it's needed.
Reps – do for 5 minutes.

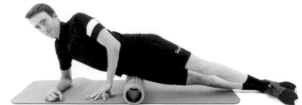

5.21 KINESIO TAPE FOR THE LOWER BACK

This can help gently alleviate mild back discomfort both on the bike and off the bike. You'll need to get someone else to help apply this tape for you.

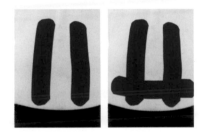

- Cut three pieces of tape – two at 20–25 cm and one at 15–20 cm.
- Bend forwards at the waist and run two strips from the very top of the gluteal muscles up the back either side of the spine, no stretch on the tape.
- Apply the third strip horizontally over the painful level of the back, applying it like a Band-Aid with near full stretch on the tape in the middle (5 cm or so) and no stretch on the anchored ends.

5.22 THE LOWER BACK RELIEF POSITION

This position takes the most amount of stress out of the discs of the lumbar spine, allowing the postural muscles of the lower back to relax helping to relieve tension and discomfort.

- Lie on your back with your hips and knees at 90 degrees with your legs resting up on a chair or sofa.
- Keep your arms by your side with your palms facing upwards.
- Focus on your breathing when in this position, it's not as important to brace as you lie there relaxing.
Reps – do for 15 minutes.

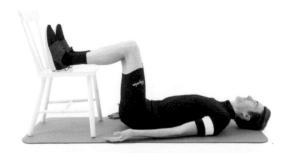

6 Legs

6.1
THE QUAD STRETCH

A common stretch you should be familiar with but with a slight twist. Quads commonly get tight through cycling so this stretch will help loosen them preparing them for riding.

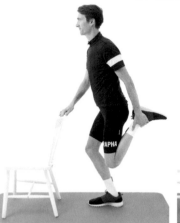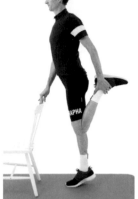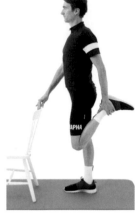

- Maintaining a straight back, lean forwards grab just above the ankle and move the leg behind you as you reach the opposite arm above your head.
- As you stand tall, go up on to your tiptoes

of the standing leg to get a deeper stretch and help activate the calf muscles at the same time.
- Hold for 1–2 seconds.
- Lower the leg and repeat on the other side.
Reps – repeat 10 times.

6.2 THE SIDE SHIFT SQUAT

Will help loosen the hip joint and gently stretch the muscles on the inside of the legs (adductors). Will also help engage some of the pelvic stabiliser muscles such as the glute medius in particular.

- Adopt a wide stance, keep your lumbar spine straight, stick your bum out backwards and hands forwards to counterbalance and keep the weight of your body more on the heels.
- Lower your body on one side.
- Hold this squatted position for 1–2 seconds,

stay low and shift the weight to the opposite leg over a three second period. One repetition.
- Don't let the knee come further forward than the ankle on the squatting side to prevent stressing the knee too much.
Reps – repeat 10 times.

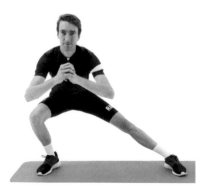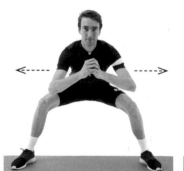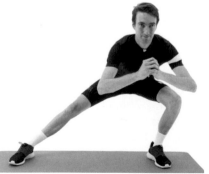

6.3 PATELLA TRACKING SIT TO STAND

Can help support and improve patella tracking function at the same time as working on the glutes and quad muscles – key muscles used in cycling.

- Perch towards the edge of a chair with your feet on the floor. (The higher the chair the easier to begin with).
- Transfer the weight to the leg of the injured knee.
- Keeping your lower back straight and gently hinging forwards from the hips, keep your arms out in front of you, and on one leg move from sitting to standing position, engaging your gluteal muscles as you do so.
- Once you are standing up, slowly sit back down again trying not to collapse as you do so. One repetition.
  Reps – 10 do 2 sets.

Bringing the feet closer to the chair makes the exercise easier to perform and gets a deeper activation of the muscles but adds more stress to the knee so find a starting position that is both challenging yet comfortable for the knee.

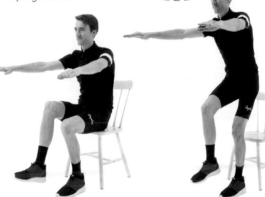

MATT SAYS:

'This simple move from sitting to standing and back down again forces you to use all the supporting muscles around your knee and begins to facilitate proper tracking of the patella, reintroducing this movement in a controlled manner while activating your core.'

6.4 CALF STRETCHES

Helps reduce the pull and tension on the Achilles tendon by stretching these muscles. It's important both the major calf muscles are stretched as they can equally become tightened and shortened and affect Achilles function. One will often feel tighter than the other.

1. Gastrocnemius (superficial muscle)

The classic age-old 'pushing the wall over' stretch.

- Lean forwards against a wall with the injured leg back and straightened and the front leg bent.
- Keep your rear heel on the floor and the foot slightly turned out.
- Lean further into the wall as you feel a stretch in the calf muscle of the rear leg.
- Once you feel the stretch, hold this position for 20 seconds.
  Reps – repeat 3 times.

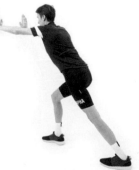

2. Soleus (deep muscle)

This stretch gets the deeper of the two calf muscles.

- Lean forwards against a wall with the injured leg back and both knees bent.
- Keep your rear heel on the floor and the foot slightly turned out.
- Lean further into the wall and slightly increase the flex in the rear knee until you can feel a stretch in the lower calf muscle of the back leg.
- Once you feel the stretch, hold this position for 20 seconds.
  Reps – repeat 3 times.

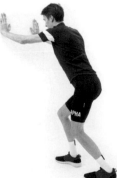

6.5 ACHILLES ISOMETRICS

This exercise can reduce symptoms in the reactive phase of Achilles tendon problems in addition to starting to build strength in the calf muscles. Using your own body weight reduces the risk of overloading the Achilles, although this exercise may initially feel uncomfortable when you do it. The superficial contraction aims to engage the gastrocnemius muscle, and the deep calf exercise aims to engage the soleus calf muscle. To begin with, do this exercise on both legs to help share the load. As you progress and your calf strength improves, move on to doing the exercise on just the injured leg.

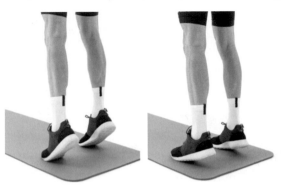 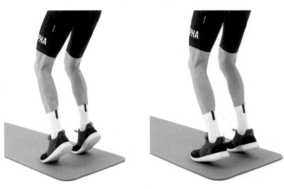

1. Superficial muscle
- Raise up on to your tiptoes as high as you can with straight legs, and then come half the way back down and hold this position for 40 seconds.
- **Reps – repeat 3 times.**

2. Deep muscle
- Raise up on to your tiptoes as high as you can with the knees slightly bent, and then come half the way back down and hold this position for 40 seconds.
- **Reps – repeat 3 times.**

6.6 CALF STRENGTHENING

Start at stage one and progress through, moving from one stage to the next once you can complete that given stage while maintaining proper form. Don't worry if there's *mild* discomfort as you do them, try and push through that.

These exercises should be performed five days a week to build calf strength and can be repeated up to twice a day. If you find you have too much discomfort, have an extra day off between exercises. You can always go back to doing the isometric exercises on this day as it can help reduce the symptoms in the Achilles.

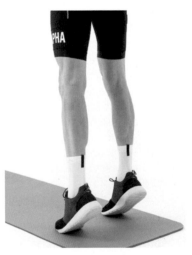

STAGE ONE – two legged heel raises
SUPERFICIAL MUSCLE
- Begin standing.
- Keep your knees extended throughout the exercise.
- Raise up on to your heels on both feet as high as you can over 1 second.
- Lower your heels to the ground over one second. One repetition.
- **Reps – repeat 15 times. Do 2 sets.**

DEEP MUSCLE

- Begin seated with knees bent at 90 degrees and feet on the floor.
- Raise both heels as high as you can over 1 second.
- Lower the heels to the ground over 1 second. 1 repetition.
  Reps – repeat 15 times. Do 2 sets.

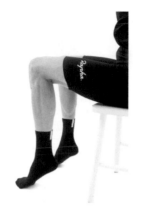

STAGE TWO – two legged stair heel raises

SUPERFICIAL MUSCLE

- Begin standing with your heels hanging over the edge of a stair.
- Raise up on to your heels on both feet as high as you can over 1 second.
- Keep your knees extended throughout the exercise.
- Lower your heels as far as you can past the horizontal over 1 second. 1 repetition.
  Reps – repeat 15 times. Do 3 sets.

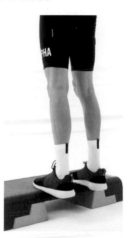
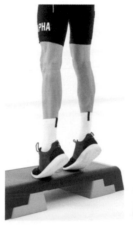
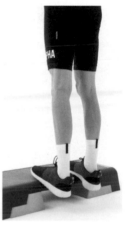

DEEP MUSCLE

- Begin standing with your heels hanging over the edge of a stair with the knees slightly bent.
- Raise up on to your heels on both feet as high as you can over 1 second.
- Keep your knees bent throughout the exercise.
- Lower your heels as far as you can past the horizontal over 1 second. 1 repetition.
  Reps – repeat 15 times. Do 3 sets.

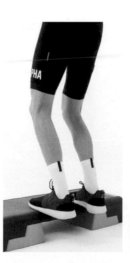
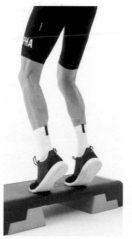
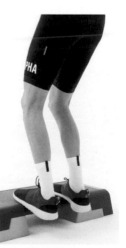

STAGE THREE – single leg heel raises

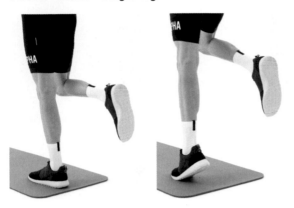
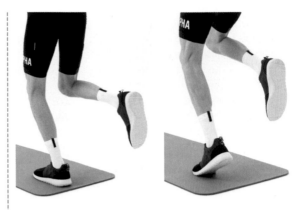

SUPERFICIAL MUSCLE
- Begin standing on the injured leg.
- Keep your knee extended throughout the exercise.
- Raise up on to your heel as high as you can over 1 second.
- Lower your heel to the ground over 1 second. This is 1 repetition.
  Reps – repeat 15 times. Do 2 sets.

DEEP MUSCLE
- Begin standing on the injured leg with the knee slightly bent.
- Keep your knee bent throughout the exercise.
- Raise up onto your heel as high as you can over one second.
- Lower your heel to the ground over one second. One repetition.
  Reps – repeat 15 times. Two sets.

STAGE FOUR – single leg stair heel raises

Get to here and you are hopefully on your way to having a good enough strength in your calves to support your Achilles back on the bike.

SUPERFICIAL MUSCLE
- Begin standing on the injured leg with the heel over the edge of a stair.
- Keep your knee extended throughout the exercise.
- Raise up on to your heel as high as you can over 1 second.
- Lower your heel as low as you can past the horizontal over 1 second. This is 1 repetition.
  Reps – repeat 15 times. Do 2 sets.

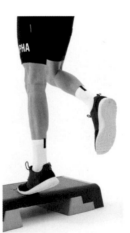
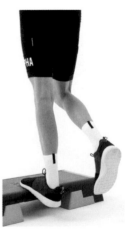

Once 2 sets becomes comfortable, increase to 3 sets.

DEEP MUSCLE

- Begin standing on the injured leg with the knee slightly bent and the heel over the edge of a stair.
- Keep your knee bent throughout the exercise.
- Raise up on to your heel as high as you can over one second.
- Lower your heel as low as you can past the horizontal over 1 second. This is 1 repetition. **Reps – repeat 15 times. Do 2 sets.**

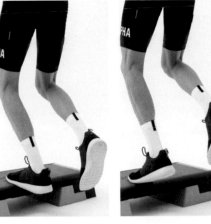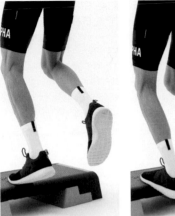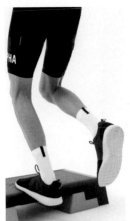

Once 2 sets becomes comfortable, increase to 3 sets.

STAGE FIVE – single leg stair heel raises with weight

Stage five is exactly the same as stage four but now you can add some weight to the exercise to increase the load. Either holding weights of 5 kg in each hand or you can place 10 kg of weights in a backpack and build up from there.

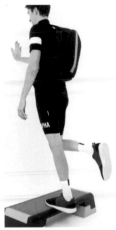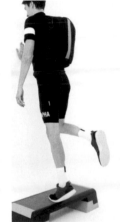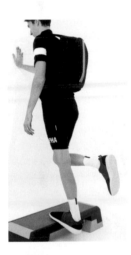

Superficial heel single leg stair heel raises with weight

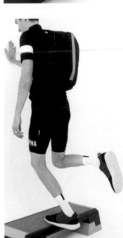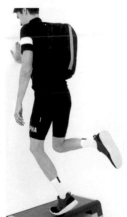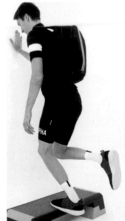

Deep heel single leg stair heel raises with weight

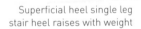

Strength maintenance

Continue these exercises for a sixth to eighth week period. Once you're at phase four or five and have been there for a couple of weeks, you can cut back doing the exercises to three times per week as you will have improved calf strength sufficiently to better support your Achilles tendon and it now only needs to be maintained. Continue the exercises for the next three months to help maintain calf muscle strength as you get back into your cycling.

6.7 THE CALF MUSCLES FOAM ROLL (GASTROCNEMIUS AND SOLEUS)

Rolling the calf muscles will support normal foot and knee function while cycling, helping the fluidity the of the pedal stroke which makes the foot feel lighter while riding.

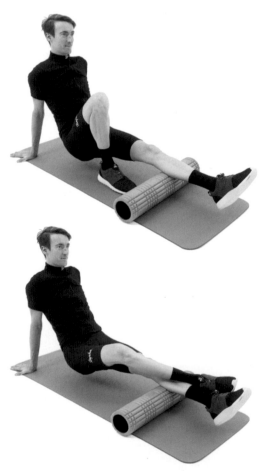

- Place one or both legs on the roller on the muscle above the Achilles tendon.
- Slowly roll up the calf muscles, scanning until you feel a tender spot.
- When you have a tender spot, stop on top of it for 10 seconds or until pain has reduced by about 75 per cent.
- With the pressure still on the tender spot, roll the foot around in circles for 15 seconds.
- Continue scanning the calf for tender spots and repeat procedure.
- For deeper penetration into the calf muscles, repeat the same procedure with one leg resting on top of the other (see picture to the right).
- Scan from bottom to top and then the reverse direction, changing the angle of the leg to target different parts of the muscle – for example, rolling the calf in slightly targets the gastrocnemius muscle and, in the midline, it will be more the soleus.

Reps – continue until less tenderness on initial scan or up to 5 minutes.

6.8 THE SHIN FOAM ROLL (TIBIALIS ANTERIOR)

This muscle is responsible for pulling the toes up during the recovery phase of the pedal stroke so gets continuous repetitive usage, making it an often overlooked muscle even during regular massage. Rolling this muscle will support normal foot function while cycling, helping the fluidity of the pedal stroke.

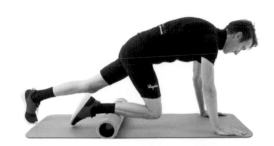

- Place one or both legs on the roller just above the ankle on the muscle at the front of the shin.
- Slowly roll up the muscle scanning until you feel a tender spot.
- When you have a tender spot, stop on top of it for 10 seconds or until the pain has reduced by about 75 per cent.
- With the pressure still on the tender spot, roll the foot around in circles for 15 seconds.
- Continue scanning the calf for tender spots and repeat procedure.
- Work your way from bottom to top and then the reverse.
  Reps – continue until less tenderness on initial scan or up to 5 minutes.

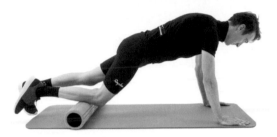

6.9 THE QUADS FOAM ROLL (VASTUS MEDIALIS AND LATERALIS)

The quadriceps group of thigh muscles get extremely overworked when cycling, so rolling them out can provide great relief. Be sure to roll up the inside and outside of the thigh as it's a large muscle – you'll need to change the angle of your body to do so.

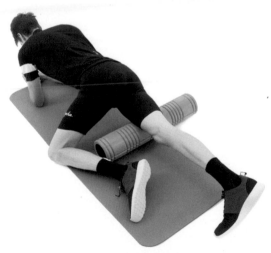

- Place a leg on the roller just above the kneecap while you adopt a 'plank' like position.
- Slowly roll up the muscle, scanning until you find a tender spot.
- When you have a tender spot, stop on top of it for 10 seconds or until pain has reduced by about 75 per cent.
- With the pressure still on the tender spot, rotate the leg over it, and bend and straighten the knee to break up the tension in the muscle.
- Continue to roll up the quad, scanning for tender spots and repeat the procedure.
- Work your way from bottom to the top of the muscle and then back down.
  Reps – do for 5 minutes.

6.10 KINESIO TAPE FOR THE KNEE

Easy to apply yourself, kinesio tape can help relieve general knee discomfort while cycling and is useful if you're coming back from injury. It can be used in the early stages of knee discomfort too to help offload the nee and provide support.

- Place the knee at a 90-degree angle and measure and cut the first piece of tape in length from the mid-thigh to just below the kneecap.
- Anchor the tape at the mid-thigh, preferably underneath the bib shorts.
- Stick the tape down with no extra stretch until just above the kneecap where the remainder of the tape should be cut in two down the centre.
- Run the split sides either side of the knee to join at the top of the shin bone in the centre. You can slightly stretch these pieces to reach.

- Cut a second piece of tape approximately 20cm in length.
- Tear the piece in the middle and expose the sticking surface like a Band-Aid and pull it tight.
- Stick the second piece over the lower half of the kneecap so that half of the top part of the tape covers the lower half of the kneecap.
- Peel off the sides of the rest of the tape and run them up either side of the thigh in a U-bend fashion.

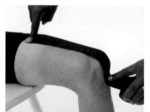 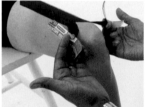 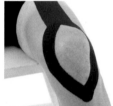 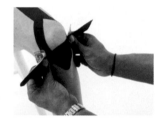

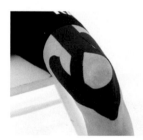

MATT SAYS:

'When you stand up, the skin in the middle of the kneecap will probably be all loose, wrinkled and baggy-looking. Don't be surprised, this means the tape has been put on correctly.'

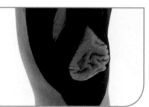

6.11 KINESIO TAPE FOR THE ACHILLES TENDON

Easy to apply yourself this helps support the Achilles tendon, reducing discomfort in this area when you ride.

- Flex the foot to gently stretch the Achilles tendon.
- Apply a small – 10 cm – piece of tape horizontally over the painful area of the Achilles like a Band-Aid, applying full stretch on the tape in the centre and none on either end.
- Apply a second piece of tape anchored from the sole of the foot up the back of the Achilles tendon to just above the tendon.
- Split the tape down the midline and with a slight stretch apply either ends of the rest of the tape up either side of the calf muscle.

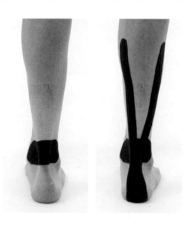

The pain-free cyclist warm-up

For a thorough warm-up before you ride, to get the body warm and loose and ready to get out on your bike, run through the following exercises we've handpicked from the rehab toolkit to get the job done. We've listed the exercises in the order we recommend, but don't worry, they can be performed in any order. There's really no excuse to skip it now! In these instances, one repetition of each exercise will suffice, though there's nothing stopping you doing more.

When returning from injury, it's important to keep an eye on your body and how it is feeling. If any of these exercises cause symptoms, skip them and move on to the next one.

EXERCISE	EX. NO.	PAGE
1. Lumbar spine movement	5.1	182
2. The bridge	5.10	185
3. The cat and camel	5.2	182
4. Upper back mobility	1.2	164
5. The child's pose	5.3	183
6. The bird dog	5.16	189
7. The plank	3.3	175
8. The stand tall and reach stretch	3.1	175
9. The founder	5.13	187
10. The hand walk	4.3	181
11. The moving leg cradle	5.9	185
12. The moving knee hugs	5.8	185
13. The quad stretch	6.1	192
14. The low lunge	4.1	180
15. The side shift squat	6.2	192
16. The squat	4.4	181

One cycle – 12 minutes

The pain-free cyclist streamlined warm-up

Just want to get out on the bike right? Sometimes it's just not practical to do a thorough warm-up before you ride. Many cyclists will rush a warm-up, or ignore it altogether, so we've designed a streamlined warm-up, that'll take no longer than five minutes to complete but will get your body ready to ride.

EXERCISE	EX. NO.	PAGE
1. The plank	3.3	175
2. The bridge	5.10	186
3. The stand tall and reach stretch	3.1	174
4. The founder	5.13	187
5. The squat	4.4	181

Once cycle – 4-5 minutes

The pain-free cyclist warm-down

Start your recovery from cycling and regeneration of the muscles and joints by warming down the body appropriately and running through this handful of exercises when you get off the bike:

EXERCISE	EX. NO.	PAGE
1. The foundation lunge	4.1	180
2. The foundation woodpecker	5.14	188
3. The cat and camel	5.2	182
4. The founder	5.13	187
5. The sitting glute and lower back stretch	5.7	184
6. The sphinx	5.5	183
7. The knees to chest hug	5.4	183

One cycle – 5-6 minutes

The pain-free cyclist core exercises

 We've discussed the benefits of doing core exercises enough, now it's time to put words into action. Start your core work with these exercises we've selected from the rehab toolkit. Gradually build up the reps or time spent doing each exercise, always remembering to maintain good form while doing the exercises. By the time you get here you'll be familiar with many of these exercises, which will make the transition from injury to core-strengthening run more smoothly. If you don't have time to do them all in one go, cycle through the exercises picking up where you left off in your next session to make sure you get through the routine.

EXERCISE	EX. NO.	PAGE
1. Lumbar spine movement	5.1	182
2. Upper back mobility	1.2	164
3. The bridge	5.10	185
4. The cat and camel	5.2	182
5. The plank	3.3	176
6. The side plank	3.4	177
7. The bird dog	5.16	189
8. The stand and reach stretch	3.1	175
9. The founder	5.13	187
10. The woodpecker with rotation	5.15	188
11. The squat	4.4	181

One cycle - 10 minutes

The pain-free cyclist advanced core exercises

After 6–8 weeks or so of performing the core exercises, you should notice improvements in your robustness and mobility and feel 'stronger' but without necessarily being able to put your finger on *why*. Well, it's because your core strength has improved. Once you've mastered each of the initial core exercises, you should move on to the advanced exercises. Tag these on to your existing progamme unless otherwise recommended and you'll have a comprehensive set of core exercises to help further support your cycling.

These advanced exercises are harder to perform, so take your time and don't expect to be able to necessarily do them all at the first attempt. Remember, the key to improvement is gradual progression.

EXERCISE	EX. NO.	PAGE
1. The single leg bridge	5.11	186
2. The marching bridge	5.12	186
3. The plank to side plank (replaces the plank and the side plank)	3.5	176
4. The foundation eight point plank	3.6	177
5. The hard bird dog (replaces the bird dog)	5.17	189
6. Abdominal curl downs	3.7	177
7. The foundation back extensions	5.18	190
8. The press-up	3.2	175

One cycle - 12 minutes

MATT SAYS:

'Core exercises shouldn't be a chore, nor should they be an afterthought. They should be a significant part of your cycling training. And now you know how to do them, there's no excuse.'

Self-massage foam rolling routine

You've been working hard on the bike, seeing improvements and reaping the rewards of your training. Give your body an added recovery boost by spending 20–30 minutes at least once a month running through a full routine of foam rolling exercises. Your body will thank you for it, you'll feel refreshed and once you've done it, your cycling will be reinvigorated.

FOAM ROLL AREA	EX. NO.	PAGE
The shin	6.8	199
The calf muscles	6.7	198
The quads	6.9	199
The glutes and piriformis	5.19	190
The tensor fascia latae	5.20	191
Upper back tennis ball release	1.9	168
Pectoral muscle tennis ball release	3.8	179

One cycle

CYCLING NIRVANA

Emilia Fahlin   SWEDEN | 2013 SWEDISH NATIONAL CHAMPION

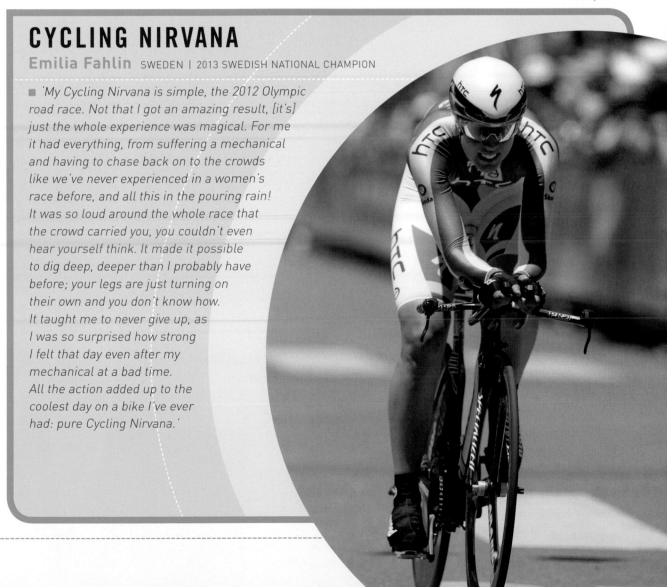

■ 'My Cycling Nirvana is simple, the 2012 Olympic road race. Not that I got an amazing result, [it's] just the whole experience was magical. For me it had everything, from suffering a mechanical and having to chase back on to the crowds like we've never experienced in a women's race before, and all this in the pouring rain! It was so loud around the whole race that the crowd carried you, you couldn't even hear yourself think. It made it possible to dig deep, deeper than I probably have before; your legs are just turning on their own and you don't know how. It taught me to never give up, as I was so surprised how strong I felt that day even after my mechanical at a bad time. All the action added up to the coolest day on a bike I've ever had: pure Cycling Nirvana.'

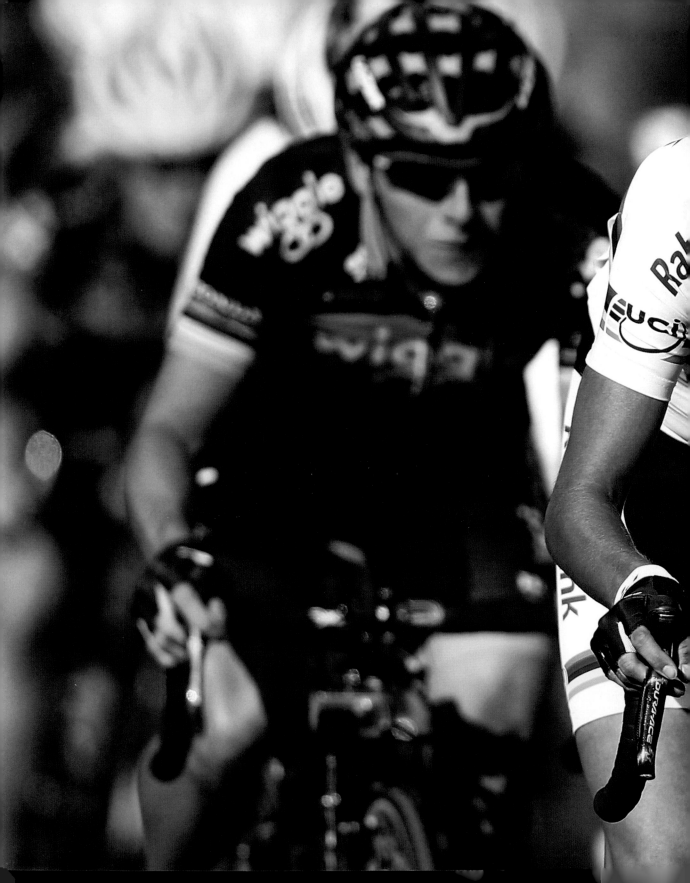

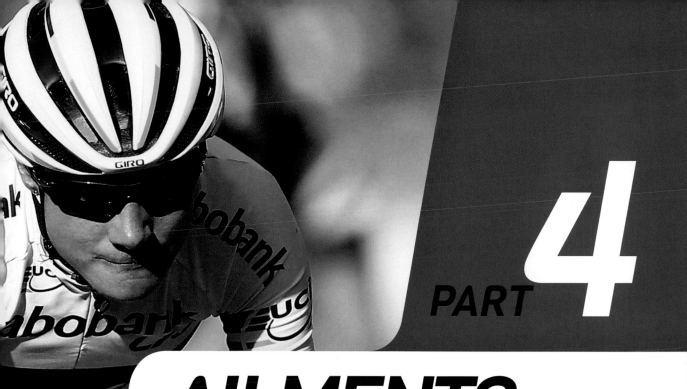

PART 4

AILMENTS

We've addressed the major injuries that you'll more commonly encounter while bike riding, now it's time to go through some of the minor, and perhaps less significant issues. We use the term 'minor' loosely, for there's nothing minor about saddle sores, as any cyclist will tell you.

A lot of the issues we'll discuss will already have been disregarded by many cyclists. To some, they aren't significant problems, and many presume they will sort themselves out. However, it is this flippant attitude that causes problems. These ailments need to be taken seriously.

It doesn't matter if it's a collarbone fracture or a bout of flu, you should have a basic understanding of what is happening in your body, the effects it can have on cycling and how to address it.

You know the 'heavy stuff' now; don't let these little pests be the ones that bring your cycling to a standstill.

19 OVERTRAINING

> ❝*I would rarely regret taking an extra day off. By pushing yourself extremely hard, you have very little to gain but lots to lose. It's a very fine balance, which is why you have to learn and be aware of the signals your body uses to tell you it's too much.*❞

Timmy Duggan RETIRED US PRO AND 2012 US NATIONAL CHAMPION

Many cyclists believe that the more training they do, the better they will get. It makes sense, but it doesn't tell the whole story. Overtraining has many labels, however, it was best described way back in 1988 by a group of elite coaches and sport scientists of the US Olympic Committee. They stated that overtraining is: 'a syndrome that results when excessive, usually physical, overload on an athlete occurs without adequate rest. The excessive overload placed on the performer results in decreased performance and the inability to train.'

■ *'When I was riding for the US U23 team, it was full gas all the time and I didn't have the volume in my legs to be able to train like that. It was too much too soon as I was only 19 years old. I started to notice I was having huge drop-offs in performance, for no real apparent reason, but I continued to push it as I was a rider trying to make it and it ended up being months before I could train properly. Eventually my blood values started to drop off and then they realised I was overtrained. I ended up taking a month off the bike then came back, started to train easily but it was still too much. The Tour de Lavenir came around in September 2007 but I still wasn't ready until* the next season. I eventually ended up taking six months off and it wasn't until the 2008 season that I was good to go again. The main thing for me is that you have to listen to what your body is telling you and you need to remain flexible and aware to not become overtrained.'

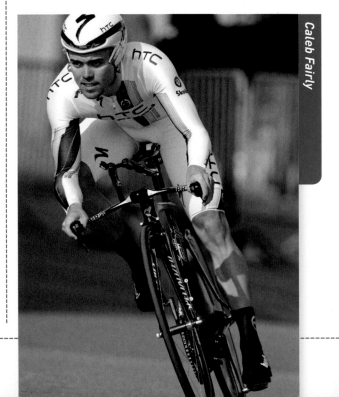

Caleb Fairly

Not just your performance

It's important to understand that overtraining doesn't just affect you on the bike; it affects your general health – you're not going to be feeling great and it can affect your sleep and how often you get sick. It's not just your performance that will suffer.

Trends show that overtraining syndrome is more commonly seen in endurance events such as cycling and people more susceptible to it are usually highly motivated, goal-orientated individuals who tend to be focused, conventional and conservative. Sound like you? Cycling requires hard, long efforts, over structured weeks in order to see improvements. It's far easier to overdo it on the bike than in some other sports. Cycling can be an extremely addictive sport, and as you strive to get fitter, ride faster and even lose more weight, the obsession can start to take over. But without rest, you will blow out.

We've talked about rest and recovery earlier in the book and it's these periods of rest where you become a better cyclist as your body adapts to the stresses of training. Overtraining syndrome isn't just caused by a lack of rest and recovery from training. Overtraining is determined by the *accumulation* of all the stresses placed on an individual and how they cope and when they don't cope, it results in a state of fatigue and significant drops in performance that don't improve after a few days of rest. Social and psychological factors play an important role too, for example, your work or home life can add to stress.

Knowing when to stop

The biggest problem amateur cyclists face, especially those who race, is to know when to back off training, or when they're pushing it too hard. Overtraining is difficult to identify yourself which is one of the reasons keen amateurs can

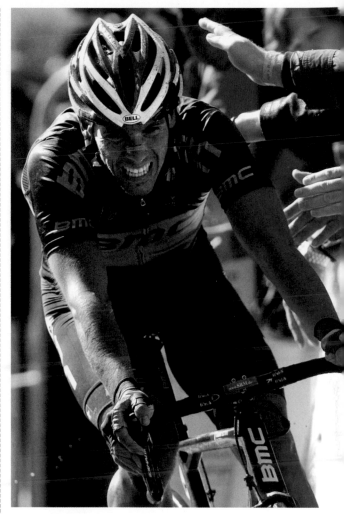

ABOVE Pushing too deep can set your performance back

benefit from having a coach. It really helps to have someone to sit down with you and review what you have done.

Prior to overtraining syndrome developing, there's usually a period of overreaching, which to an extent is an effect of training that provides the cornerstone to improving fitness. When you push the body then give it the rest it requires, you'll push your boundaries, overreach slightly and get fitter. But when the same training session is repeated over and over again *without* appropriate rest then it's a problem and the more serious state of overtraining syndrome can develop.

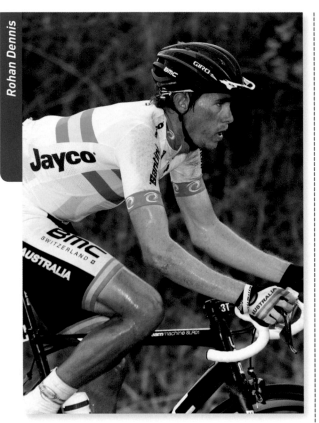

Rohan Dennis

Where does the 'balance' lie?

Overtraining syndrome is likened to a downward spiral. It's something that catches up on you without you knowing, and is very difficult to get out of. It normally develops over a period of time, usually a few weeks or months. There's a balance, and if you go too far one way, problems can occur. Recognising the early signs can help you to identify this condition more quickly and stop overtraining before it becomes a serious issue.

- **A decrease in performance:** Of course we all have 'off days' on the bike, when things sometimes don't click. However, if you're having trouble completing your normal workout, such as your everyday training route, failing to hit certain numbers, or even struggle to get up the hill you climb every day, then it could be that you are overtraining. If you feel you are getting weaker, or your endurance in general is deteriorating, then this could be another sign.
- **Frequently falling ill:** When we excessively exercise, our immune system becomes increasingly vulnerable. While a cold or cough is nothing really to worry about, if the frequency of sickness and infection rises, and constantly develops into something more serious, or it takes longer to shake them off, then you could have fallen into the trap.
- **Aches and pains:** Sometimes you might ache after a particular strenuous bout of cycling. The delayed onset of muscle soreness (DOMS) is expected after a hard workout on the bike, but if your muscles and joints feel particularly stiff, and the pain doesn't seem to be subsiding, then it may be more than that.
- **Change in sleeping patterns:** Struggling to fall asleep after a long ride could be a sign that you have overdone it. This is because the body is still reacting to the stress that it has been put under through training and your sympathetic nervous system is stimulated, meaning your parasympathetic nervous

■ *'Leading into the Australian nationals and the 2013 Tour Down Under, I felt overtrained which left my immune system vulnerable and that's why I think I came down with suspected viral meningitis. At the end of October 2012, I broke my collarbone which kept me off my bike a while and then I started worrying about form for January as I wanted to make a good first impression for my start as a pro. I consequently trained super hard in November and December and in hindsight I completely wrecked myself and overdid it. I don't think my body was strong enough at the time to do the training I was doing. While I felt good at the time I was training, I over-exerted myself and think I was on the wrong edge of the fine line of pushing myself too far.'*

Doing too much when the body isn't ready, or pushing too hard without adequate rest can significantly hamper performance and health. So how should you make sure this never happens?

SPOTTING THE SIGNS

Cadel Evans RETIRED AUSTRALIAN PRO AND 2011 TOUR DE FRANCE WINNER

■ 'For me, the first signs are when my concentration levels either on or off the bike drop, the quality of my sleep gets worse and my appetite drops. These are the fluctuations that I'm looking for. At the end of a Grand Tour, these signs are not uncommon and you have to soldier on, but if I'm training, then I'll take a couple of days' rest and will usually recover.

I would say though, the signs vary between people and are personal to the individual. One of the characteristics of great riders is not the ability to just do lots of training, but train enough to get the improvement, listen to their body and stay on the limit without exceeding it and getting overtrained and falling ill.

You need a strong head to get through that and that will come with experience. Listening to your body and learning your signs are important.'

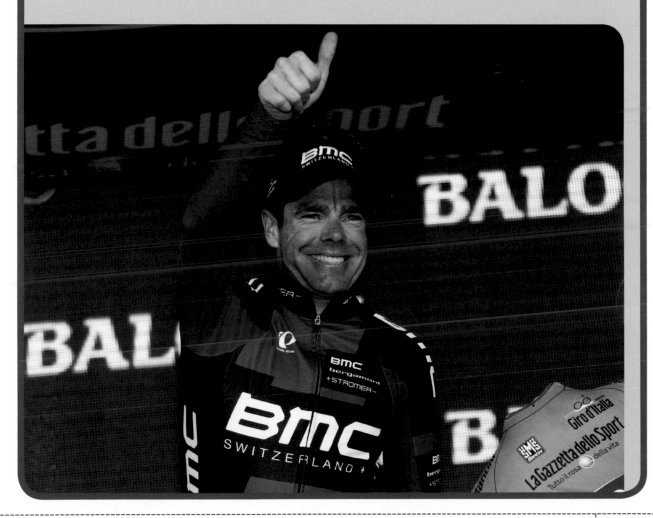

system (for recovery) has to work extra hard to combat the body's reaction to exercise, both physically and emotionally.

- **Prolonged lack of motivation:** If you don't want to ride, and you can't find a reason, then you need to be wary. A constant lack of motivation to not only ride, but to do anything, could be a sign that you have overdone it.

The chances are, one of these will apply to you and if so, don't panic. Anyone can be affected by one of these symptoms. However, if you do happen to have the majority of the symptoms, then chances are you have fallen victim to overtraining syndrome. Now it's a case of dealing with it.

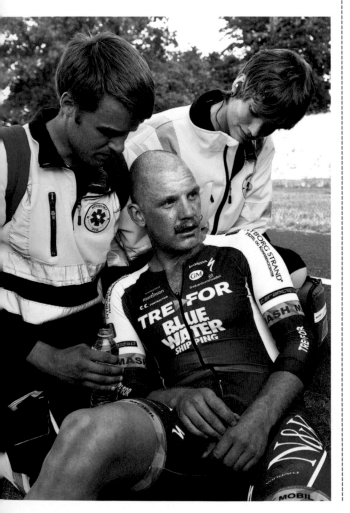

Getting through

Once you have ruled out medical issues and your doctor can help you with this, you then need to rest. That doesn't mean you should completely refrain from riding, but forget about long rides or riding at high intensity, in fact anything more than a recovery ride (see page 66). Usually, in the early stages, a few days off the bike will help.
But if after this you haven't seen an improvement in your energy levels or mood, then you need to give yourself at least a two-week rest away from cycling and maybe start to think of other contributory factors. Remember, other stresses in your life need to be looked at and addressed too, such as your work commitments, social life and even worries like paying bills, as all these can contribute to overtraining syndrome.

In extreme cases refrain from exercise until you feel fresh both physically and mentally. Begin with the initial two-week rest period and extend it if this hasn't made the difference. OK, taking a break from cycling isn't what you want to hear – especially if you have a race or sportive coming up – but you'll benefit in the long run. Some cyclists are reluctant to take a break, fearing they'll lose their fitness which they have worked so hard for. But it's important to see the big picture as pushing yourself too hard when you're not physically capable could set you back months – remember Caleb and Rohan's story?

Prevention is most important

Remember, gradual, structured increases in your training complemented by proper nutrition and appropriate rest will best help prevent overtraining syndrome becoming an issue. Listen to your body, understand what it is telling you and don't be afraid to take a break.

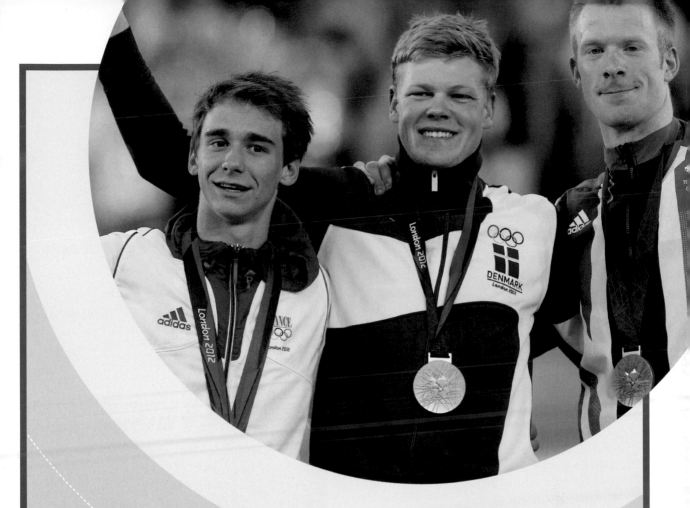

CYCLING NIRVANA

Lasse Norman Hansen DENMARK | 2012 OLYMPIC OMNIUM CHAMPION

■ 'At the Olympics in 2012 I was racing the omnium. Going into the final event, four riders were in the frame to win. I had had my ups and downs throughout the whole event, been in the lead, lost it, crashed at 50 km/h and got back on, it was an emotional rollercoaster.

The final event was the kilo: 1000 m of flat out effort to determine the medals and I was going off last, still bruised from the crash earlier that day. I'd watched my competitors go and I knew I had to beat my own personal best and

the Danish record to win but I was confident. I even made a joke to the Danish Chef de Mission five minutes before I went on the track.

I took 1.1 seconds off my own PB and got a Danish record. I crossed the line, looked up and knew I'd won and I was Olympic champion. My Cycling Nirvana actually came 30 minutes later when I got presented with my medal and felt the weight of it around my neck. That feeling will never leave me.'

20 SICKNESS

> *Everyone gets sick; it's just the way it is. I had my fair share of it over my career both leading up to and even during some big races. Not everyone treats it properly, and that's where cyclists come unstuck. Providing you know what to do when you get ill, and take the adequate rest you need, then it shouldn't be an ongoing problem.*

David Millar RETIRED BRITISH PRO CYCLIST AND TOUR DE FRANCE STAGE WINNER

No one wants to get sick, and, for cyclists, getting ill has the ability to put a significant dent into your fitness levels. The average adult will suffer between 2–5 colds a year, the majority lasting no more than 4–5 days, but in around 25 per cent of cases, symptoms can last up to four weeks. As little as ten days without training can result in a drop in fitness, so you can see how illness can affect your ability to maintain fitness if you're not careful.

■ *'The one thing that I have had to really teach myself is to listen to my body,'* says Namibian pro cyclist, Dan Craven. *'It seems like such an obvious thing to do, but the mind always has its own objectives and it doesn't necessarily come naturally. I see it over and over and over again with other people too; when they know how their body feels, but they try and tell themselves something else – and the fear that missing a few days of training is going to ruin their fitness. So instead they go out and ruin their health, thus having to take more time off and then really ruining their fitness. If the body is not working well, it does not matter what the mind wants. A rest day is not going to ruin anything. But pushing it can.'*

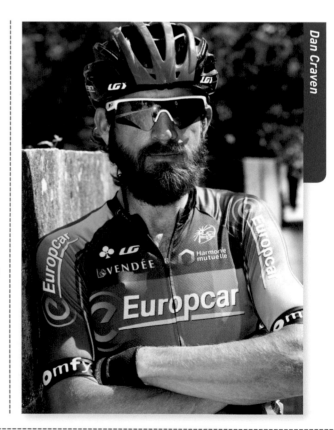

Dan Craven

The common cold

Upper respiratory tract infection (URTI), more commonly known as the common cold, is typically a viral infection of the nose and upper airways. The common symptoms are a congested, runny nose and frequent sneezing. You may generally feel under the weather and even develop a mild headache or sore throat. Thankfully these symptoms usually don't last more than 3–4 days, and provided that your symptoms occur no lower than in your throat, as in it hasn't developed into a chest infection, then it shouldn't stop you from riding your bike. If symptoms move onto your chest, then it's time to see your doctor.

Treatment

There's no treatment that will shorten the length of a cold. Many believe that taking vitamin C helps but a thorough review of the literature available in 2013 concluded vitamin C doesn't reduce the incidence of colds or URTIs. However, for people under extreme stress, and who aren't consuming enough vegetables and fruit, supplementation does appear to offer some health protective benefits.

It's advised that you don't exceed more than 1000 mg of vitamin C a day, as it can cause stomach pains, and in such large doses, can pass straight through the body – which is why urine will often be bright yellow not long after taking supplements.

Echinacea extracts are also a popular choice among those who have caught a cold but over the years, their benefits have been largely disproven. A 2014 review of the literature concluded that while echinacea may be more effective at treating colds than a placebo, the evidence is weak and did not show significantly that it can reduce the likelihood of illnesses occurring.

So, perhaps vitamin C and echinacea aren't the way to go, but there are a few things you can try to limit the severity of colds.

- **Fluids:** Colds can promote sweating, so it's important you do not become dehydrated. It can also be hard to eat when you are ill. If you are struggling to eat, a carbohydrate drink, such as a bottle of Lucozade, will help you to keep energy levels up and maintain hydration.
- **Steam inhalation:** Putting your head over a basin of hot water may help clear your nose and nasal passages, but it's only a temporary effect. A blocked nose isn't due to a build-up of mucus, it's due to the blood vessels in your nose becoming inflamed and hardened.
- **Oral zinc sweets:** Zinc lozenges are considered possibly effective for reducing the length of the common cold but are not useful for preventing colds.

Is vitamin D the answer?

Vitamin D is forever being advocated as a cold killer. But how effective is it?

In 2009 it was established that people with the lowest blood vitamin D levels reported significantly more cases of cold and flu.

But in 2013 a study concluded that vitamin D did not reduce the severity of URTIs in healthy adults, although they acknowledged that supplementation of vitamin D for deficient individuals may be beneficial. The research on the effectiveness of vitamin D for treating colds is hazy. However, you should strive to consume adequate amounts to maintain health, because a lack of vitamin D can cause other issues as well, such as softening of the bones, and is even linked to chronic pain and depression.

Sunlight is the best source of vitamin D, but it is also found in food such as oily fish, eggs, and fortified fat spreads and breakfast cereals.

For those living in the UK, the summer sun is strong enough to produce vitamin D, but during winter the skin isn't able to make sufficient vitamin D from the sun as it isn't strong enough. This is why, during the colder months, it's even more important to get vitamin D from food sources or supplementation, although current UK guidelines recommend that adults take no more than 25 micrograms (1000 IUs) per day.

Infection

If after a week your cold hasn't subsided, it's possible that your body has succumbed to a secondary bacterial infection. Severe muscle pains and sore throats are classic signs that your cold may have progressed. A fever may also be present. A fever is an important part of the body's defence and is telling you that your body is fighting an infection. However, one that rises too high is extremely dangerous, so it's best to try and keep it down. If you have a fever, you should stop riding your bike and see your doctor. A doctor may prescribe you antibiotics for the infection or advise you to rest and wait for it to pass. At this point your immune system is already fighting to combat your illness – for example, your heart rate will be naturally raised as it attempts to circulate more oxygen and immune cells to the parts of the body that need it – so exercise will only make things worse and delay recovery. Don't worry about your fitness levels as your health is your priority at this time.

A good rule of thumb to follow: when you get sick, for every day ill, take two days to recover.

GETTING SICK

Cadel Evans RETIRED AUSTRALIAN PRO AND 2009 WORLD CHAMPION

■ 'I had a virus in 2012 which was making me ill, which was more frustrating than any injury I've had. I raced for seven months before I knew what was wrong with me. I knew I wasn't right because I was just so exhausted all the time; training, racing everything and in the end it took the specialists some time to get to the bottom of it as all the initial tests came back negative and I continued to train and race. At the 2012 Tour de France I finished 7th which was a fantastic result considering what I was dealing with but I should've been contending to defend my win from 2011.

At the time I still didn't know what was wrong with me. Eventually I was diagnosed with a virus that was causing a form of chronic fatigue. It was good to finally find out what was wrong, as I knew it wasn't in my head. I was told to have two months of complete rest, no bike riding at all, which as a stage racer was frustrating but I knew I had to be rational about it and take the time to recover.'

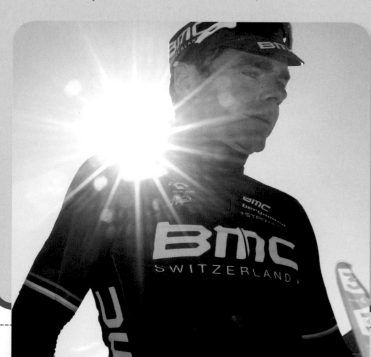

Immunity

Your immune system is designed to fight infection, so it helps to have one that is strong and healthy. However, it's difficult to just strengthen the immune system as it's a complex system that requires a number of factors such as a healthy balanced diet, good hygiene and adequate sleep.

Exercise and nutrition helps immunity

Cycling is a great way to naturally protect the body from picking up infections. During moderate bouts of cycling, immune cells circulate through the body more quickly, enabling them to kill bacteria and viruses that enter the body. Exercise may help by flushing pathogens (things that cause sickness) out from the lungs so decreasing the chance of them getting *into* the body and causing a cold, flu or other airborne illness. Also, the temporary rise in temperature from exercise may prevent bacterial growth, allowing the body to fight infection more easily.

However, the 72 hours *after* heavy exercise can leave your immune system vulnerable, and it's important you do your best to avoid picking up bugs even more during this time. This is one of the reasons that protein intake is advocated

Prevention

Just like injuries, the best form of treatment is prevention and it's a case of doing the simple things right. According to research, around 80 per cent of contagious diseases are transmitted by touch. So thoroughly wash your hands before and after eating, and when you leave the bathroom.

Hand sanitizer gels are more effective at killing bacteria and viruses than soaps, and they don't dry out the hands as much so are a great option to carry around with you.

Sleep

Sleep is the time your body most significantly switches into recovery mode and a lack of sleep can suppress the immune system, creating a negative effect on the body's production of certain white blood cells that play a central role in your body's immune system response. 6–8 hours sleep is recommended. Napping during the day also has a positive effect on the immune system. See page 54 for tips on good sleeping habits.

immediately following high intensity exercise. According to research, cyclists who consume a high protein diet reported fewer URTI symptoms compared to those on a lower protein diet. Recommendations of 1.4 to 1.8 of protein per kg of body weight per day is advised to help maintain a healthy immune system during periods of more intense training, for example, riding 3–4 times a week with efforts of moderate to high intensity.

A final thought

Bacteria, viruses and parasites are around us constantly, it's *how* your body reacts to them that will be the key to how frequently you get ill. Getting sick is unavoidable and often it comes down to luck. But if you follow the right precautions, eat the right foods and keep fit, you can skew the odds in your favour and keep your immune system as healthy as possible.

When you get ill, don't try and be a hero and push through as you may dig yourself a bigger hole. Take a break from your cycling and concentrate on getting back to full health. You may be tempted to go out and ride, after all, 'what harm can one ride do?' Well, as we've shown from the likes of Dan and Cadel, a lot of harm can be done. Don't let a cold ruin your season. It's really not worth it.

21 SADDLE SORES

How you sit on a saddle can either irritate or alleviate saddle sores; for example, sitting on the tip of your saddle is one way to certainly aggravate them. But once they come on, or you feel it coming on, backing off the bike or taking a couple of days rest usually gets them right.

Jack Bobridge AUSTRALIAN PRO CYCLIST AND AND TOUR DOWN UNDER STAGE WINNER

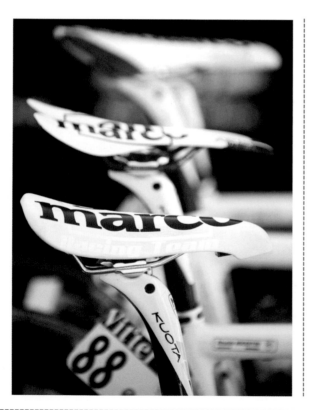

Saddle sores are nothing more than a nuisance content on making your life on the bike a misery. However, the good news is that so long as you know what is causing them and how to treat them, you can deal with them appropriately.

If left untreated, saddle sores will bring any cyclist to a standstill, and could cause extreme pain. In some extreme cases, they could even become infected.

What are they?

The term 'saddle soreness' includes many symptoms ranging from bruises to blisters, right the way through to full-fledged boils. The majority of saddle sores are born out of skin abrasions or irritation to skin follicles, caused by friction in your chamois (cycling shorts). During the course of a ride, it can get hot, moist and sweaty in your bib shorts. Bacteria thrive in conditions like these, and if they start to fester, they can become a real nuisance. Over time they will enlarge, redden and

LEFT The root cause of saddle sores!

harden into a painful boil. At this time, it's extremely painful to sit down on the saddle, and as you can imagine, almost impossible to ride your bike.

Saddle sores aren't something you may often hear about – after all, it's not something you'd broadcast – but they do occur.

■ *'I'd say rather frustratingly, that saddle sores are very common,'* says Australian pro cyclist, Nathan Haas. *'I probably get a proper saddle sore about twice a year. There's no real method to the management. Now I'm at the point that as soon as I get one I take three days off the bike and this will usually settle it. If I don't stay off my bike and they get bad, it can become hard to sit straight on the saddle because of the pain, so you end up sitting skewed on the bike. Do this for too long and it leads to injuries elsewhere and that's the last thing you want.'*

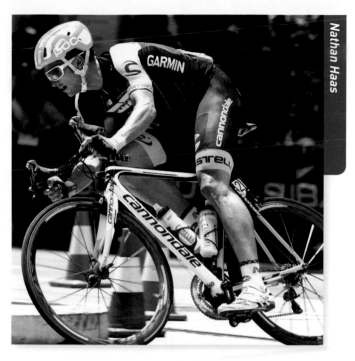

Nathan Haas

As Nathan points out, these sores aren't just painful, they can also lead to other problems as the body compensates to adjust for the pain. For example, if the pain makes it uncomfortable to place your whole body weight down on the right side of the saddle, you may lean towards the left in order to alleviate the pain or vice versa. As we mentioned at the beginning of the book, all the muscles are interconnected, and the body is stubborn. It doesn't like to be pushed and pulled into positions it's not comfortable with. And if you continue to ride, compensating for something like a saddle sore, placing excess pressure on another part of the body that it isn't used to, it could result in a muscular imbalance and injury.

Treatment

- **Get out of your dirty cycling clothing.** Hot, moist environments are a breeding ground for bacteria. Dirty shorts may also start to build dirt and grit, which can cause skin abrasions. The moment you finish your ride,

change into something else and remember to wash them, as soon as possible.
- **Clean it.** If you notice a saddle sore, apply antiseptic cream to help prevent infection. Clean and dry it immediately.
- **Stop riding!** Riding on already developed sores can lead to further problems like infection. Taking a break will help settle the sores. As Nathan points out, 2–3 days off the bike will help them clear more quickly.
- **Hot compress.** In most cases boils will clear by themselves. However, applying hot compresses will make them mature more quickly: place a very warm flannel on the area at regular intervals for a few minutes.
- **Medical advice.** If they get worse – get bigger or infected – seek medical advice as it may need to be lanced, or cut out. Unfortunately, this will mean time off the bike, as the wound will need to heal.

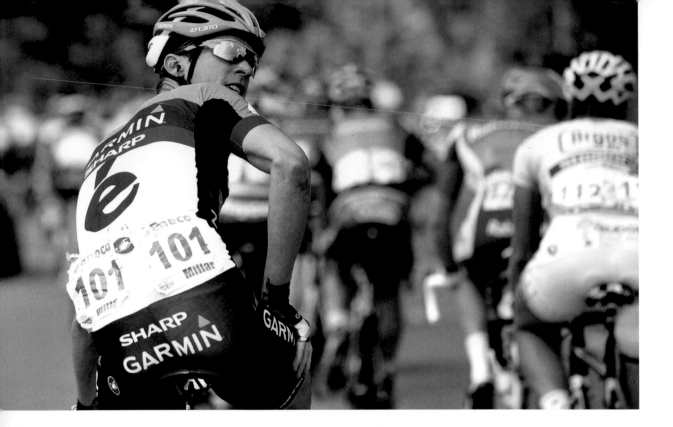

Prevention

As with most things we have touched on, prevention will go a long way towards stopping these sores from developing.

- **Before each ride:** ensure you have a clean, dry pair of bib shorts on: You want to limit the likelihood of germs spreading and the best way to achieve this is through clean, dry shorts.
- **Buy a decent pair of bib shorts with a good chamois:** the chamois is the padding inside the shorts. Good bib shorts are not only more comfortable, but modern synthetics are softer on the skin and less likely to cause friction and abrasions. They'll also allow breathing, which will keep the region cooler and minimise sweating. A well-made pair of bib shorts will have the chamois sewn into them, which will prevent the seat from chafing. Women should opt for a one piece or a curved 'baseball' cut. This will eliminate the

seams on the midline, reducing friction and potential abrasions over the genital area. The majority of bike stores will sell specific bib shorts for women.
- **Soften the ride:** a softer, more comfortable ride will help reduce friction. Try and keep to a rhythm that is settled and doesn't require rocking, or moving. A proper bike fit and strong core will help minimise movement by improving stability on the bike.
- **Chamois cream:** will help minimise friction between you and the saddle, and protect the skin from breaking. Find out what works for you. Some people's skin is more sensitive than others and it may cause a rash.

 If you get repetitive saddle sores, it may be a case of looking at other factors, such as the saddle itself.

Saddle height

Incorrect saddle position can significantly increase the likelihood of saddle sores developing. If it's too high, you may be placing a lot of force on to to your sit bones and perineum. This pressure could cause bruising. If it's not level, you may slide forward or back. Constantly shuffling and rocking from side to side while pedalling will cause a lot of friction, which will result in skin abrasions. The width of the saddle is also very important and this should be set up in accordance to the rider's sit bones (ischial tuberosities). A saddle that is too narrow will cause the sit bones to 'hang' over the sides, where your soft tissues will bear the load and it may create pinching of the skin, which in turn will result in sores. On the other hand, a saddle that is too wide could cause chafing on the inner thighs. If you are experiencing problems, which you think could be saddle-related, return to your bike fitter to see if they can find a suitable replacement.

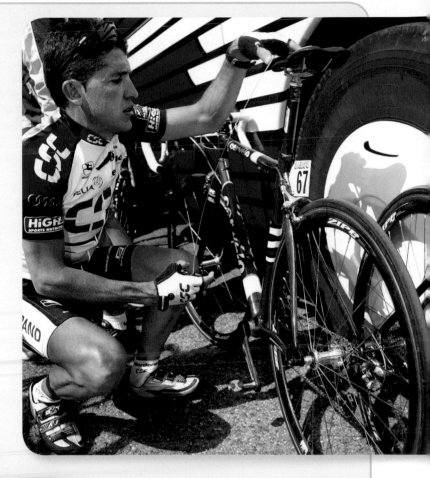

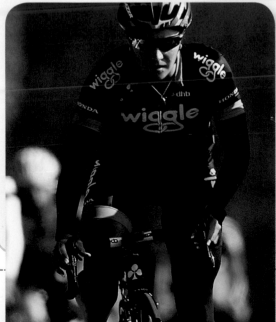

'Ladies, make sure you buy female-specific bib shorts as the chamois designed for women will greatly improve comfort, relieve friction and reduce the chance of saddle sores '

Rochelle Gilmore
RETIRED AUSTRALIAN PRO AND
JAYCO BAY CLASSIC WINNER

22 GENDER SPECIFIC ISSUES

> *If it starts stinging when you pee, or worse you're getting blood in your urine, there is something wrong! These are warning signs that are precursors to potentially bigger problems so should be heeded.*

Steve Cummings BRITISH PRO CYCLIST AND TOUR MÉDITERRANÉEN

These might not be classed as injuries but they are a serious topic that causes concern among the cycling community. There are a number of issues that affect the genders specifically and here's where we'll discuss them, the causes, how to manage them and most importantly, how to treat them.

Erectile dysfunction

Let's not sugar-coat it, for men the biggest concern related to cycling is erectile dysfunction. Riding for long periods of time exerts high pressure on the perineum, the area between the genitals and the anus, an area packed full of nerves and blood vessels. Excess prolonged pressure on this area can damage the nerves and temporarily impede blood flow, potentially causing tingling and numbness around the genital region both on and eventually off the bike that can lead to erectile dysfunction. This issue is known as pudendal nerve entrapment (PNE), 'Alcock's' or 'cyclist's syndrome.' Leading urologist Irwin Goldstein famously stated: 'There are only two kinds of male cyclists – those who are impotent and those who will be impotent.' Strong words, so should you be concerned? Getting numbness

or tingling around the genital area is a warning sign that something isn't right. If you get these symptoms on three consecutive rides, you need to stop and investigate why.

Management

We don't want to scare male cyclists and it's worth highlighting that there are other diseases such as diabetes, kidney disease and alcohol abuse that cause a greater proportion of erectile dysfunction in the real world. We're merely letting you see what's down the road if certain symptoms are ignored. But there's no denying that cycling can cause significant complications regarding erectile dysfunction and the majority of the research indicates the pressure that is placed on the perineum as the contributing factor. So it's worth understanding how to limit this pressure.

The first thing to realise is that there are three main points of contact between you and the saddle. One and two are the ischial tuberosities, also known as your 'sit' bones. The third is the soft tissue between your legs, the perineum. The sit bones are able to withstand pressure, the soft tissue is not. This is the problem area and in order to reduce this pressure, the first place to look at is your saddle:

SADDLE CHECKS

- One that's too narrow with a thin nose means a huge amount of pressure is placed on your perineum, which can compress the area and cause numbness. A wider saddle may help distribute weight across a greater area and reduce pressure.
- Research has also shown that a saddle with a cut out centrepiece or one with a shorter nose can help alleviate pressure. But be aware that shorter nosed saddles may lead to less control over the bike, due to the thighs not being in full contact with the saddle.
- It's important to ensure the saddle is level. While a saddle that tilts slightly forwards (nose down) may ease pressure on the perineum, it may cause problems elsewhere, such as the lower back. Some male cyclists prefer a saddle with 1–2 degrees of backward tilt. However, more than four degrees will create more pressure on your perineum.
- A saddle too high and you may find your legs stretching to turn the pedals, which will increase pressure. Reaching too far on your handlebars will also encourage you to slide forwards on your saddle, which again, will put a lot of strain on the soft tissue.
- Correct clothing will also help. For example, a good quality pair of bib shorts will aid comfort, and reduce the impact between your body and the saddle. However, a thicker pair of padded shorts doesn't mean a softer ride. In fact, too much padding may make the problem worse.
- To alleviate pressure, you can always ride out of the saddle for short periods, giving your backside a break, but this certainly isn't a long-term solution!

Women's issues

A number of studies have highlighted cases of women cyclists reporting feelings of numbness, skin infections and chronic swelling after lengthy spells on the bike. It's been reported that female cyclists who position their handlebars lower than the bike's seat are at a risk of decreased anterior vaginal and labial sensation because of increased pressure on the area. Female saddle injuries can also include swelling and chafing of the female genitalia as well as potential damage to the urethra. Fortunately in most cases these issues can be rectified.

If you are suffering from increased pressure or discomfort of your genitalia, it's worth taking a look at your saddle shape. The naturally wider hips women have can result in the sit bones overhanging a narrow saddle, which can lead to painful pressure on soft tissue. If it's possible, opt for women-specific saddles, which are wider and shorter than men's and may help reduce discomfort. Also, opting for one with a cut-out in the centre can help offload pressure. The majority of bike shops will sell saddles designed for women.

'Girls, get a saddle that you can ride as comfortable as possible on. When you start to spend more time on the bike you wanna be able to sit alright on the bike! Having the best one possible for your own preference can make a big difference in riding the bike!'

Emilia Fahlin
2013 SWEDISH NATIONAL CHAMPION

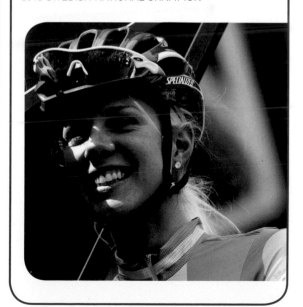

Urinary tract infections

Female cyclists are more prone to urinary tract infections (UTI) than men because of how close the urethra – where urine leaves the body – sits to any possible bacterial contamination of the chamois. If you develop itching, burning, increased frequency of urination or blood in the urine, you may have developed a UTI and should see your doctor for urinalyses and antibiotics to treat it.

Candida vaginitis

This unusual sounding delight (commonly known as thrush) is also common in female cyclists due to fungal spores that live in moist chamois. Ladies, it's *even more* important to keep your bib shorts as clean and completely dry as possible in between rides. If you get vaginal itching or discharge, or discomfort with intercourse or riding, then go see your doctor.

Treatment: labial swelling and pain

- Keep clean – wash with plenty of water.
- DO NOT douche, as it can predispose you to developing a yeast infection as you clean out normal vaginal flora (friendly bacteria).

 Ice as needed for the swelling, twice a day for ten minutes.

Over-the-counter medication

Take ibuprofen as indicated for pain and swelling, and additional paracetamol can be taken if ibuprofen alone is not enough. See pages 62–63

UTIs in men

UTIs in men are rare and should *always* be reported to a doctor. Symptoms include pain/burning with urination, blood in the urine or semen, pain in perineum or lower abdomen or back, with possible addition of fever or chills. UTIs in men can develop into a prostate infection which can be serious, but this usually only occurs in older men.

A final word

Many factors contribute to perineal and genital symptoms, and it's a case of experimenting with what works and what doesn't. First thing to do is to get your bike fit right!

We don't want to distract people from riding their bikes, and issues such as impotency and swelling of the female genitalia is a real concern for many; you're not alone. If problems persist and bike fit doesn't remedy the situation quickly, or you continue to get symptoms off the bike, see your doctor as the next step.

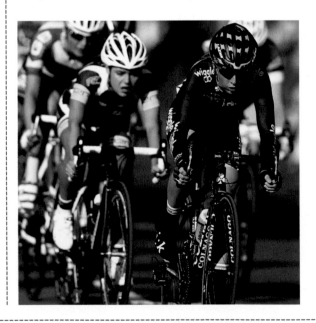

CYCLING NIRVANA

Fabian Wegmann GERMANY |
THREE-TIME GERMAN NATIONAL CHAMPION

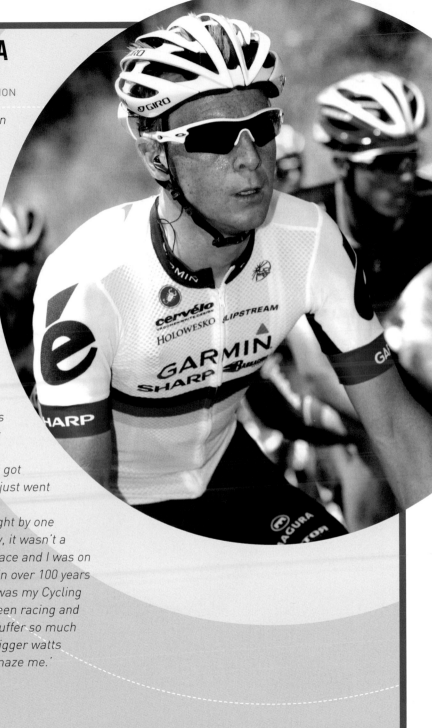

■ 'The 2006 Giro Lombardia, I had an amazing feeling from the beginning. Everyone was going hard from the start. I even crashed in the first 80 km but this time I didn't panic. I felt strangely calm.

It was one of those days when you can do whatever you want and ride on your limit all day. Sometimes it doesn't feel possible to go deep enough but this day I could go so hard, I could go deep on the main climb and even though I got dropped it wasn't by that much.

Paolo Bettini attacked on the small climb at the finish, I went all in, caught him on the descent. It was over 80 km/h on a technical descent and that's fast but I felt confident as I knew the roads. On the last climb I got slightly dropped but I didn't crack, I just went at my speed.

With a kilometre to go I got caught by one from behind. I finished third that day, it wasn't a win, but it's a "cycling monument" race and I was on the podium. I was the first German in over 100 years to be on the podium at that race. It was my Cycling Nirvana. This is the difference between racing and training; in racing, you can always suffer so much more and push that much harder, bigger watts and bigger gears, it never fails to amaze me.'

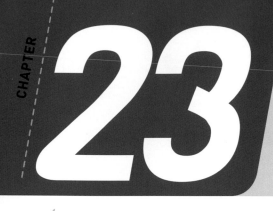

23

ROAD RASH

'Road rashes are an all too common occurrence for anyone involved in cycling. Coming down and getting it during a race can be a nightmare. You've lost a lot of skin, are probably banged up and on top of that it messes up one of the most important aspects of recovery, sleep.'

Matthew White FORMER AUSTRALIAN PRO AND TOUR DOWN UNDER STAGE WINNER

From time to time, you will fall off your bike and when that time comes and you slide along the ground you'll probably experience road rash. Road rash occurs when the top layers of skin are quite literally scraped away by another surface, more often than not the road. While some crashes are extremely dangerous and can cause severe traumatic injury such as broken bones and deep abrasions, a lot of falls result in shallow abrasions, which don't break the deeper layer of the skin and little blood is lost. That's not to say there's no pain. In fact, it is often agony. Welcome to a bugbear of every keen cyclist, this is road rash.

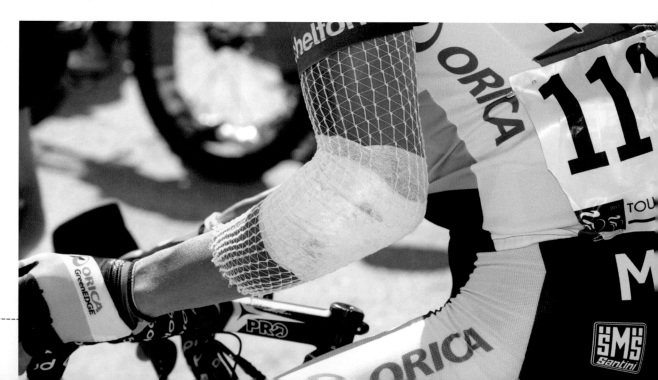

Not a pretty sight

In a lot of road rash incidences, it's not necessarily the impact of the crash that is most painful, but rather the process of dealing with its consequences over the coming days. For example, as the area turns sticky, gets hot and starts to throb, it can be very hard to sleep at night, and hurts to get dressed – and that's before you've even thought about riding your bike.

Take Rohan Dennis for example. During the Australian national time trial championship in 2014, he was literally swept off his bike by what he described as a 'mini tornado,' but it was the days after that proved the bigger challenge.

■ *'I was into my ride motoring along at 50 km/h when I suddenly saw a big dust storm on the left side of the road,'*

'As a junior I was always told to power through crosswinds, so I powered into it, then the wind changed just as I hit it. I was on the TT bars in the tuck position, the bike got blown out from underneath me, and I landed on the road still in the exact same tuck position. I had road rash all over my body from knuckles, palms of hands, forearms, elbows, right shoulder, both knees and my hips: it was bad.

That was in January and the road rash was that bad and that deep that by mid-March the deeper cuts were only just healing up. Sleeping was a nightmare because I couldn't lie on either side as I would stick to the bed and yelp with pain. Anytime I was asleep and rolled over I was in immediate pain and it woke me up. The thing a lot of people don't think about is that cleaning the wounds every day in the shower is agony.'

OPPOSITE Bike crashes are hard to avoid, unfortunately!

Tetanus

A concern when you get road rash is tetanus infection. Although rare, it's caused by bacteria found in dirt on the road, which can contaminate a wound as you scrape along the ground when you come off a bike. It's a serious problem and not something to ignore. Tetanus is a toxin to the nerves so if it gets into the body it will cause symptoms including muscle spasm and stiffness, difficulty swallowing and spasms of the jaw muscles (aka lockjaw), and will need medical treatment. Have you been vaccinated in the past five years? If not, you're more vulnerable to tetanus when you crash so it's worth speaking to your doctor about getting vaccinated.

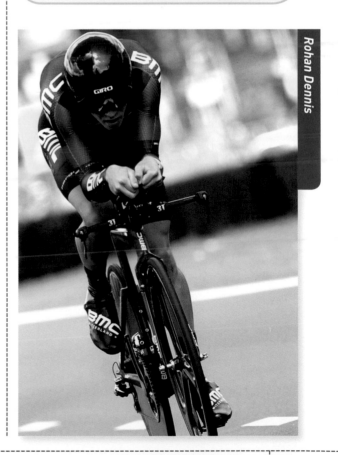

Rohan Dennis

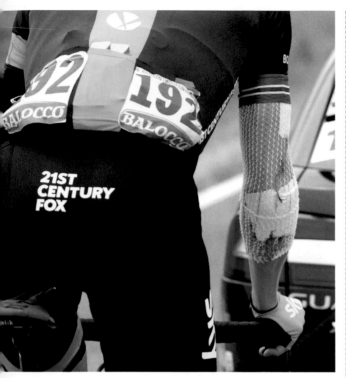

ABOVE Make sure you dress road rash properly

Take action

As skin is ripped away at the point of impact, the blood vessels are exposed, and the presence of dirt and other bacteria increases the chance of infection.

At the time of the crash, you need to check for deep lacerations, before cleaning the area immediately. If after 10 minutes your cut hasn't stopped bleeding, or you notice that it is particularly deep, then you may need stitching up. If this is the case, go to hospital.

There's no need to panic at the sight of road rash but in most cases, it looks worse than it is. Over time it will heal and scab over as new skin forms underneath.

Getting air to a wounded area is a good thing and will help to dry it out and avoid further infection, but it will need to be covered when you are wearing clothes, allowing you to put pressure on to it without it sticking or ripping the scab off.

Treatment

- Wash the area as you normally would when you cut yourself; use warm water and soap. If the road rash is particularly heavy, and has dirt in it, use a soft brush or sponge to clean out all of the debris. You may need to scrub hard and beware, it's going to hurt, but getting the wound absolutely clean first time is *the* most important thing.
- If you have been injured particularly badly, swelling may occur. Clean the area, dress it and then apply a cold compress to reduce swelling.
- As the wound is dried, apply an antibiotic ointment to a dressing, then layer the dressing on top of the wound.
- With any open break in the skin, you have to dress it. Dressing will protect the wound and help keep pathogens out, reducing the risk of infection. It will also help to prevent friction irritation from clothes.
- It's a good idea to change the dressing on a daily basis, or every few days at least, in the early stages so you can keep an eye on the wound to make sure it's healing properly.
- If you have not had a tetanus shot in the preceding five years, visit your doctor for a vaccination.

CYCLING NIRVANA

Johan Vansummeren   BELGIUM | 2011 PARIS-ROUBAIX WINNER

■ *'I knew already in the Forest of Arenberg that it felt easy. I'd just done one of the hardest sections and I'd felt fine. I then immediately attacked the peloton and caught the breakaway. It was a two minute gap which we closed within 10 km, we were going full gas and caught the first group. Luckily I could then rest when*

I got to the front group. I relaxed and everyone started attacking before the Carrefour de l'Abre – on normal roads, not even on the cobbles. By the time we got to 22 km to go, there were three of us left. Then we turned into the Carrefour de l'Abre. I remember I took a corner so fast halfway through the sector then accelerated. At that

time, I felt that good I figured there can't be anyone on my wheel; I could feel there was nobody behind me.

Coming out of that sector I had a 10–15 second gap. You know it could be your chance. I was in a mental fury and going so hard the last 15 km was like a daze. At 5 km to go there's a bridge that I always feel tired after and this time I didn't. But this time from 5 km to go I knew my tyre was losing air as I could feel the rim bouncing against the cobbles.

Turning into the velodrome felt so overwhelming and special, I didn't really think enough to enjoy it. My fiancée was there on the finish line, which was amazing. Working hard for that race my whole career, the one moment that summarises Cycling Nirvana is entering the velodrome solo: you can hear the noise, feel the atmosphere, it's electric. It's like a wave that carries you round. That was a super day. You only get a few days like that in your career.'

24 RIDING TWISTED

In the same way that some people have one foot slightly bigger than the other, one leg may also naturally be longer than the other. This is known as a 'structural' leg length discrepancy and may be 'normal' for that individual. However, overuse of the pelvis and lower back muscles after extended periods of time on the bike, or a fall off, can lead to a transient asymmetry in the pelvis, causing a 'functional' leg length discrepancy. This is riding twisted. This can be improved through exercises (see page 230) or manual treatment, reducing the sensation of 'riding twisted'.

Telltale Signs

- Continued fidgeting on the bike to get comfortable or feeling of 'reaching' for the pedal with one leg.
- Excessive rocking from side to side and potential development of lower back tightness or discomfort.
- Premature fatigue for no apparent reason as one leg is working far harder than the other.

How it affects your ride

1 Drop in performance as you're not getting optimal power through the pedals when you're not sitting straight on the bike.
2 Muscular imbalances can occur as your body compensates for poor biomechanics, which can lead to injuries developing from 'nowhere', such as knee problems or lower back pain.

MATT SAYS:

'The biggest thing I'm consulted for by cyclists of all levels, is riders feeling like they're "riding twisted". This is by no means a scientific term. Put simply it means they don't feel like they're sitting straight on the bike. This is often caused by asymmetry in the pelvis that causes one leg to be slightly longer than the other and affects comfort on the bike. This leads to a sensation of unequal power being produced from the left and right leg and is noticed even more when cycling for a while and are getting tired, one leg often fatiguing more quickly than the other

This isn't really an injury, nor is it an ailment. But there's no section in the book called "the aggravator" or "the robber of performance"; ask the pros and that's exactly what it can be, the difference between a good day or a bad one, winning or finishing in the grupetto. Whatever you call it, it has the potential to cause downright misery and can lead to injury elsewhere due to the uneven energy transference through the legs.'

THE FRUSTRATION OF RIDING TWISTED

Charly Wegelius

FORMER BRITISH PRO CYCLIST AND HIGHEST PLACED BRITISH FINISHER, 2007 TOUR DE FRANCE

■ *'It's like getting up in the morning and finding out your jeans don't fit you anymore – that's the simple way to describe it. They fitted yesterday, and now they don't – that's how it hits you on the bike.*

There are two parts to it as far as I see it. There's the physical aspect, which is like having the tap closed off to your muscles. You know you have the energy but you frustratingly can't get it out. Let's say you're twisted on your bike, and you only have 80 per cent of your potential available to access. That's when the second part, the mental side kicks in. Even though you have 80 per cent available, you don't use it, as you end up spending so much time tormenting yourself, wondering how you can get straight on the bike.

It does your head in. It's like losing your wallet and spending all your time and energy looking for it, when you know there are 100 other more important things you can do at that time without your wallet. It preoccupies your mind.

You can fidget on the saddle and temporarily feel better as you are using slightly different muscles, but you'd be kidding yourself as eventually it would drift back to feeling twisted.

In the end I found an osteopath who lived near me who probably extended my career by four years: it worked for me. I'd do exercises, movements and core work just to try and stay straight and that ended up being my best insurance to keep everything on track.'

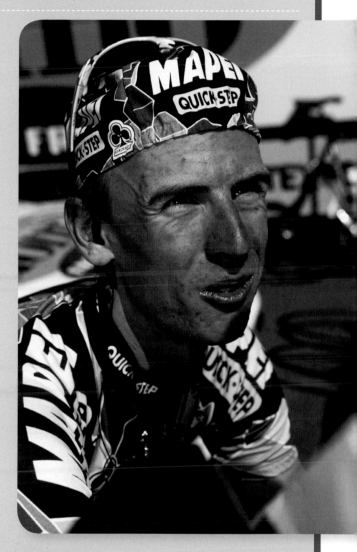

Getting it fixed

These selected exercises from the rehab toolkit will loosen the muscles around the pelvis and help improve symmetry on the bike. Repeat these at least once a day for a two-week period and do them before and after each ride during this time too.

After two weeks begin the pain-free cyclist core exercises (see page 202). Strengthening the core will improve pelvic stability and help symmetry on the bike.

If you still feel 'twisted' after three weeks or so, or to speed up your improvement, see an expert such as a chiropractor, osteopath or physio as they have the skill set to get to the bottom of the problem quickly.

RECOMMENDATIONS TO IMPROVE PELVIC SYMMETRY

EXERCISE	EX. NO.	PAGE
The stand tall and reach stretch	3.1	175
The low lunge	4.1	180
The foundation lunge	4.2	180
Lumbar spine movement	5.1	182
The cat and camel	5.2	182
The child's pose	5.3	183
The knees to chest hug	5.4	183
The sitting glute stretch	5.7	184
The founder	5.13	187
The bird dog	5.16	189
The glutes and piriformis foam roll	5.19	190
The tensor fascia latae foam roll	5.20	191
The quad stretch	6.1	192

MATT SAYS:

'I'm not a huge fan of changing the bike fit around; putting in things like shims, or heel lifts should be the absolute last resort. I think they're done too early before basic principles have been explored and finding out how much you can improve the body beforehand to help the symmetry and balance.'

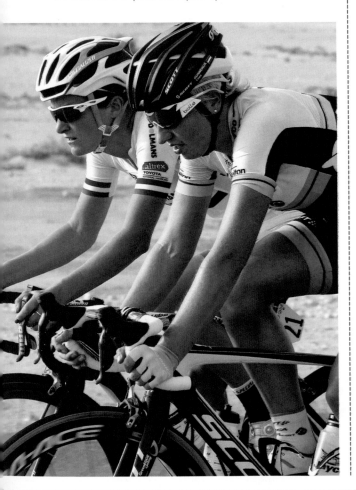

GET IT SORTED

Christian Vande Velde

RETIRED AMERICAN PRO CYCLIST AND TOP FIVE TOUR DE FRANCE FINISHER

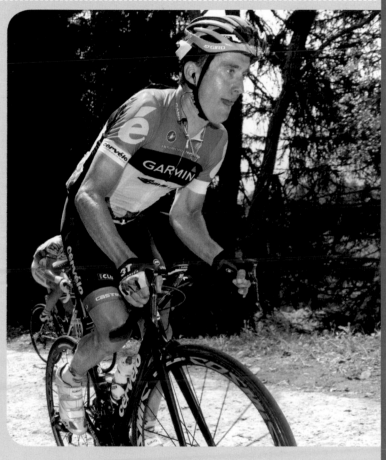

■ 'I've always had a slight issue in the lower vertebra of my back but managed it well. However, there was a time in the middle of my career when I let it get way out of control. It took the best part of three years to really put it behind me. And even to this day I need to make sure I strengthen and stretch my lower back and hips to allow me to remain supported properly when I ride.

For two years I literally rode with one leg not working properly due to irritation in my lower back causing imbalance in my pelvis muscles, and I developed some seriously bad habits. This feeling of riding out of balance was mostly due to a torsion or twist in my pelvis and was one of the most frustrating times during my long career and affected my performance on a daily basis. It would lead to some muscles overworking while others I couldn't get to work.

It's not like a knee injury that keeps you off the bike. It plays with your mind as you think you can push through it and that it will come right. I got there in the end – through the help of strength exercises and chiropractic care – but when it was bad it was so frustrating. It felt like I had a V12 engine driving a beaten up stock car chassis.

If I knew as a younger rider what I know now, I'd tell my younger self to take time off the bike, do the work needed away from the bike and it would all get better far quicker than trying to bulldoze through it and hoping it would get better.'

CYCLING NIRVANA

Sir Bradley Wiggins GREAT BRITAIN | FIRST BRITISH TOUR DE FRANCE WINNER

■ 'From the moment I left the start ramp at the final time trial into Chartes at the 2012 Tour de France, it felt like I always imagined it would feel. I always ride to power when I do a time trial and I left the start with a number in my head. I was aiming to hold 450 watts, and for the first ten minutes I was above that holding between 460–470 watts, which felt surprisingly easy. I liken a time trial effort to a 2000 m rowing race when in the first 500 m of the race they put in a big effort to get out up to speed and get the boat ahead of all the others. After that, in a rowing race, the aim is to then maintain that pace and keep your boat ahead of your rivals before emptying the tank and giving it all you have got to the finish. Well, the first time check at 13 km was like my first 500 m of a rowing race and when I got there I still felt great and I hadn't actually had to begin to dig in yet. When I got to the first time check I was told by Sean Yates (my director) that I was 12 seconds up. It was at that time I knew in myself, this is it, that nobody was going to beat me that day as they would have to hold above 450 watts for the rest of the ride as that is at least what I was going to do.

The rest of the time trial seemed to go in slow motion, almost like an out-of-body experience where I imagined myself in the helicopter above looking down on myself. I was going fast and I was going deep but I remember vividly seeing faces on the side of the road of people I recognised. I remember seeing a bloke hopping up and down, jumping, going mad shouting as I got closer to him and then realising it was an old friend of mine, all while in this deep concentration.

I plugged on maintaining my power whenever I checked it on my bike computer, and at each time check, I was up on the previous one. I was going harder and harder but felt better and better. As the race continued I tried to nudge up my power to 470–480 watts, playing a game with myself to see how far I could go.

You're suffering, but you are still so aware of what is going on. As I came into the last few kilometres I remember having all these flashbacks, going back over my career. I remember in my head people saying after I was 4th in the 2009 Tour de France "he's a flash in the pan, Sky had wasted their money signing me"; all these thoughts.

As I came over the finish line I punched the air and screamed. That was a Cycling Nirvana moment, that was when all the tension of all the previous three weeks and the months leading up to that Tour came out and I will never forget that feeling.

Ten days later, was the London Olympic time trial. My London ride was amazing, and almost a carbon copy of my Tour de France time trial. Seeing a million people wearing "Wiggo" sideburns, lining the road and hearing everyone screaming at me along the route, was a magical experience. Unlike at the Tour, when I finished the Olympic time trial I was in a kind of a daze; I didn't know if I was leading or what was going on so there were no immediate sensations. Having won the Tour I really felt like I had nothing to lose and I really gave it everything. When I found out I had won I felt all the emotions come flooding back. It was only, however, when I went out to face the press, receive my medal and sat on the throne that it really hit me and that was a huge Cycling Nirvana moment for me.

I remember sitting there, everyone going mad, and I thought that having won the Tour de France in Paris on one weekend and wining Olympic Gold in my home town in London 10 days later that was the pinnacle, and I couldn't help but think at the time "it doesn't get any better than this".'

BIBLIOGRAPHY

ADIT, G. A., Camargo, C. A. and Mansbach, J. M., 'Association between serum 25-hydroxyvitamin D and upper respiratory tract infection in third national health and nutrition examination survey', *Archives of Internal Medicine*, (2009), p. 169.

AKUTHOTA, V., Garvan, C., Lindberg, K., Plastaras, C., Press, J. and Tobey, J., 'The effect of long-distance bicycling on ulnar and median nerves: an electrophysiologic evaluation of cyclist palsy', *American Journal of Sports Medicine*, 33 (8) (2005), pp. 1224–1230.

AMINAKA, N., Pietrsimone, G.G., Armstrong, C.W., Meszaros, A., and Gribble, P.A. (2011). Patellofemoral pain syndrome alters neuromuscular control and kinetics during stair ambulation. *Journal of Electromyography and Kinesiology.* Aug 21(4) 645-51.

ARMSTRONG, C., 'Evaluation and management of concussion in athletes: recommendations from the AAN', *American Family Physician*, 89 (7) (2014), pp. 585–587.

ASPLUND, M. D. and St Pierre, P., 'Knee pain and bicycling', *The Physician and Sports Medicine*, 32 (2004), pp. 23–30.

BARTON, C. J., Lack, S., Malliaras, P., and Morrissey, D. (2013). Gluteal muscle activity and patellofemoral pain sydrome: a systematic review. *British Journal of Sports Medicine.* Mar 47(4):207-14

BEELEN, M., Berghuis, J., Bonaparte, B., Ballak, S. B., Jeukendrup, A. E. and van Loon, L. J., 'Carbohydrate mouth rinsing in the fed state: Lack of enhancement of time-trial performance', *International Journal of Sport Nutrition and Exercise Metabolism*, 19 (2009), pp. 400–409.

BERNADO, N. D., Barrios, C., Vera, P., Laiz, C. and Hadala, M., 'Changes in sports injuries incidence over time in world-class road cyclists', *International Journal of Sports Medicine*, (Epub ahead of print, 2014).

BERNADO, N. D., Barrios, C., Vera, P., Laiz, C. and Hadala, M., 'Incidence and risk for traumatic and overuse injuries in top-level road cyclists', *Journal of Sports Science*, 30 (10) (2012), pp. 1047–1053.

BENARDOT, D., 'Fluids and electrolytes', *Advanced Sports Nutrition* (Human Kinetics, 2006), pp. 75–100.

BRUKNER, P. and Khan, K., 'Pain in the Achilles region', *Clinical Sports Medicine*, (2012), pp. 776–805.

BRUKNER, P. and Khan, K., 'Shoulder pain', *Clinical Sports Medicine*, (2012), pp. 342–376.

BRUKNER, P. and Khan, K., 'Sports concussion', *Clinical Sports Medicine*, (2012), pp. 272–289.

BURKE, L., 'Nutrition for recovery after training and competition', *Clinical Sports Nutrition*, (2010), pp. 358–392.

CARTER, J. M., Jeukendrup, A. E. and Jones, D. A., 'The effect of carbohydrate mouth rinse on 1-h cycle time trial performance', *Medicine & Science in Sports & Exercise*, 36 (2004), pp. 2107–2111.

CLARSEN, B., Krosshaug, T. and Bahr, R., 'Overuse injuries in professional road cyclists', *American Journal of Sports Medicine*, 38 (12) (2010), pp. 2494–2501.

CLIFFT, J. K., Coleman, F. A. and Malone, C. B., 'Vascular disorder in a competitive cyclist: a case report', *Physiotherapy Theory and Practice*, 30 (7) (2014), pp. 517–520.

COYLE, E. F. and Hemmert, A. R., 'Effects of detraining on cardiovascular responses to exercise: role of blood volume', *Journal of Applied Physiology*, 35 (2014), pp. 119–126.

CRANE, J. D., Ogborn, D., Cupido, C., Melov, S., Hubbard, A., Bourgeois, J. M. and Tarnopolsky, M., 'Massage therapy attenuates inflammatory signalling after exercise-induced muscle damage', Science Translational Medicine Journal 4 (2012), pp. 119–119ra13.

ELLIS, R., Hing, W. and Reid, D., 'Iliotibial band friction syndrome – a systematic review', *Manual Therapy*, 12 (3) (2007), pp. 200–8.

FAIRCLOUGH, J., Hayashi, K., Toumi, H., Lyons, K., Bydder, G., Phillips, N., Best, T. M. and Benjamin, M., 'The functional anatomy of the iliotibial band during flexion and extension of the knee: implications for understanding iliotibial band syndrome', *Journal of Anatomy*, 208 (3) (2006), pp. 309–316.

FARRELL, K. C., Reisinger, K. D. and Tillman, M. D., 'Force and repetition in cycling: possible implications for iliotibial band friction syndrome', The Knee International Journal 10 (1) (2003), pp. 103–109.

FERNANDEZ-GARCIA, B., Alvarez Fernandez, J., Vega Garcia, F., Terrados, N., Rodriguez-Alonso, M., Alvarez Rodriguez, E., Rodriguez Olay, J. J., Llaneza Coso, J. M., Carreno Morrondo, J. A., Angeles Menendez-Herrero and M., Maria Gutierrez J., 'Diagnosing external iliac endofibrosis by postexercise ankle to arm index in cyclists', *Medicine & Science in Sports & Exercise*, 34 (2) (2002), pp. 222–227.

FRADKIN, A. J., Zazryn, T. R. and Smoliga J. M., 'Effects of warming-up on physical performance: a systematic review with meta-analysis', *The Journal of Strength and Conditioning Research*, (2010), pp. 140–148.

GANIO, M. S., et al., 'Effect of caffeine on sport-specific endurance performance: a systematic review', *The Journal of Strength and Conditioning Research*, (2009), pp. 315–324.

GARDNER, A., Iverson, G. L and McCrory, P., 'Chronic traumatic encephalopathy in sport: a systemic review', *British Journal of Sports Medicine*, 48 (2) (2014), pp. 84–90.

GODEK, S. F., Bartolozzi, A. R., Burkholder, R., Sugarman, E. and Dorshimer, G., 'Core temperature and percentage dehydration in professional linemen and backs during pre season practice', *Journal of Athletic Training*, 41 (2006), pp. 8–17.

HARVIE, D., O'Leary, T. and Kumar, S., 'A systematic review of randomized controlled trials on exercise parameters in the treatment of patellofemoral pain: what works?', *Journal of Multidisciplinary Healthcare*, 4 (2011), pp. 383–392.

HEALEY, K. C., Hatfield, D. L., Blanpied, P., Dorfman, L. R. and Riebe, D., 'The effects of myofascial release with foam rolling on performance', *The Journal of Strength and Conditioning Research*, 28 (1) (2014), pp. 61–68.

HEMILÄ, H and Chalker, E., 'Vitamin C for preventing and treating the common cold' (The Cochrane Library, 2013).

HERBERT, R. D., de Noronha, M. and Kamper, S. J., 'Stretching to prevent or reduce muscle soreness after exercise', *Cochrane Database System Review*, 6 (7) (2011).

HERMAN, S. L. and Smith, D. T., 'Four week dynamic stretching warm-up intervention elicits longer-term performance benefits', *Journal of Strength and Conditioning*, 22 (2008), pp. 1286–1297.

HUMPHRIES, D., 'Unilateral vulval hypertrophy in competitive female cyclists', *British Journal of Sports Medicine*, (2002), pp. 462–464.

HYOON, M. W., Johnson, N. A., Chapman, P. G. and Burke, L. M., 'The effect of nitrate supplementation on exercise performance in healthy individuals: a systematic review and meta-analysis', *International Journal of Sports Nutrition and Exercise Metabolism*, (2013), pp. 522–532.

JEUKENDRUP, A. E., 'Carbohydrate and exercise performance: the role of multiple transportable carbohydrates', *Current Opinion in Clinical Nutrition and Metabolic Care*, 13 (4) (2010), pp. 452–457.

JEUKENDRUP, A. E., 'The new carbohydrate intake recommendations', *Nestlé Nutrition Institute Workshop Series* (Epub 16 April, 2013).

JEUKENDRUP, A. E., 'A step towards personalised sports nutrition: carbohydrate intake during exercise', *Sports Medicine*, (2014), pp. 25–33.

JONES, G., 'More than just a game: research developments and issues in competitive anxiety in sport. The psychology of concentration in sport performance', British Journal of Psychology (2011), pp. 2044–8295.

KAY, A. D. and Blazevich, A., 'Effect of Acute Static Stretch on Maximal Muscle Performance: A Systematic Review', *Medicine & Science in Sports & Exercise*, 44 (2012), pp. 154–164.

KEELMAN, M., 'Under recovery and overtraining: Different concepts – similar impact?', *Human Kinetics*, (2002), pp. 219–229.

KOYACS, E. R., Schmahl, R., Senden, J. and Brouns, F., 'Effects of high and low rates of fluid intake on post-exercise rehydration', *International Journal of Sport Nutrition and Exercise Metabolism*, 12 (2002), pp. 14–23.

KUIPERS, H. and Keizer, H., 'Overtraining in elite athletes. Review and directions for the future', *Sports Medicine*, (1998), pp. 79–92.

LEE, H. K, Hwang, I. H., Kim, S. Y. and Pyo, S. Y., 'The effect of exercise on prevention of the common cold: a meta-anaylsis of randomised controlled trial studies', *Korean Journal of Family Medicine*, (2013), pp. 119–126.

MACDONALD, G. Z., Button, D., Drinkwater, E. and Behm, D., 'Foam rolling as a recovery tool after an intense bout of physical activity', *Medicine & Science in Sports & Exercise*, (2014), pp. 131–412.

MARGONATO, V., Casasco, M. and Veicsteinas, A., 'Effects of stretching on maximal anaerobic power: the roles of active and passive warm ups', *The Journal of Strength and Conditioning Research*, 22 (2008), pp. 794–800.

MARTETSCHLÄGER, F., Gaskill, T. R. and Millett, P. J., 'Management of clavicle non-union and malunion', *Journal of Shoulder and Elbow Surgery*, 22 (6) (2013), pp. 862–868.

MASCAL, C.L., Landel, R., abd Powers. (2003). 'Management of patellofemoral pain targeting hip, pelvis and trunk muscle function: 2 case reports', *Journal of Orthopaedic and Sports Physical Therapy*. Nov 33(11): 747-60

MAUGHAN, R. J., 'Impact of mild dehydration on wellness and on exercise performance', *European Journal of Clinical Nutrition*, 57 (2003), S19–23.

MAUGHAN, R. J., 'Fluid and carbohydrate intake during exercise', *Clinical Sports Nutrition*, (2010), pp. 330–357.

MCCRORY, P., Meeuwisse, W. H., Aubry, M., Cantu, B., Dvorák, J., Echemendia, R. J., Engebretsen, L., Johnston, K., Kutcher, J. S., Raftery, M., Sills, A., Benson, B. W., Davis, G. A., Ellenbogen, R. G., Guskiewicz, K., Herring, S. A., Iverson, G. L., Jordan, B. D., Kissick, J., McCrea, M., McIntosh, A. S., Maddocks, D., Makdissi, M., Purcell, L., Putukian, M., Schneider, K., Tator, C. H. and Turner, M., 'Consensus statement on concussion in sport: the 4th International Conference on Concussion in Sport held in Zurich', *British Journal of Sports Medicine*, 47 (2013), pp. 250–258.

MOUNTAIN, S. J., Sawka, M. N. and Wenger, C. B., 'Hyponatreamia associated with exercise: risk factors and pathogenesis', *Exercise and Sports Sciences Reviews*, (2001), pp. 113–117.

MUELLER, S. M., Gehrig, S. M., Frese, S., Wagner, C. A., Boutellier, U. and Toigo, M., 'Multiday acute sodium bicarbonate intake improves endurance capacity and reduces acidosis in men', *International Society of Sports Nutrition*, (2013), pp. 10–16.

PARTIN, S. N., Connell, K. A., Schrader, S., LaCombe, J., Lowe, B., Sweeney, A., Reutman, S., Wang, A., Toennis, C., Melman, A., Mikhail, M. and Guess, M. K., 'The bar sinister: does handlebar level damage the pelvic floor in female cyclists?', *The Journal of Sexual Medicine*, (2012), p. 1367.

REES, J. D., Maffulli, N. and Cook, J., 'Management of tendinopathy', *American Journal of Sports Medicine*, 37 (9) (2009), pp. 1855–1867.

RES, P. T., Groen, B., Pennings, B., Beelen, M., Wallis, G. A., Gijsen, A. P., Senden, J. M. and van Loon, L. J., 'Protein ingestion before sleep improves post exercise overnight recovery', *Medicine & Science in Sports & Exercise*, (2012), pp. 1560–1590.

SAIGAL, R. and Berger, M. S., 'The long-term effects of repetitive mild head injuries in sports', *Neurosurgery*, 4 (2014), pp. 49–55.

SALAI, M., Brosh, T., Blankstein, A., Oran, A. and Chechik, A., 'Effect of changing the saddle angle on the incidence of low back pain in recreational bicyclists', *British Journal of Sports Medicine*, 33 (6) (1999), pp. 398–400.

SANNER, W. H. and O'Halloran, W. D., 'The biomechanics, etiology, and treatment of cycling injuries', *Journal of the American Podiatric Medical Association*, 90 (7) (2000), pp. 354–376.

SAWKA, M. N. and Burke, L., 'Exercise and fluid replacement', *American College of Sports Medicine*, (2007), pp. 377-390

SCHULZ, S. and Gordon, S., 'Recreational cyclists: the relationship between low back pain and training characteristics', *International Journal of Exercise Science*, 3 (3) (2010), pp. 79–85.

SCHWELLNUS, M. P. and Derman, E. W., 'Common injuries in cycling: Prevention, diagnosis and management', *South African Family Practice*, 47 (7) (2005), pp. 14–19.

SFORZO, G. and Braun, W., 'Delayed onset of muscle soreness', *American College of Sports Medicine*, (2011), pp. 114-119

SILBERMAN, M. R., 'Bicycling injuries', *Current Sports Medicine Reports*, 12 (5) (2013), pp. 337–345.

SINCLAIR, J., Bottoms, L., Flynn, C., Bradley, E., Alexander, G., McCullagh, S., Finn, T. and Hurst H. T., 'The effects of different durations of carbohydrate mouth rinse on cycling performance', *European Journal of Sport Science*, (2014), pp. 259–264.

SLANE, J., Timmerman, M., Ploeg, H. L. and Thelan, D. G., 'The influence of glove and hand position on pressure over the ulnar nerve during cycling', *Clinical Biomechanics*, 26 (6) (2011), pp. 642–648.

TATOR, C. H., 'Chronic traumatic encephalopathy: how serious a sports problem is it?', *British Journal of Sports Medicine*, 48 (2) (2014), pp. 81–83.

THACKER, S. B., Gilchrist, J. and Stroup, D. F., 'The impact of stretching on sports injury risk: a systematic review of the literature', *Medicine & Science in Sports & Exercise*, (2004), pp. 443–449.

TOMARUS, E. K. and MacIntosh, B., 'Less is more: standard warm-up causes fatigue and less warm-up permits greater cycling output', *Journal of Applied Physiology*, (2011), pp. 228–35.

TUFANO, J. J., Brown, L. E., Coburn, J., Tsang, K., Cazas, V. and LaPorta, J., 'Effect of aerobic recovery intensity on delayed-onset muscle soreness and strength', *The Journal of Strength and Conditioning Research*, (2012), pp. 2777–2782.

VAN TASSEL, D., Owens, B. D., Pointer, L. and Moriatis Wolf, J., 'Incidence of clavicle fractures in sports: analysis of the NEISS database', *International Journal of Sports Medicine*, 35 (1) (2014), pp. 83–86.

VÖLK, M. K., Barrett, B., Kiefer, D., Bauer, R., Woelkart, K. A. and Linde, K., 'Echinacea for preventing and treating the common cold' (The Cochrane Library, 2014).

WALL, B. A., Watson, G., Peiffer, J., Abbiss, C., Siegel, R. and Laursen, P., 'Current hydration guidelines are erroneous: dehydration does not impair exercise performance in the heat', *British Journal of Sports Medicine*, (2013), pp. 385–391.

WITVROUW, E., Mahieu, N., Danneels, L. and McNair, P., 'Stretching and Injury Prevention', *Sports Medicine*, (2004), pp. 443–449.

WOODMAN, T. and Hardy, L., 'The relative impact of cognitive anxiety and self confidence upon sport performance: a meta analysis', *Journal of Sports Sciences*, 21 (2011), pp. 443–457.

INDEX

ACKNOWLEDGEMENTS

Thank you to all the riders who have featured throughout the book. Without your advice, insight and Cycling Nirvanas, this book wouldn't have worked.

Thanks to Charlotte Croft and Nick Ascroft at Bloomsbury, and a special thanks to Sarah Cole and the rest of the Bloomsbury team for both holding and bringing the book together. Thanks to the photographers Eddie Macdonald and Grant Pritchard and to David Luxton for getting the show on the road.

Our particular thanks goes to Daniel Lloyd for agreeing to spend an entire day (and a half) in a hot, sweaty photo studio being pushed and pulled apart for the benefit of demonstrating our exercises. Thanks to Danny Murphy for saving the day with the fill in shots and to Eric Goodman and all the guys at Foundation Training for their passion, assistance and permission to advocate and deliver some of their excellent work.

To all the MDs and physios – you know who you are – for unreservedly letting us pick your brains. Big thanks to Rapha for supplying the kit used throughout the exercise demonstrations. Our overwhelming thanks to Graham Watson, whose mark is stamped all over this book, for kindly allowing us to use his iconic photography. Special thanks to Sir Bradley Wiggins for providing the Foreword, putting injury into context and believing in this project.

Finally unreserved thanks to Alix for having the patience and being on call 24/7, yet will never get any official recognition for her work and to Gemma for keeping Rob sane when it seemed like this project would never end.

PICTURE CREDITS

All inside images © Graham Watson with the exception of the following: pp. 159–200 © Grant Pritchard and Eddie MacDonald; pp.29, 31 and 53 © Shutterstock.com; p.8 © Maxisport/Shutterstock.com; p.18 © PhotoStock10/Shutterstock.com; pp.2–3 © Yoshikazu Tsuno/AFP/Getty Images; pp.7 (top) and 205-6, 31, 48, 97, 155, 219, 221 and 222 © Bryn Lennon/Getty Images; p.7 (bottom) © Asron Ontiveroz/The Denvor Post via Getty Images; p.15 © Kristof Van Accom/Getty Images Europe; p.19 (top) © Miguel Riopa/AFP/Getty Images; p.20 © Universal Images Group Editorial/Getty Images; p.28 © Nigel Roddis/Getty Images Europe; pp.37 and 115 © Aaron Ontiveroz/Getty Images; pp.39 and 41 © Doug Pensinger/Getty Images; p.46 (left-hand image) © Adrian Dennis/AFP/Getty Images; p.50 (left-hand image) © Javier Soriano/Getty Images; p.50 (right-hand image) © Jasper Juinen/Getty Images; p.52 © Pascal Pavani/Getty Images; p.62 © artparadigm/Getty Images; p.64 © Grant Pritchard; pp.65 and 216 © Lionel Bonaventure/Getty Images; pp.81-1 © Karim Jaafar/Getty Images; pp.98 and 112 © Joel Saget/Getty Images; p.109 © Jung Yeon-JE/Getty Images; p.110 © Daniel Petty/Getty Images; p.122 © Scott Mitchell/Getty Images; pp.130–1 © Jan Greune/Look-foto/Getty Images; p.139 © Chris Bolin/Getty Images; p.142 © Press Association Images; p.151 © BSIP/Getty Images; p.158 © GibsonPictures/Getty Images; p.161 © Ruth Jenkinson/Getty Images; p.210 and 219 © Lars Ronbog/Getty Images; p.230 © Francois Nell/Getty Images Europe.

AQA English Language B

A2

Mark Saunders
Felicity Titjen

A2 Series Editor
Mark Saunders

ornes

Published in 2009 by:
Nelson Thornes Ltd
Delta Place
27 Bath Road
CHELTENHAM
GL53 7TH
United Kingdom

11 12 13 / 10 9 8 7 6 5 4

A catalogue record for this book is available from the British Library

ISBN 978 0 7487 9852 0

Cover photograph by Photolibrary
Illustrations include artwork drawn by Harry Venning, Peters and Zabransky UK Ltd and Pantek Arts
Page make-up by Pantek Arts, Maidstone, Kent
Printed in China by 1010 Printing International Ltd

Acknowledgements

The authors and publishers wish to thank the following for permission to use copyright material:

p7 Fig. 4, Taken from the resource 'What's in a name? An introduction to language study at AS level' © 2005 www.teachit.co.uk; p8, Pamela Grunwell for material from Pamela Grunwell, *PACS: Phonological Assessment of Child Speech*, NFER-Nelson (1985); p10 Jane Hale for Rachel's first words; p11 Fig. 6, Fotolia; p13, Continuum International Publishing Group for an extract from Clare Painter, *Into the Mother Tongue: A Case Study in Early Language Development* (1984); pp16,18 and 20, Cengage Learning Services Ltd for Tables 1, 12 and 14 from Jean Stilwell Peccei, *Child Language* (1999); p17 Fig. 10, iStockphoto; p18, Laura Grimes; p19, Cengage.com for an extract from Victoria Fromkin, Robert Rodman and Nina Hyams, *An Introduction to Language*, 8E. Copyright © 2007 Heinle/Arts & Sciences, a part of Cengage Learning, Inc.; p20, Amanda Coultas; pp21 and 22, Jess Darby; p22, Jean Berko Gleason © 2006; pp25 and 26, Amanda Coultas; p26 Fig. 14, Fotolia; p27, Laura Grimes; p28, Amanda Coultas; p29 Fig. 15, Fotolia; p30, Penguin Books Ltd for extract from David Crystal, *Listen To Your Child: A Parents' Guide to Children's Language* (1986). Copyright © David Crystal 1986; p30, Jess Darby; p37 Fig. 16, Fotolia; p37 Fig. 17, Fotolia; p39, Julia Donaldson and Axel Scheffler, The Gruffalo, Macmillan Children's Books, 1999; p43, Oxford University Press for material from Roderick Hunt and Alex Brychta, *Oxford Reading Tree: Stage 8: Storybooks (Magic Key): Victorian Adventure* (1990); p47 Fig. 18, Fotolia; p63 Fig. 20, Fotolia; pp64 and 65, Jess Darby; p68, Oxford University Press for material from Roderick Hunt and Alex Brychta, *Stage 8: More Magpie Workbooks: Flood!* (2003); p73 Fig. 3, iStockphoto; p74 Fig. 4, Alamy; p77, Oxford University Press for definition of 'Nice' from Oxford English Dictionary, eds J. Simpson & E. Weiner (1989); p79, Penguin Books Ltd for extract from Richard Curtis and Ben Elton, *Blackadder: The Whole Damn Dynasty*, Michael Joseph (1998). © Richard Curtis and Ben Elton 1987; p79 Fig. 6, BBC Motion Gallery; p84, The Random House Group Ltd for material from Ainsley Harriott, *Meals in Minutes*, BBC Books (1998); pp87 and 92, University Librarian and Director, The John Rylands University Library, The University of Manchester for material from John Gabriel Stedman, *Narrative of a Five Years' Expedition Against the Revolted Negroes of Surinam*, 1796; p85 Fig. 8, iStockphoto; p87 Fig. 9, Fotolia; p91, Nicholas Culpeper, *The English Phyfitian Enlarged*, 1676; p92 Fig. 10, Alamy; p93, Darren McClelland, Rodney and Inge for material from www.travelblog.org; p94, Hester Thrale Piozzi, *Observations and Reflections Made in the Course of a Journey Through France, Italy and Germany*, 1789; p95, Cambridge University Press for material from David Crystal, *The Cambridge Encyclopedia of the English Language*, 2nd edition (2003); p98, DC Thomson & Co Ltd for material from 'The Cathy and Claire page' from *Best of Jackie Magazine*, Prion Books (2005); p100 Fig. 11, Fotolia; p101, British Library Newspapers for pages from the *Leedes Intelligencer*, 19 May 1761 and *The Times*, 10 January 1806. © British Library Board; p102, The Press for material from the *Yorkshire Evening Press*, 2 May 1945; p105, Palgrave Macmillan for material (bulleted list) from Dennis Freeborn, *Varieties of English* (1993); p106, DC Thomson & Co Ltd for material from 'The Four Marys' in *Bunty* Book (1963); and 'The Four Marys' in *Bunty* Book (2001); p108 Fig. 12, Fotolia; p109 Fig. 13, Alamy; p111, Universal Press Syndicate for Lynn Johnston, 'For Better Or For Worse', 22 April 2007. Copyright © 2007 Lynn Johnston; p113, Jean Aitchison, The Language Web, The Power and Problem of Words – The 1996 BBC Reith Lectures (1996); p115 (top), Ingrid Tieken-Boon van Ostade for material from Ann Fisher, *A Practical New Grammar with Exercises of Bad English*, 1789; p115 (bottom), unable to trace; p117, Solo Syndication for material from John Humphrys, 'I H8 text speak', *The Daily Mail*, 24 September 2007; p121, Trustees of the Keep Military Museum for Private Honey, 'Camp Before Sebastapol, Nov 20 1854'; p122, Georgina Foss; p128 Fig. 2, Fotolia; p130 Fig. 3, Fotolia; p134 Fig. 5, Alamy; p134 Fig. 6, Alamy; p136 Fig. 7, Fotolia; p141 Fig.10, Alamy; p149 Fig. 13, Silly Pig, by Sue Graves © Parragon Books Ltd, 2004; p150, Parragon Books Ltd for material from Sue Graves, *Silly Pig Has An Idea* (2004); p153, Cambridge University Press for material from Jenny Cheshire, *Variation in an English Dialect. A Sociolinguistic Study* (1982); p154, Joanna Przedlacka for material from www.phon.ox.ac.uk; p157 Fig. 14, Fotolia; p168 Fig. 1, Fotolia; p170, Beverley D'Silva for material from her article, 'Mind your language', *The Observer*, 10 December 2000; p171, British Broadcasting Company with Ian Peacock and Michael Rosen for material from Word of Mouth, BBC Radio 4; p172 Fig. 3, Alamy.

Every effort has been made to contact the copyright holders and we apologise if any have been overlooked. Should copyright have been unwittingly infringed in this book, the owners should contact the publishers, who will make the corrections at reprint.

Contents

AQA introduction

Nelson Thornes has worked in partnership with AQA to ensure this book and the accompanying online resources offer you the best support for your GCSE course.

All resources have been approved by senior AQA examiners so you can feel assured that they closely match the specification for this subject and provide you with everything you need to prepare successfully for your exams.

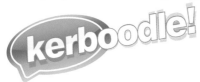

These print and online resources together **unlock blended learning**; this means that the links between the activities in the book and the activities online blend together to maximise your understanding of a topic and help you achieve your potential.

These online resources are available on **kerboodle!** which can be accessed via the internet at **http://www.kerboodle.com/live**, anytime, anywhere. If your school or college subscribes to this service you will be provided with your own personal login details. Once logged in, access your course and locate the required activity.

For more information and help visit **http://www.kerboodle.com**

Icons in this book indicate where there is material online related to that topic. The following icons are used:

💡 Learning activity

These resources include a variety of interactive and non-interactive activities to support your learning.

✅ Progress tracking

These resources include a variety of tests that you can use to check your knowledge on particular topics (Test yourself) and a range of resources that enable you to analyse and understand examination questions (On your marks…).

🔎 Research support

These resources include WebQuests, in which you are assigned a task and provided with a range of weblinks to use as source material for research.

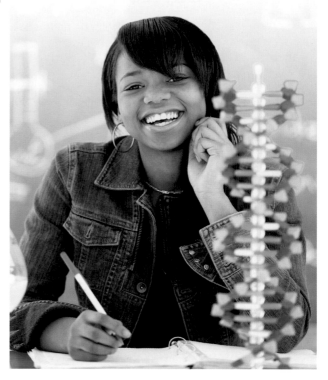

📝 Study skills

These resources support you and help develop a skill that is key for your course, for example planning essays.

🔍 Analysis tool

These resources feature text extracts that can be highlighted and annotated by the user according to specific objectives.

How to use this book

This book covers the specification for your course and is arranged in a sequence approved by AQA.

Its structure mirrors the specification exactly: it is split into two units (Unit 3 Developing language and Unit 4 Investigating language), each of which is divided into Sections A and B. Each section begins with an introduction to the topics that will be covered and concludes with exam (Unit 3) or coursework (Unit 4) preparation. At the back of the book you will find feedback on the activities and exercises, and a glossary of key terms.

The features in this book include:

Learning objectives

At the beginning of each section you will find a list of learning objectives that contain targets linked to the requirements of the specification.

■ Key terms

Terms that you will need to be able to define and understand.

■ Research points

Linguistic research that has been carried out in the area you are studying.

Thinking points

Questions that check your understanding of the research point.

■ Activities

Classroom, Language around you and Extension activities all appear throughout. Coursework activities appear throughout Unit 4.

■ Links

Links to other areas in the textbook which are relevant to what you are reading.

■ Data response exercises

Questions based on given data.

■ Further reading

Suggestions for other texts that will help you in your study and preparation for assessment.

AQA Examiner's tip

Hints from AQA examiners to help you with your study and to prepare for your exam.

AQA Examination-style questions

Questions in the style that you can expect in your exam. AQA examination questions are reproduced by permission of the Assessment and Qualifications Alliance.

Nelson Thornes is responsible for the solution(s) given and they may not constitute the only possible solution(s).

■ Transcription conventions

In order to make analysis of transcripts easier and more predictable for you, the AQA specification follows particular conventions that you need to be aware of. This information is provided to help you interpret the data, exploring some of the reasons for these features in the light of the specific contexts of the speech. You should refer to this key for all the transcripts provided in the book.

Key:

(.) indicates a normal pause

(2.0) Numbers within brackets indicate length of pause in seconds

Words between vertical lines are spoken simultaneously

:: indicates elongated sounds

Underlining indicates a stress placed on this syllable

Capital letters indicates volume

Other contextual information is in italics in square brackets

Phonemic symbols are set within square brackets

■ Weblinks in the book

As Nelson Thornes is not responsible for third party content online, there may be some changes to this material that are beyond our control. In order for us to ensure that the links referred to in the book are as up-to-date and stable as possible, the websites are usually homepages with supporting instructions on how to reach the relevant pages if necessary.

Please let us know at **kerboodle@nelsonthornes.com** if you find a link that doesn't work and we will do our best to redirect the link, or to find an alternative site.

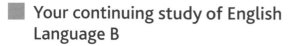

Introduction to this book

Your continuing study of English Language B

Your AS Level studies have, no doubt, whetted your appetite for linguistics, and given you a fresh perspective on the language that surrounds you each and every day. You are now a seasoned linguist, and I am sure that you are enjoying your new-found insight: maybe you can't help analysing the differences in the way your male and female friends interact in conversation with you, or perhaps you are now conscious of the orthographical choices you make when you text with your mobile phone. There are many ways in which a wider awareness of language enhances your life – and, at A Level, you are about to extend these horizons even further.

You will now know that the way you approach texts and language at Advanced Level is quite different from your GCSE experiences of textual analysis, original writing, investigation and discussion. You have put your natural interest in language to work on the study of linguistics, and that can indeed be a weird and wonderful world.

Midway along the path from GCSE English, through to AS Level, and then A Level study, you are now much better acquainted with the challenges involved. The AS level course gave you the opportunity to build on your original writing abilities and skills of textual analysis. In the A Level units, you will deepen your knowledge and understanding of these areas and add new approaches, including that of language investigation, and an increasingly academic approach to working with existing research and theory.

At A Level, the skill of textual analysis remains a fundamental part of the AQA GCE English Language B experience. The knowledge of word classes, grammatical structures, semantics, graphological elements and phonology you developed during your AS Level studies will underpin the analytical work that you undertake in the A Level units. Of course, the adverbs, clauses and syllables you can spot in the language remain the same as they were before; only now you will need to bring them into your work with increasing frequency and confidence, and understand the way that these different layers of language interact in complex situations – like those you will encounter in learning about child language acquisition, or in pursuing your own language investigation.

The opportunity to produce some of your own writing is also retained at A Level, although it is given more of a supporting role in relation to the more dominant newcomer, the language investigation. Your original writing will definitely be a work of non-fiction this time, taking up the voice of a particular aspect of language and allowing you to articulate your own understanding and thoughts on the issues involved. The editorial know-how that you developed in Unit 2 will stand you in good stead when producing this text, as you work to blend the intellectual quality of your discussion of the topic, with a creative eye and ear for what works in the varied and vivid language of the media.

However, it is the language investigation in Unit 4 that perhaps most profoundly epitomises the nature and spirit of A Level English study. The debates that you have engaged with at AS Level surrounding the interrelation of gender, power and technology with language are joined by new voices from the Unit 3 Developing language material. From the veritable linguistic feast that these serve up, you will be able to start to take out your own samples of language use and begin to experiment with your own tastes and ideas. The project that ensues will be a piece of true, independent scholarship. You will be able to take social variables (for example, gender, age, ethnicity, social class) and linguistic variables (for example, the glottal stop, sentence types or slang) that you have encountered elsewhere in the course, and measure and test them in ways of your own devising, writing up your findings academically, for posterity – and even for coursework!

How is English Language B assessed at A Level?

You will already be familiar with the assessment breakdown at AS Level, and there is still coursework at A2 Level, which amounts to 40 per cent of the A Level marks. Again, there is a good balance of the ways in which you will be assessed, and the coursework helps you to embark upon the sort of independent study and exploration that A Level work makes possible.

The Unit 3 examination counts for the remaining 60 per cent of the A Level marks. One important thing to remember is that the marks you get in the AS and A Level each count equally towards your overall grade. Therefore the percentage for each unit is halved in the final analysis: AS Unit 1 exam becomes 30 per cent, Unit 2 coursework 20 per cent; the A2 Unit 3 exam counts for 30 per cent, and the Unit 4 coursework, 20 per cent of the final outcome.

The same four assessment objectives (AOs) used in your AS units continue into the A2 units. The way that your coursework and examinations are marked is governed by these AOs, and you'll find plenty of detail in this book to help you understand exactly what they mean for Units 3 and 4. The four AOs used in 'Spec B Lang' help to emphasise the importance of communicating your ideas clearly, using linguistic approaches well, placing the language examples that you deal with in context, and developing your creative abilities. Just as with your AS Level units, it is a good idea to get to know the way that these AOs are shared out in the A Level units, to help you make sure your work fits them as well as possible.

What does each unit cover?

The units presented in this textbook are carefully designed to meet the expectations that the AQA examination board has of what you can achieve as an A Level student. The two units at AS Level, fully covered in the AS Level book, introduced you to a wide range of skills, all of which can be built upon at A Level. The main areas of analytical writing, textual analysis, language debates, and even your own original writing are all developed in the content of Units 3 and 4.

The Unit 3 examination, 'Developing language', looks at two very different ways in which the English language can be seen to develop: the personal, somewhat miraculous development of the way that children acquire language on the one hand; and, on the other, the way that the English language as a whole has changed over time, and is developing still.

You may well remember (or have been told by your parents) anecdotes of how you learned to speak. Your study of language acquisition will help you to make some sense of this most beguiling of linguistic enquiries – how do we all learn something as complex as language apparently so intuitively and simply? After understanding some of the main approaches adopted by researchers, this unit takes the issue further, tackling the wider issues of literacy and the way in which reading and writing are mastered by children.

On a larger scale, studying language change will take you on a tour of several hundred years of linguistic history and chart the path of English right through to the present day. This added dimension of time will bring you into contact with texts that reveal some of the many different faces of English over time, and the character of a language that has made its ability to morph and adapt a definitive virtue – one that has enabled it to survive and grow so successfully.

In the Unit 4 coursework, you get the chance to investigate a particular area of the language in more detail. To prepare for this unit, look back over the topics that you have studied at AS and A Level, and choose something you have nurtured a real interest in. This can be an excellent way to explore an area that you may want to go on to study further (for example, journalistic writing from your coursework from Unit 2), or even forge a career in (for example, the language of technology from Unit 1, or supporting children's literacy, from Unit 3).

As well as producing an investigative project, Unit 4 also affords the opportunity to add your own voice to the area of language you have chosen to focus on. You will be asked to produce a media text of some kind, designed to communicate ideas related to your investigative topic – be it in the form of a careful article giving detailed advice, or a spirited editorial debating a heated language issue.

Where could it take you?

So, what *does* the future hold for a linguist? English Language is certainly a subject very well regarded by Higher Education institutions, and because you are studying the thing that you will probably use the most whatever you do in life – your language – it easily complements any educational course you might follow, and provides a new perspective on most conceivable professions.

At university, there is a considerable range of English-related courses available, that directly build on one or more aspects of your work at AS and A Level, from creative writing through to speech therapy. However, outside the wider school of English, your knowledge and skills will share ground with the many subjects within the social sciences, and particularly with psychology, sociology and law-related courses. Even further afield, it is not difficult to see the value of a sophisticated understanding of English in areas of design, business, computer science – in almost anything you could imagine, really.

When you come to begin a career, you will find linguistic study will make you an attractive, skilled and flexible employee in most services and industries. Whether it is the increased insight you can bring to analysing written or spoken language, or your ability to control and shape your own communication, abilities of this nature will prove a real benefit to you. Even some of the specific topics you will have studied may find their niche: maybe the language and technology work you have done at AS Level will give you an overview of the impact of technology as you start out as a software designer. Or perhaps the section on language acquisition will help you get to grips with work in childcare and with very young children. You never know, you might even want to start teaching English yourself and pass your ideas on!

■ The English Language B series

All of which brings me back to a quick reminder about the Nelson Thornes English Language series. The examination boards have all produced entirely new courses for 2008, with the A Level units rolling out in 2009; AQA have worked exclusively with Nelson Thornes to produce a series of books designed to be an ideal companion and guide to your journey through our language. In addition to these texts, there are support materials for your teachers, and online e-learning resources, which help to create a multi-dimensional and truly blended learning experience. The work that has gone into this collection has been carried out by teachers and examiners who have taught linguistics in schools, colleges and online, with AQA and students, for many years, and have just the right mix of experience and subject knowledge to bring the course to life for you.

The English language holds something for everyone, and I am sure that the step you have taken to embark upon AS and A Level English Language is one that you will enjoy and one which will offer you genuine challenge and personal satisfaction. Use this book to help you, but be prepared to follow your nose too – language is such a tremendous and ever-changing thing, it would be impossible for one book to cover everything. Then, maybe, come back to the book to keep you right on track as you prepare for your exams, your coursework, and success. Finally, let me wish you the very best in your life as a linguist – it should be fun.

Developing language

- AO1 Select and apply a range of linguistic methods, to communicate relevant knowledge using appropriate terminology and coherent, accurate written expression (15 per cent of the A Level mark).

- AO2 Demonstrate critical understanding of a range of concepts and issues related to the construction and analysis of meanings in spoken and written language, using knowledge of linguistic approaches (10 per cent of the A Level mark).

- AO3 Analyse and evaluate the influence of contextual factors on the production and reception of spoken and written language, showing knowledge of the key constituents of language (5 per cent of the A Level mark).

Key terms

Multimodal texts: texts that combine word, image and sound to produce meaning.

By the time you have reached A2 you already know some key concepts and theories surrounding language study, and you may be wondering how the A2 course uses this knowledge. In Unit 3, this is achieved by focusing on two main topics:

- the acquisition of language by children
- the development of and changes in English over time.

Your study of the language used in particular social contexts and the genres of speech, writing and **multimodal texts** first explored in Unit 1, along with your practical experience of writing in Unit 2, are directed in your second year to questions about language development in specific contexts. Detailed breakdowns of the key knowledge required for each section of the unit are provided in each section and topic of this book, but by concentrating on two specific areas you will engage with some of these important questions about language acquisition and development:

- How do children first acquire spoken language and learn to read and write?
- How and why has English changed in both spoken and written forms?

The focus of your A2 is on synopticity, offering opportunities to look at the English language as a whole through your investigation of language in Unit 4, and here, in Unit 3, building on your existing knowledge and understanding with new theories and concepts to test out and evaluate. Above all, this unit is data-based. You will explore real-life texts to illustrate how children encounter language and develop the sophisticated skills they need in order to become effective communicators, and the ways in which English speakers have changed the nature of English to reflect their society and the influences on it. Enjoy the challenges of interpreting children's skilful use of English as they develop communication abilities, and engaging with English in its different forms and varieties over the last three centuries.

The examination tasks

You will be assessed through one written paper of $2\frac{1}{2}$ hours, where you will answer two questions based on a selection of data relating to the topics: one on Language acquisition (Section A) and one on Language change (Section B). You will be able to choose from two questions for each topic. Further advice about how to maximise potential marks is contained in the Examination preparation and assessment topics on pages 62–69 (Section A) and pages 119–123 (Section B), but keep the assessment objectives in mind as you study each topic. Being aware of these will help you prepare for the final examination, focusing you on effective ways to approach the texts you study by:

- demonstrating your linguistic awareness
- applying relevant theories and ideas about the language used
- thinking about important contextual factors.

A Language acquisition

Introduction

In this section you will:

- learn the stages of early spoken language development and children's acquisition of literacy skills, focusing on early reading and writing, from birth to age 11

- evaluate the different theoretical views about child language acquisition

- assess the importance of contextual factors in governing early language and literacy development

- apply and select appropriate linguistic methods, key concepts and relevant contextual factors to data about young children's speech and writing.

Key terms

Idiolect: an individual's own 'linguistic fingerprint'.

Register: a variety of language appropriate to a particular purpose and context.

Section A of Unit 3 concerns the acquisition of language by children up to the age of 11 years. The three particular areas of focus are spoken language and the beginnings of reading and writing. The first topic will help you develop your knowledge of early speech development, the second will cover reading, and the third will cover writing.

What is language acquisition and why is it an important area of study? Well, the understanding of how we, as speakers and communicators, first acquired the ability to use words, string them together in a meaningful way and convey our thoughts and feelings to others must be at the heart of all language study. In fact, it might seem strange that you didn't study this at AS. However, all your AS knowledge about speech and writing modes, the social contexts of language use and the concepts of language use, such as **idiolect** and **register**, will underpin your A2 study of child language. Child language acquisition is a truly synoptic topic, combining all the linguistic areas that you are already able to use in analysing texts, and using them to examine children's speech and literacy development.

Above all, language acquisition relates to all of our experiences. We have all acquired language and learnt to read and write. You might remember humorous anecdotes about your early speech, and your parents may have kept your early attempts at writing because they found them amusing or touching. This might seem quite remote to you now as a competent, adult user of language, but younger family members, interactions in your job role, or seeing children in the social environment should make you a keen observer of language development.

Surprisingly, language acquisition remains a hotly debated topic amongst linguists. Despite the amount of research on all aspects of language acquisition, linguists can't explain every developmental feature. Many opposing views jostle for acceptance, and evaluating these ideas will encourage you to be inquisitive about language development. You could already be thinking about how children acquire language – is it a 'taught' skill or is it just within all humans to communicate through speech? We record our ideas in written form and enjoy reading what other people have written, but are reading and writing instinctive?

Responding to unseen data involving children's speech and literacy development is a compulsory topic area. A sound knowledge of these areas will assist you in making informed choices about the right question to choose in the examination. Opportunities to practise examination questions and to get advice about what you can do to maximise your mark potential are given at the end of this section, and you might be inspired to investigate children's development further for your A2 coursework (covered in Unit 4).

Developing speech

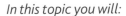 Key terms

Phoneme: the smallest contrastive unit in the sound system of a language.

Phonetics: the study of the sounds used in speech, including how they are produced.

Lexis: the vocabulary of a language.

Semantics: the study of meaning.

Syntax: the way words are arranged to make sentences.

Morphology: the area of language study that deals with the formation of words from smaller units called morphemes.

Phonology: the study of the sound systems of language and how they communicate meaning.

Discourse: a stretch of communication.

Pragmatics: the factors that influence the choices that speakers make in their use of language – why we choose to say one thing rather than another.

Child language skills

Children learn an enormous amount of language very quickly. While learning to say so much, they are also learning many motor skills, such as walking. Therefore, it's important not to criticise them for not talking like adults.

Look at what they have to learn:

- To create individual **phonemes** and phonemic combinations (**phonetics**).

- To use a vocabulary of words and understand their meanings (**lexis/semantics**).

- To combine words in a variety of sentence constructions, changing word formations to express different word classes (**syntax/morphology**).

- To use prosodic features such as pitch, loudness, speed and intonation to convey meaning (**phonology**).

- To structure interactions with others (**discourse**).

- The subtleties of speech such as politeness, implication and irony (**pragmatics**).

This demonstrates why language acquisition study is so important. Children's acquisition of language combines all the linguistic methods used throughout the course – it is the start of the synopticity that your A2 study is all about.

What are the main stages of language development?

As a starting point, an outline of the main stages of development will help you to understand how children acquire language and the ways that sounds (phonology) lead to words (lexis) and then to forming sentences (syntax). You can begin to grasp the complex processes involved in language development.

Later on you will evaluate the different theoretical debates; you might agree with some of the arguments more than others. However, to understand what aspects of speech are acquired by the age of 5 it is important to interpret transcripts of young children's speech. Nobody disputes that the ability to acquire language is universal (i.e. possible by all children in all speech cultures), but there is disagreement about the significance and role of certain factors that influence speech development.

Be aware that the stages outlined offer only approximate timescales. Most parents worry about the milestones their children reach, making comparisons between children in all aspects of their development. Obviously a lack of speech development can indicate particular learning difficulties, but most parental worry is unfounded, as children pass all the developmental thresholds and become successful adult language users.

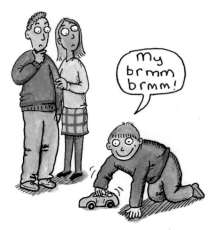

Fig. 1 *Not all children develop speech at the same rate, but most end up as successful adult language users*

Tables 1 and 2 chart the key linguistic stages of development.

Table 1 *The pre-verbal stage*

Stage	Features	Approx. age (months)
Vegetative	Sounds of discomfort or reflexive actions	0–4
Cooing	Comfort sounds and vocal play using open-mouthed vowel sounds	4–7
Babbling	Repeated patterns of consonant and vowel sounds	6–12
Proto-words	Word-like vocalisations, not matching actual words but used consistently for the same meaning (sometimes called 'scribble talk'). For example, using 'mmm' to mean 'give me that', with accompanying gestures such as pointing, supporting the verbal message	9–12

Table 2 *Lexical and grammatical stages of development*

Stage	Features	Approx. age (months)
Holophrastic/ one-word	One-word utterances	12–18
Two-word	Two-word combinations	18–24
Telegraphic	Three and more words combined	24–36
Post-telegraphic	More grammatically complex combinations	36+

During the post-telegraphic stage the acquisition of the key literacy skills of reading and writing starts to develop. This is covered separately in the Developing reading and Developing writing topics later on in this section.

■ Classroom activity 1

Think how children's communication skills develop. Using Tables 1 and 2, create a table like the one below to suggest at what stage lexis, grammar, phonetics/ phonology, pragmatic and discourse skills might develop. For example:

1 Why might phonology be one of the first skills acquired? What are children practising in the pre-verbal stage?

2 When will syntactical awareness develop and how do you think word order might be important?

Stage	Lexis/ semantics	Phonology	Grammar	Pragmatics/ discourse
Pre-verbal				
Holophrastic/ one-word				
Two-word				
Telegraphic				
Post-telegraphic				

You can see that language is acquired very quickly in a child's life; this is a factor that influences some schools of thought about the ways that children learn to communicate.

Research point

Noam Chomsky, an American linguist, believes that learning takes place though an innate brain mechanism, pre-programmed with the ability to acquire grammatical structures. He calls this the **Language Acquisition Device (LAD)**. To him, it is also significant that human languages, although they might seem different, share many similarities, which he describes as **universal grammar**.

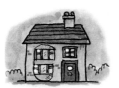

casa/maison/house/
haus/huis

mano/main/hand

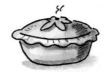

torta/pie/tarte/tarta/
pastel

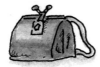

sacchetto/bag/sac/
bolsa/sacola

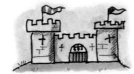

château/schloss/castelo/
castello/castillo/castle

Fig. 2 *Children all round the world are thought to develop language skills in similar stages and at a similar rate*

Supporting this is evidence that children from all around the world develop at a similar rate in similar stages of development. That all children can acquire complex grammars by an early age, regardless of their environment or intelligence, points to an innate learning device – although the actual nature of this has never been pinpointed.

Thinking points

From your experience of learning other languages, what similar features do you think human languages have?

💡 Developing phonology

Producing sound is crucial for any child's language development. From an early age using their vocal cords gets the attention needed for their basic survival and emotional needs. The 'cooing' and 'babbling' stages mark the beginnings of prosodic features. Pitch and tone encode meaning for a listener/receiver of a verbal message; this links to pragmatic development, as prosody is important for social interaction. Crucially, early developments allow the child to increase the variety of sounds produced (**phonemic expansion**) and then reduce the sounds to only those they need for their own language (**phonemic contraction**), showing that children have, at this stage, the potential to learn any language.

Key terms

Language Acquisition Device (LAD): the human brain's inbuilt capacity to acquire language.

Universal grammar: the explanation that all world languages share the principles of grammar despite surface differences in lexis and phonology. Sometimes called linguistic universals.

Phonemic expansion: the variety of sounds produced increases.

Phonemic contraction: the variety of sounds is reduced to the sounds of the main language used.

Table 3 *Stages of phonological development*

Stage	Features	Examples	Approx. age (months)
Vegetative	Sounds of discomfort or reflexive actions	Crying, coughing, burping, sucking	0–4
Cooing	Comfort sounds Vocal play	Grunts and sighs become vowel-like 'coos' Laughter starts Hard consonants and vowels produced Pitch (squeals and growls) and loudness (yells) practised	4–7
Babbling	Extended sounds resembling syllable-like sequences Repeated patterns	Sounds linking to own language Reduplicated sounds ('ba-ba') and non-reduplicated (variegated) such as 'agu'	6–12
Proto-words	Word-like vocalisations		9–12

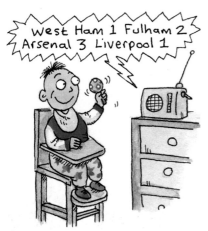

Fig. 3 *Early responses to football scores*

Research point

Linguists have been interested in whether young children can understand the effects of intonation. Intonation is important because it gives a listener clues to the meanings of a speaker's message. We often use pitch to signal our feelings (rising pitch might show excitement) or to give the listener notice that we are giving up our turn to speak (a rising intonation indicates a question).

Alan Cruttenden (1974) compared adults and children to see if they could predict football results from listening to the scores, finding that adults could successfully predict winners by the intonation placed on the first team, but children (up to age 7) were less accurate.

Thinking points

1. Why did Cruttenden use football scores?

2. Why do you think young children are less able to interpret intonation?

Key terms

Consonant: a speech sound that is produced when the vocal tract is either blocked or so restricted that there is audible friction.

How are sounds produced?

Sounds are produced by air from the lungs passing across the vocal cords. The production of **consonant** sounds is affected by:

■ the manner of articulation (how the airstream is controlled)

■ the place of articulation (where it occurs); to make sounds we can use our lips, tongue, teeth and the roof of our mouth, or combine these

■ if the sound is voiced or unvoiced (by vibrating or not vibrating the vocal cords).

Sounding phonemes out loud helps you to hear how and where they are produced. The IPA chart shows the types of sounds produced (consonants, **vowels** and **diphthongs**), but the manner in which sounds are produced is also relevant to children's phonological development.

Consonants	Vowels
p as in **p**et, ca**p** and s**p**ort	ɑː as in b**ar** and f**a**ther
b as in **b**ox and cra**b**	iː as in f**ee**t and sp**ea**k
t as in **t**ap, s**t**ory and co**t**	ɪ as in qu**i**ck
d as in **d**og and co**d**	ɛ as in fr**ie**nd and s**ai**d
tʃ as in **ch**ampion, fea**t**ure and ca**tch**	ɜː as in h**ea**rd and th**i**rd
dʒ as in **g**erm, **j**et and do**dge**	æ as in sp**a**t
k as in **c**aravan, **k**ick, s**k**y, **qu**easy	ʌ as in dr**u**nk and t**ou**gh
g as in **g**arden, da**gg**er and lo**g**	ɒ as in sp**o**t and w**a**sp
f as in **f**it, cou**gh**, **ph**at and bee**f**	ɔː as in t**au**ght, p**o**rt and s**aw**
v as in **v**ein and gi**v**e	ʊ as in f**u**ll
θ as in **th**imble and four**th**	uː as in m**oo**n, tr**ue**, thr**ough** and gr**ew**
ð as in **th**is and smoo**th**	ə as in wat**er** and **a**bove
s as in **s**auce, hi**ss** and **c**inema	eɪ as in pr**ay**, sl**eigh**, gr**ey** and f**a**de
z as in **z**ero, ho**s**e and row**s**	aɪ as in fr**y**, h**igh** and sp**i**der
ʃ as in **sh**op, lo**ti**on, ma**sh** and **s**ugar	ɔɪ as in j**oy** and t**oi**let
ʒ as in lei**s**ure and bei**ge**	əʊ as in g**o**, bl**ow** and t**oe**
h as in **h**air	aʊ as in c**ow** and Sl**ough**
m as in **m**ould, nu**mb** and ja**m**	ɪə as in h**ear**, p**ier** and w**e're**
n as in **n**ight and loa**n**	ɛə as in c**are**, fl**air** and wh**ere**
ŋ as in mi**ng**er and cli**ng**	ʊə as in t**our**
l as in **l**augh and be**l**ow	juː as in b**eau**tiful and st**u**dent
ł as in mi**lk** and te**ll** (Cockney)	
r as in **r**eady and co**rr**upt	
w as in **w**all	
j as in **y**awn	
ʔ as in bu**tt**er and bo**tt**le (Cockney)	
ʍ as in **wh**ich (Scottish)	
x as in lo**ch** (Scottish)	

www.teachit.co.uk

Fig. 4 *IPA symbols for standard English*

■ Key terms

Vowel: a sound made without closure or audible friction.

Diphthong: a vowel in which there is a perceptible change in quality during a syllable.

AQA Examiner's tip

Becoming familiar with the IPA chart and its phonetic symbols may help you analyse children's phonological development in more depth. However, the IPA will be printed on the exam paper if phonetic transcriptions are present, so you don't need to learn it!

Table 4 *The different types of sounds produced*

Types of sound	Voiced	Unvoiced
Plosives are created when the airflow is blocked for a brief time (also called 'stop consonants')	b, d, g	p, t, k
Fricatives are created when the airflow is only partially blocked and air moves through the mouth in a steady stream	v, ð (as in thy), z, ʒ (as in leisure)	f, θ (as in thigh), s, ʃ (as in ship), h
Affricatives are created by putting plosives and fricatives together	dʒ (as in judge)	tʃ (as in church)
Approximants are similar sounds to vowels	w, r, j	
Nasals are produced by air moving through the nose	m, n, ŋ	
Laterals are created by placing the tongue on the ridge of the teeth and then air moving down the side of the mouth	l	

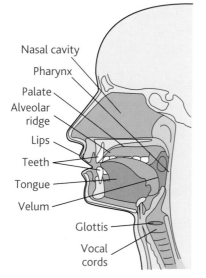

Nasal cavity
Pharynx
Palate
Alveolar ridge
Lips
Teeth
Tongue
Velum
Glottis
Vocal cords

Fig. 5 *The human vocal apparatus*

Classroom activity 2

The table below shows the sounds acquired by age.

Table 5 *Phonological acquisition sequence*

Age (months)	Phoneme
24	p, b, m, d, n, w, t
30	k, g, h, ŋ
36	f, s, j, l
42	tʃ dʒ, v, z, ʃ, r
48+	θ, ð, ʒ

Pamela Grunwell's *sequence from* Phonological Assessment of Child Speech, *1987*

Use this sequence and the information you have on the types of sounds produced to answer these questions:

- ■ In what order do the sounds appear?
- ■ What reasons can you find for this order?

Types of early phonological 'mistake'

One feature of child language acquisition is that children master language by making mistakes until they fully acquire the skills. This 'trial and error' approach is taken by some linguists as evidence that learning is taking place, but as you have seen, phonological development seems also to depend on physical ability to produce sounds.

In phonology the following patterns have been observed.

Table 6 *Early phonological errors*

Term	Explanation	Examples
Deletion	Omitting the final consonant in words	do(g), cu(p)
Substitution	Substituting one sound for another (especially the 'harder' sounds that develop later, such as ʃ)	'pip' for 'ship'
Addition	Adding an extra vowel sound to the ends of words, creating a CVCV pattern	e.g. doggie
Assimilation	Changing one consonant or vowel for another (as in the early plosive sounds 'd' and 'b')	'gog' for 'dog'
Reduplication	Repeating a whole syllable	dada, mama
Consonant cluster reductions	Consonant clusters can be difficult to articulate, so children reduce them to smaller units	'pider' for 'spider'
Deletion of unstressed syllables	Omitting the opening syllable in polysyllabic words	'nana' for 'banana'

Research point

Researchers have looked at children's phonological errors to see how they link to their understanding of words and ideas, as well as their ability to imitate the language surrounding them. In a famous study Jean Berko and Roger Brown (1960s) found that a child who referred to a plastic inflatable fish as a 'fis', substituting the s sound for the sh, couldn't link an adult's use of 'fis' with the same object.

Child: A fis **Adult:** Is this your fis? **Child:** no

Child: A fis **Adult:** is this your fish? **Child:** yes, my fis

Thinking points

1 Why do you think that the child only responded to the adult's correct pronunciation of the noun 'fish'?

2 What does this suggest about a child's ability to imitate adult speech?

Developing lexis

Once children can produce sounds effectively they can use these skills to form 'real' words that others can recognise. By the first-word stage (usually around 12 months) they have already contracted their sounds to those of their main language. Initially, **proto-words** have meaning for the child and their carers, but are less effective with others. So a child needs to acquire the vocabulary that will help them be understood by a wider audience. Together with vocabulary building, a child needs to learn the meanings (semantics) of words in order to link objects and ideas.

Key terms

Proto-word: an invented word that has a consistent meaning.

Table 7 *Rate of lexical development*

Age	Number of words
12 months	50
24 months	200
36 months	2,000

Key terms

Holophrase: a single word expressing a whole idea.

Holophrases and one-word utterances are likely to develop either alongside or after proto-words. The differences between one-word utterances (usually a label for objects) and holophrases (where a word contains an entire sentence meaning) will be covered in more detail when investigating grammatical development.

The first 50 words

Here is a data set of one child's first 50 words.

Data set: Rachel's first words

Jasper	no	my	cuddle
socks	yes	toast	biscuits
Daddy	yeah	Marmite	cat
shoes	ta	jam	wassat
juice	poo	ball	bubbles
bye-bye	book	hot	Laa-Laa
more	duck	cup	jump
hello	quack quack	spoon	nice
hiya	woof	bowl	two
Nana	please	Mummy	eyes
Grandad	bot-bot	bang	weeble

Jane Hale, AQA June 2007

Classroom activity 3

Before you look at the categories identified by researchers, try to group the words in different ways. For example, group the references to people or animals, or group by word classes such as proper nouns. What conclusions can you draw from the types of words used by Rachel?

💡 *Categorising first words*

Katherine Nelson (1973) identified four categories for first words:

■ naming (things or people)
■ actions/events
■ describing/modifying things
■ personal/social words.

She found that 60 per cent of first words were nouns (the naming group). Verbs formed the second largest group, and were used with actions or location words like 'up' and 'down'. Modifiers came third. Personal/social words made up about 8 per cent of the sample. Re-categorising your earlier list of Rachel's words according to Nelson's groups would probably produce the following:

Naming		Action	Social	Modifying
Jasper	woof	more	bye-bye	more
socks	bot-bot	poo	hello	my
Daddy	Marmite	book	hiya	hot
Shoes	jam	quack-quack	no	nice
juice	ball	woof	yes	two
Nana	cup	bang	yeah	
Grandad	spoon	cuddle	ta	
poo	bowl	jump	please	
book	Mummy		wassat?	
duck	cuddle			
quack-quack	cat			
biscuits	Laa-Laa			
bubbles	weeble			
eyes				

This data shows that first words are often proper or concrete nouns. Children can link a word and the referent (the object it describes) quite easily as they can usually see it, or see a visual representation in a book. The social and interactive nature of many of these words also indicate the importance of interacting with others, suggesting that pragmatic awareness (see page 23) is vital to early language development. The reduplicative ('quack-quack') and diminutive **vocative** ('Mummy') show the bridge between phonological and lexical development.

Early vocabulary contains **content words** (from word classes such as nouns, verbs and adjectives). **Function words** (determiners, prepositions and auxiliary verbs) have a grammatical rather than a semantic function, and are acquired later.

■ Research point

You have already considered some theories about language acquisition. Chomsky's focused on grammatical development and doesn't explain children's acquisition of words and their associated meanings. Some psychologists and linguists believe that language is acquired through **social interaction**, and this would seem true with lexical and semantic development. This view started from B.F. Skinner's views that children imitate and copy adults and, as they get either positive or negative reinforcement for their verbal behaviour, they are conditioned into using the right language. Attention and praise are often given as **positive reinforcement** for the right naming word or for politeness, with **negative reinforcement** resulting from their frustration at not being understood or being denied positive comments. However, recent researchers have looked at the role and importance of interaction to help children acquire language, rather than simply taking a **behaviourist** standpoint.

Thinking points

1. What do Rachel's first words show about her early social experiences?

2. How might her first words encourage the view that other people help children to acquire language?

■ Key terms

Vocative: a form (especially a noun) used to address a person.

Content word: a type of word that has an independent 'dictionary' meaning, also called a lexical word.

Function word: a word whose role is largely or wholly to express a grammatical relationship.

Social interactionists: those who believe that child language develops through interaction with carers.

Positive reinforcement: when a behaviour is rewarded, including verbal praise to encourage this behaviour to be repeated.

Negative reinforcement: when an undesirable behaviour is unrewarded with the intention that it will not be repeated.

Behaviourists: those who believe that language is acquired through imitation and reinforcement.

■ Link

There is more information about positive and negative reinforcement in the 'Developing speech' topic on page 42.

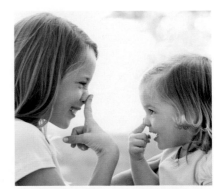

Fig. 6 *Some experts believe that language is acquired through social interaction*

Overextension: a feature of a child's language where the word used to label something is 'stretched' to include things that aren't normally part of that word's meaning

Underextension: a feature of a child's language where the word used to label is 'reduced' to include only part of its normal meaning.

Developing meanings

It is common for children to **overextend** a word's meaning. Children link objects with similar qualities and may, for example, apply the word 'dog' to all four-legged household pets. Less frequently children **underextend** a word by giving it a narrower definition than it really has, for example a child might use 'duck' for fluffy cartoon ducks, and not for the brown ones in the local pond.

Eve Clark's study of first words found that children base overextensions on:

■ the physical qualities of objects

■ features such as taste, sound, movement, shape, size and texture.

Children's first words connect to their experiences of the world, dominated by the senses. Think how babies and toddlers delight in touching objects and putting them in their mouths.

In other research, Leslie Rescorla divided overextensions into three types, as set out in Table 8.

Table 8 *Types of overextension*

Type	Definition	Example	% of overextension
Categorical overextension	The name for one member of a category is extended to all members of the category	Apple used for all round fruits	60%
Analogical overextension	A word for one object is extended to one in a different category; usually on the basis that it has some physical or functional connection	Ball used for a round fruit	15%
Mismatch statements	One-word sentences that appear quite abstract; child makes a statement about one object in relation to another	Saying 'duck' when looking at an empty pond	25%

Another linguist, Jean Aitchison, connects children's lexical and semantic development. Her developmental stages are shown in Table 9.

Table 9 *Aitchison's stages of children's linguistic development*

Number	Stage	Description
1	Labelling	Linking words to the objects to which they refer, understanding that things can be labelled
2	Packaging	Exploring the labels and to what they can apply. Over/underextension occurs in order to eventually understand the range of a word's meaning
3	Network-building	Making connections between words, understanding similarities and opposites in meanings

Once children expand their vocabulary they use network-building to sort the words. An aspect of this stage is an understanding of **hyponymy**, the links between lexical items that divides into **hypernyms** and **hyponyms**. If you take 'clothes' as the hypernym, you could list all the hyponyms a child could use for specific items of clothing they wear: socks, shoes, coat, vest, pants, T-shirt, jumper, jeans, trousers, top, gloves, hat, wellies etc. When they have a larger vocabulary (18 months onwards), they may use these more accurately and precisely to identify individual items of clothing. Synonymy appears too, offering different ways to name the same object. Rachel (page 10) used the noun 'duck' and the onomatopoeic 'quack-quack' to refer to the same animal.

This example of overextension demonstrates the child's exploration of labels. The child uses the word 'moon' for 'stars' as a categorical overextension – both being bright objects in the night sky. The adult provides a new word ('stars') and the packaging process begins. In a few months this child may know a host of words associated with outer space.

Transcription conventions are given on page v.

Context: adult and child are looking at a night scene in a picture book.

Child:	moon
Adult:	moon yes
Child	moon (.) moon (.) more (.) more
Adult:	more
Child:	more moon
Adult:	[*suddenly realising that he is pointing at stars in picture*] oh these are stars (.) these are little stars (.) stars in the sky

Clare Painter, Into the Mother Tongue: A Case Study in Early Language Development, *1984*

As in this interaction, it has been found that parents are more likely to use the specific words for objects (hyponyms) than the general word (hypernym); this encourages children to network-build and increases their vocabulary as they acquire new words for particular objects.

Research point

Jean Piaget was a 20th-century Swiss psychologist whose views about children's cognitive development have been very influential.

He emphasised that children are active learners who use their environment and social interactions to shape their language. Rachel's use of 'wassat' (page 10) shows that she wanted more labels to describe the objects around her and used this word to be an active learner.

Piaget linked linguistic development with an understanding of the concepts surrounding the word's meanings, suggesting that children cannot be taught before they are ready. His four developmental stages are shown in Table 10.

Key terms

Hyponymy: the hierarchical structure that exists between lexical items.

Hypernym: a superordinate, i.e. a word that is more generic or general and can have more specific words under it.

Hyponym: a more specific word within a category or under a hypernym.

Table 10 *Piaget's stages of children's linguistic development*

Stage	Age (years)	Key elements
Sensorimotor	Up to 2	The child experiences the physical world through the senses and begins classifying the things in it; lexical choices, when they appear, tend to be concrete rather than abstract Object permanence develops – the concept that objects exist when out of sight
Pre-operational	2–7	Language and motor skills develop and become more competent Language is egocentric – either focused on the child or used by the child when no one else is around
Concrete operational	7–11	Children begin thinking logically about concrete events
Formal operational	11+	Abstract reasoning skills develop

Eve Clark's more recent research found that common adjectives ('nice', 'big') are among children's first 50 words, but spatial adjectives ('wide'/'narrow', 'thick'/'thin') are acquired later. Try explaining what 'wide' means, and you will see why a child might have difficulty with its meaning!

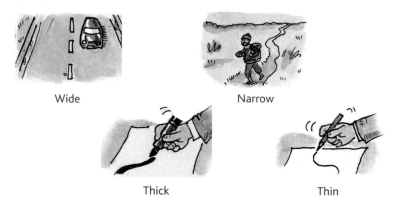

Wide   Narrow

Thick   Thin

Fig. 7 *Why might a child have difficulty in learning to use spatial adjectives?*

Thinking points

1. Using Piaget's ideas, what reasons can you give for the adjectives that children use first?

2. Why do you think children find spatial adjectives more difficult to understand and use?

Developing grammar

Acquiring greater lexical and semantic understanding requires grammatical skills to combine words into complete and increasingly complex utterances. A 24-month-old with a 200-word average vocabulary, in the two-word stage, is limited in the ways those words can be joined. Compare this with a 36-month-old, with a 2,000-word vocabulary, and you can see the connection between grammatical progression and the number of words at a child's disposal.

The two areas of grammar are syntax and morphology.

■ Syntactical advances allow children to:

1) order words into phrases and clauses
2) make different types of utterances (simple, compound, complex) for different functions apart from declarative (interrogative and imperative require different word order).

■ Morphological advances allow children to:

1) add inflections to words creating tense, marking distinctions between adjectives, showing possession and making plurals (**inflectional morphology**)
2) experiment with language by adding prefixes and suffixes to make up words and to convert words from one word class to another (**derivational morphology**).

When linguists calculate the **mean length utterance (MLU)** for children, they look at the individual morphemes that children use rather than adding up the number of words. Why do you think this is a more effective way to analyse children's grammatical development?

💡 **Table 11** *Stages of children's grammatical development*

Stage	Descriptors	Grammatical constructions	Age (months)
One-word/ holophrastic	One-word utterance		12–18
Two-word	Two words combined to create simple syntactical structures	Subject + Verb Verb + Object	18–24
Telegraphic	Three or more words joined in increasingly complex and accurate orders	Subject + Verb + Object Subject + Verb + Complement Subject +Verb + Adverbial	24–36
Post-telegraphic	Increasing awareness of grammatical rules and irregularities	Instead of saying 'runned' using 'ran'	36+

From a theoretical perspective, it is useful to look at Chomsky here. His view of acquisition is built on the universal features of all language (for example nouns and verbs) along with phonological aspects (vowels and consonants). These are termed 'linguistic universals'. Children, to Chomsky, are equipped to discover the grammar of their language because they have an innate grammar. This, to him, means that acquiring language must be about more than just imitating adult speakers.

One-word/holophrastic stage

The one-word stage provides the building blocks for syntax to develop. You saw that first words are mainly nouns used to label and name objects. The term 'holophrastic' means 'whole phrase' and is used to describe words that don't simply fulfil the naming purpose, but behave more like a short utterance. To show the variation between young children's first words, here are two siblings' first words.

The child in Figure 9 said 'duck' first because it was linked to a favourite picture book. For a few months the mother and child had been reading over and over again an interactive book where a yellow duck could be

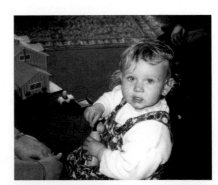

Fig. 8 *First word 'duck'*

15

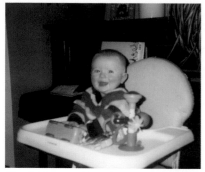

Fig. 9 *First word 'stuck'*

found hiding on each page. Before finally saying the word the little girl has been pointing to the hidden duck when asked to by her mother, eventually using the noun 'duck' to describe it. So this child's first word named an object.

Figure 9 shows the child whose first word was 'stuck'. What did 'stuck' mean to him? It could have been a statement, as he used it when sitting in his highchair. However, it was often accompanied by actions as he struggled to climb out of the highchair. It probably meant 'I want to get out!' Rising intonation on the word 'stuck' could indicate that it was a request to be lifted out, or stress on the word could show his frustration at being trapped. At first he used this word only when in his highchair, but later used it when shut in anywhere he did not want to be, so it could be described as a holophrase.

Having only one word makes meaning a matter of interpretation, relying on others successfully decoding your meaning. At this stage the carer's role is important as they try to make sense of early words through trial and error ('Are you hungry?', 'Did you want this teddy?'). Context, too, is central to understanding children's needs; the meaning of proto-words or holophrases can be deduced from the fact that the child uses them in a particular place or when holding a certain toy. Children also use other linguistic clues, such as prosodic features ('juice?'), to make their intentions clearer, showing the importance of having acquired and practised phonological skills early on.

Do you know what your first word was? If so, did it name an object or was it a holophrase? Why did you use this word?

Two-word stage

This stage marks the beginning of syntactical development. Once two words are joined the child can explore different combinations and learn correct English word order. Roger Brown's 1970s study of two-word sentences found that children from all cultures and countries make the same relationships between grammatical concepts.

Table 12 *Types of meaning relations in two-word utterances*

Meaning relation	Explanation	Example	Context
agent + action	Did someone (the do-er) perform an action?	Daddy kick	Dad kicks ball
agent + affected	Does someone do something to an object (done-to)?	Me ball	Child kicks ball
entity + attribute	Is a person or object described?	Kitty big	Sees tigers in zoo
action + affected	Does an action affect an object?	Throw stick	Child throws stick
action + location	Does an action occur in a place?	Sit chair	Child sits on chair
entity + location	Is an object located?	Spoon table	Spoon is on the table
possessor + possession	Does an object have a possessor?	Daddy coat	Points to dad's coat
nomination	Is a person or object labelled?	That cake	That is a cake
recurrence	Is an event repeated?	More ball	Finds second ball
negation	Is something denied?	No ball	Has lost her ball

Classroom activity 4

Use these examples to practise applying Brown's findings. Copy and complete the table below, matching each two-word utterance with the correct meaning relation.

Example	Meaning relation
More cat (the second family cat arrives in the room)	
Daddy sit (father sits down at the kitchen table)	
No dolly (not finding a favourite toy)	
Brush hair (child brushes hair)	
Mummy key (child points to mother's car keys)	
Ball big (picking up a ball)	
There Jack (on seeing baby brother)	
Biscuit floor (child sees her biscuit on the floor)	
Sit buggy (child sits in his pushchair)	
Drop juice (child throws cup to the floor)	

Telegraphic stage

Once a child can combine three or more words they are starting to make their meanings more explicit. This is the telegraphic stage; utterances are similar to the style and construction of a telegram (or even like a text message) in that function words are left out but content words are retained. Early in the stage, verb inflections, auxiliary verbs, prepositions, determiners are all omitted. As the child moves towards the post-telegraphic stage, these function words appear accurately in utterances. Key developments take place in the construction of questions, negatives and pronouns.

Questions

Questions are a feature in early speech but, in the one- and two-word stages, they are formed by rising intonation alone ('juice', 'have book'). Only later can children successfully create yes/no interrogatives because these involve changing word order and using auxiliary verbs ('can I have book?').

Other questions require the words 'what', 'where', 'when', 'why'. These too appear fairly early on in development and are frequently used correctly at the beginning of a sentence ('where mummy?'). But inversion of the subject and auxiliary/**copula verb** does not happen until later ('where is mummy?'). They appear to be acquired in a certain order:

■ What – subject or object
■ Where – location
■ Why – reason
■ When – time

If you think about it, you can see why this order is typical. Knowing 'what' is happening ('what doing?' or 'what that?') gives a child more

Key terms

Copula verb: a verb used to join or 'couple a subject to a complement.

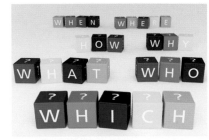

Fig. 10 *Children's questions tend to develop in the order 'what', 'where', 'why' and 'when'*

words. The 'where' stage ('where teddy?') pinpoints where objects can be found, with the 'why' stage showing some cognitive awareness (relevant later when you consider different theories about language development) and the desire to learn about their environment. 'When', the temporal aspect, is more abstract and any parent knows that children do not acquire a sense of the constraints of time until much later!

Negatives

The ability to use negation also needs syntactic awareness; researcher Ursula Bellugi identified three stages of negative formations in young children.

Table 13 *Stages of negative formation*

Stage	The child:	Example
1	uses 'no' or 'not' at the beginning or end of a sentence	No wear shoes
2	moves 'no'/'not' inside the sentence	I no want it
3	attaches the negative to auxiliary verbs and the copula verb 'be' securely	No, I don't want to go to nursery I am not

David Crystal, a respected contemporary linguist, adds another way of learning to say 'no' to Bellugi's stages. This is a more pragmatic than grammatical method of expressing what you don't want to do, as it does not use a negative word at all. It can be observed when adults don't want to be direct in disagreeing with their children – for example, using 'maybe' to mean 'no'– and is a skill that children will develop.

Pronouns

Pronouns can be difficult words to use accurately. This is because they express many things: for example, person (the people involved in a communication, I/you, and the subject/object positioning with an utterance, I/me); number (the singular or plural, I/we); gender (s/he); possession (mine).

Ursula Bellugi found three stages:

1 the child uses their own name (for example, 'Tom play')
2 the child recognises the I/me pronouns and that these are used in different places within a sentence (for example, 'I play toy', 'Me do that')
3 the child uses them according to whether they are in the subject or object position within a sentence (for example, 'I play with the toy', 'Give it to me').

In the following extract, two 4-year-olds are playing. Children of a similar age can be at different stages of pronoun development. As you have already looked at negation, look too at Ewan's stage of pronoun development.

Transcription conventions are given on page v.

> *Ewan:*   no me shopkeeper (2.0) Hollie Hollie playing
> *Hollie:* yes (.)
> *Ewan:*   don't go home yet Hollie (.)
> *Hollie:* I'd like to buy all these please (.)
> *Ewan:*   right (.) me

Laura Grimes, AQA June 2007

Ewan still uses the object pronoun ('me') in the subject position but is in Stage 2 of Bellugi's model as he uses pronouns rather than nouns. Hollie is in Stage 3 as she opts for the subject pronoun ('I'd like'), although this is at the beginning of her sentence. She is clearly well into the telegraphic stage with her ability to create a long and accurate sentence using **deixis** correctly ('these'). However, Ewan is in Stage 3 of negation with his use of the auxiliary verb ('do') and the attaching of the negative ('not') in the contracted form to it. His use of the negative in his opening utterance ('no me shopkeeper') suggests he is either responding to a yes/no question or asserting the role he wants to take in the play.

Determiners

Determiners are another function word acquired later in development. Determiners are attached to nouns and are: articles ('a', 'the'); numerals ('one'); possessives ('my'); quantifiers ('some', 'many'); or demonstratives ('this'). Look at this child's struggle to use determiners accurately, despite valiant attempts.

Transcription conventions are given on page v.

	Child:	want other one spoon Daddy
	Adult:	you mean you want the other spoon
	Child:	yes I want other one spoon please Daddy
	Adult:	can you say the other spoon
5	**Child:**	other (.) one (.) spoon
	Adult:	say other
	Child:	other
	Adult:	spoon
	Child:	spoon
10	**Adult:**	other spoon
	Child:	other spoon (.) now give me other one spoon

Victoria Fromkin, Robert Rodman and Nina Hyams, Introduction to Language, *2002*

> ### Classroom activity 5
>
> Earlier you read some different perspectives on language acquisition.
>
> ■ Skinner's view was that children acquire language through conditioning and imitation. How does the father attempt to correct the child? Does correcting children's language work?
>
> ■ Piaget's ideas centre on the understanding of concepts coming before language. How does the 'spoon' extract support his views of language acquisition?
>
> ■ Chomsky suggests that children learn the rules of language. What evidence is there here that the child has learnt some syntactical rules?

Post-telegraphic stage

This is when the remaining function words are acquired and used appropriately. The child can:

■ combine clause structures by using coordinating conjunctions ('and', 'but') and subordinating conjunctions ('because', 'although') to make complex and compound utterances

■ manipulate verb forms more accurately, for instance using the passive voice ('The car was followed by the lorry')

■ construct longer noun phrases ('the two big red buses').

Here is Olivia, who is in the post-telegraphic stage. How would you identify that she has reached this? Focus on the complexity of her utterances and verb usage.

Transcription conventions are given on page v.

> *Olivia:* I never get a chance to be the leader (.) but I got to be today
>
> *Mother:* you were the leader today
>
> *Olivia:* yeah (.) on yeah (.) I so so I been there (.) actually I need a present
>
> 5 *Mother:* you've had a good day (1.0) you've been the leader and you were star of the week
>
> *Olivia:* I know but (1.0) I need someone to get me a PRESENT
>
> *Mother:* what sort of present
>
> *Olivia:* my daddy
>
> 10 *Mother:* what (.) your daddy's going to
>
> *Olivia:*   I had a nosebleed |today |
>
> *Mother:* |oh no| (.) did you (2.0) when
>
> *Olivia:* when I was playing out after dinner time

Amanda Coultas, Prudhoe High School, AQA June 2005

Olivia uses compound sentences, using the coordinating conjunction ('but') to structure her utterances. She also uses subordinate clauses ('when I was playing out after dinner time') as an adverbial to give her mother extra information. She uses the past progressive ('I was playing') and expresses future actions ('I need someone to get me'). Pronouns ('I' and 'me') in the correct subject/object positions also indicate her competence. Her sophistication is shown with her MLU: she constructs long utterances. Obviously, some development is needed as her meanings are not entirely clear ('I so so I been there'). But even adult speech, as you know from your study at AS, is not always grammatically accurate.

Morphological development

Moving from the telegraphic to post-telegraphic stage involves understanding that not only can word order be changed but so too can words themselves. A useful starting point is to look at the two types of **morphemes**: **free** and **bound**.

Roger Brown found that morphemes are acquired in a particular order:

Table 14 *Stages of morpheme acquisition*

Present tense progressive	–ing
Prepositions	in, on
Plural	–s
Past tense irregular	run/ran
Possessive	's
Uncontractible copula	is, was
Articles	the, a
Past tense regular	–ed
Third person regular	runs
Third person irregular	has
Uncontractible auxiliary verb	they were running
Contractible copula	she's
Contractible auxiliary	she's running

*Adapted from **Jean Stilwell Peccei**, Child Language, 1999*

Key terms

Free morpheme: one that can stand alone as an independent word, e.g. apple.

Bound morpheme: one that cannot stand alone as an independent word, but must be attached to another morpheme/word (affixes, such as the plural '–s', are always bound, as is the comparative adjective inflection '–er').

Research point

Piaget's **cognitive theory** is useful to apply to Brown's findings as the increasing complexity of the morphemes acquired suggests a link between cognitive development and language acquisition. Adding '–ing' to verbs and working out that more than one of a noun requires the plural '–s' seems more straightforward than using the correct form of 'to be', which needs more understanding of tense and number.

Piaget believed that children will only acquire more complex forms of language when their intellectual development can cope, so trying to teach children before they are ready will fail because they cannot grasp the ideas involved. He advocated 'discovery learning' (learning by doing), theorising that language doesn't shape thought but that thought shapes language.

Thinking points

1. What play activities could parents and carers use that would help 'discovery learning'?

2. What toys might help children learn about language rules?

3. What links are there between children's language development and the ages they attend playschool, nursery or infant reception class?

Key terms

Cognitive theorists: those who believe that language acquisition is part of a wider development of understanding.

Virtuous error: syntactic errors made by young children in which the non-standard utterance reveals some understanding, though incomplete, of standard syntax.

Overgeneralisation: a learner's extension of a word meaning or grammatical rule beyond its normal use.

'Virtuous errors' and overgeneralisations

The phrase '**virtuous error**' is usually applied to the mistakes children make as they develop grammatically. It implies that children make choices from a linguistic basis, and therefore are logical. Because English has many irregularities, these seem 'wrong'. If you listen to children around age 3 or 4 you often hear them say 'I runned' instead of 'I ran'. A good way to respond to this virtuous error is to think how clever they are to have worked out that most verbs end with the –ed inflection. Linguists call some virtuous errors **overgeneralisations**. Another common overgeneralisation is to add the plural –s inflection to nouns ('house'/'houses') but there are of some irregular plurals ('mouse'/'mice', 'foot'/'feet'). Children go through the process of applying rules and then learn the exceptions.

Overgeneralisations are often used to support Chomsky's views about acquisition, as they show that children produce language that they have never heard an adult say. Using 'goed' instead of 'went' shows that children have worked out a syntactical rule. You have seen from the data extracts that adult correction doesn't seem to work and that children repeat their errors. However, they do learn irregular verbs, suggesting that hearing correct versions or having adults correct them might be needed as well.

Here Tom talks to his mother about stroking a chicken at a friend's house. The conversation demonstrates how children overgeneralise and why virtuous errors might happen.

Transcription conventions are given on page v.

Mother:	what did it feel like
Tom:	it feels shy (2.0)
Mother:	it felt shy
Tom:	yeah
Mother:	did you feel shy or did the chicken feel shy
Tom:	the chicken feeled shy (2.0)

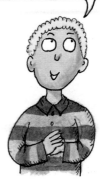

Fig. 11 *'Virtuous errors' are mistakes made by children as they develop grammatically – their choices are often logical even though incorrect*

J.A. Darby, *AQA January 2005*

Stative verb: verb that describes a state; stative verbs are not usually used in the progressive aspect, which is used for incomplete actions in progress.

Dynamic verb: a type of verb that expresses activities and changes of state, allowing such forms as the progressive.

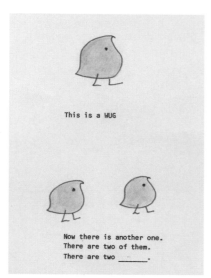

Fig. 12 *The 'wug' test*

Tom uses the present tense ('feels') to describe a previously completed action. The mother models the correct irregular past tense verb ('felt'). Later, when the mother asks Tom his feelings, and uses the present tense verb (feel) Tom now places his ideas in the past tense but overgeneralises the –ed ending and concludes that 'the chicken feeled shy'. You can see why Tom might be confused as in this context even the word 'feel' is used ambiguously as it is both an abstract concept (a **stative verb**) and a tangible action (a **dynamic verb**).

■ Research point

These overgeneralisations were famously proved by Jean Berko who, in the 1950s, conducted a study into children's pronunciation and morphological development. Part of this study was into the use of the –s plural. She gave children a picture of an imaginary creature called a 'wug' and asked them what more than one wug would be called. Three-quarters of the 4- and 5-year-olds surveyed formed the regular plural 'wugs'.

Thinking points

1 Why do you think she chose an imaginary creature?

2 What does this study suggest about how children acquire grammatical skills?

3 Could you devise a test for other morphemes acquired?

Possession

The concept of possession is another aspect of inflectional morphology that children need to acquire. Here you can see Tom (aged 2 years) grapple with the idea of 'dad's bike'.

Transcription conventions are given on page v.

Tom:	OH PLEASE	
Mother:	so what are you doing Tom	
Tom:	I sitting on the bike (.) it make noises	
Mother:	it makes noises	
5 ***Tom:***	yeah	
Mother:	what sort of noises	
Tom:	the bike (.) the dad bike	
Mother:	dad's bike	
10 ***Tom:***	yeah (.) the dad (.) dad's bike (.) dad's bike mum (.) dad's bike	
Mother:	you're not on dad's bike (.) you're on your bike	
Tom:	I am on dad's bike but I not on dad's bike	

J.A. Darby, AQA January 2005

First he terms it 'the dad bike'. After his mother's correction, he seems to copy her correctly, following a false start and self-correction ('dad's bike'). When he says that he is 'on dad's bike but I not on dad's bike' he seems to be struggling with some concepts of ownership. His dad has been mending Tom's bike and so, to Tom, has some responsibility towards it. Ideas about possession still have to be worked through; this is perhaps a limitation of his understanding rather than a linguistic one, as he copies his mother's words and uses the –s inflection accurately.

♀ Developing pragmatics

Pragmatic understanding, especially with regard to conversational skills, is crucial to children's successful language development. As a reminder, pragmatics is about:

■ implicature (what we mean rather than what we say)
■ inference (interpreting what others mean)
■ politeness (using the right words and phrases to be polite)
■ conversational management and turn-taking (knowing when to speak).

A good starting point is to use Michael Halliday's 'taxonomy'. His functions of speech are shown in Table 15.

Table 15 *Halliday's functions of speech*

Function	Where language is used to:
Instrumental	fulfil a need (e.g. 'want milk')
Regulatory	influence the behaviour of others (e.g. 'pick up')
Interactional	develop and maintain social relationships (e.g. 'love you')
Personal	convey individual opinions, ideas and personal identity (e.g. 'me like Charlie and Lola')
Representational	convey facts and information (e.g. 'it hot')
Imaginative	create an imaginary world and may be seen in play predominantly (e.g. 'me shopkeeper')
Heuristic	learn about the environment (e.g. 'wassat?')

John Dore offers another way of describing language functions that focuses more on speech acts as individual utterances (Table 16), rather than Halliday's broader approach to pragmatic functions.

Table 16 *Dore's language functions*

Function	Description
Labelling	Naming a person, object or thing
Repeating	Repeating an adult word or utterance
Answering	Responding to an utterance of another speaker
Requesting action	Asking for something to be done for them
Calling	Getting attention by shouting
Greeting	Greeting someone or something
Protesting	Objecting to requests from others
Practising	Using language when no adult is present

Both provide useful models for analysing children's utterances, explaining why a child uses language. However, it is often hard to apply them accurately without information on the context of the utterance. Imagine a child at the one-word stage using the noun 'mummy'. In Dore's categories this could be labelling. But 'mummy' could also be repeating an adult utterance as a statement, or it could be used as a greeting.

Classroom activity 6

Practise applying Halliday and Dore. Copy and complete the table below, deciding which categorisation model seems to be the most helpful in identifying language functions.

Utterance	Context	Halliday's function	Dore's function
Look at me, I superman	Child playing		
Mummy	Mummy returns home from work		
Want juice	Child is thirsty		
Put down	Father is holding child		
Me like that	Child looks at toy in a shop		
Why?	Child asks why she has to get her shoes on		
Night night daddy, love you	Being put to bed		
No	Child wants to stay at the park		

For some, pragmatic development is a key aspect of language that has to be learnt from others and supports those theorists who believe that social interactions lead to language advances rather than the 'innate' view. However, as you have seen from Halliday and Dore's model, the focus is on the child's use of language as a way to discover the world and so draws on Piaget's ideas. Indeed, where Dore sees children practising with language without needing adults present, Piaget coined the phrase **egocentric speech** to describe his observations of children talking when alone, seeing it as their way to classify their experiences and environment.

How important is politeness?

Politeness is encouraged by parents from an early age. Your own experiences of being instructed to say 'please' and 'thank you' suggest how important these words are for social interaction – these words also featured in Rachel's first 50. Politeness extends to the ways conversations are maintained, encompassing the face theory proposed by Penelope Brown and Stephen Levinson. They suggested two main aspects of face in communicative interactions:

- **Positive** – where the individual desires social approval and being included
- **Negative** – where individual asserts their need to be independent and make their own decisions.

This transcript, documenting a child's first visit to a friend's house, demonstrates young children's pragmatic awareness. Note the efforts to be polite and accommodate others' needs.

Transcription conventions are given on page v.

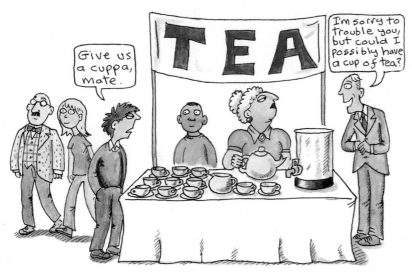

Fig. 13 *Politeness strategies in action*

Context: the children are playing downstairs and Anya has said she needs to go to the toilet.

Keri's mother:	Keri will show you where it is Anya (.) in case you don't know
Keri:	okay Anya (.) that a deal
Anya:	I remember where it is
5 ***Keri:***	no (.) I show you
Anya:	I know where mine is (.) mine's upstairs (.) cos you're supposed to have toilets upstairs aren't you
Keri's mother:	mmm
Anya:	my nan (.) em has one toilet <u>down</u>stairs
	[*they go upstairs to the bathroom*]
10 ***Keri:***	yes (.) that's it (.) it's nice my toilet (1.0) do you want a step (.) Anya
Anya:	yeah
Keri:	I get you one (.) oh (.) there one in my bedroom
	[*Keri goes to get a step which will enable Anya to climb up onto the toilet*]

Amanda Coultas, AQA January 2003

The mother's modelling of politeness directs Keri to show Anya the toilet with a face-saving phrase ('in case you don't know'); this makes Anya feel good about herself by not pointing out the obvious – that she won't know where the toilet is because it's her first visit. Keri adopts the helpful host role in her declaratives ('I show you') and ('I get you one') and in the polite interrogative ('do you want a step'). The mother's minimal response ('mmm') shows her unwillingness to correct Anya's assumptions about downstairs toilets, viewing this as rudeness. This, too, provides Keri with a politeness model. Anya, however, is demonstrating some aspects of negative face by asserting her independence and her own point of view, justifying the accuracy of her assertion that houses only have toilets upstairs with her tag question ('aren't you') to prompt agreement from Keri or her mother.

How important is context?

First, what is meant by the context? As it refers to the situation of an interaction, you should ask these questions when examining data:

■ who participates? (one or more speakers, gender)

■ what relationship exists between speakers? (family members, friends, carer and child, teacher and student)

■ what is the setting? (domestic, nursery, local environment etc.)

■ in what developmental stage is the child? (age)

■ what other factors might affect the data? (cultural influences such as books, television, social experiences).

Look at this transcript. The supporting contextual information provided is:

■ this is the first time that they have played together outside their shared time at nursery

■ they are playing at Keri's house

■ Keri is 38 months old and Anya is 44 months old.

How does this contextual knowledge affect your linguistic analysis of the language choices and the structure of the discourse?

Transcription conventions are given on page v.

Context: the children are sitting at the top of the stairs and Keri is showing Anya the contents of her jewel box.

> **Keri:**   look at my necklace grandma oh (.) look at my necklace (.) Anya
>
> **Anya:**   I have a necklace (.) a duck one and I lose my glasses (.) you know
>
> 5 **Keri:**   I lose MY glasses (.) that's only mine [pointing at necklace] (.) but we can share them
>
> **Anya:**   well I lose mine (.) mummy's going to get another ones (.) and then I'll share them (.) right
>
> **Keri:**   yeah
>
> 10 **Anya:**   when I come again I'll wear them (.) and then I'll share them
> [Anya stands up]
>
> **Keri**   you can hold my hand you want (1.0) when you jump (.) jump
>
> **Anya:**   no I can't (.) I want to walk
>
> **Keri:**   you want to hold my hand when we go downstairs
>
> **Anya:**   no
>
> 15 **Keri:**   you can go in my bedroom you want

Amanda Coultas, AQA specimen paper

Keri appears quite assertive in her control of the role-play with her choice of imperatives ('look') and assigning Anya with the role of 'grandma'. She also refuses to accept Anya's attempt to take control of the game through the suggestion that Anya loses her glasses by stressing her ownership of the role-play object ('glasses') with the possessive pronoun ('MY'). She could be making these linguistic choices because she feels it is her right to do this in her own house and extends her possession to claiming ownership of her bedroom, magnanimously allowing Anya access to it (because this is polite).

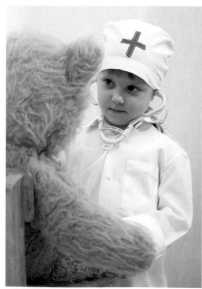

Fig. 14 *Children often role-play adult behaviours*

Because this is the first time they have played together in a domestic context, they negotiate frequently about roles and activities. Indeed, playing at each other's houses for the first time is a social development and the sign of an emerging friendship; the use of the inclusive plural pronoun ('we') indicates they are sharing experiences and want to play together. Their given ages pinpoint the likely features you could expect from children in the telegraphic stage with subject pronouns ('I'), possessive pronouns ('my') and the second person pronoun ('you') used accurately. The children are competent in using auxiliary verbs ('want' and 'can'). The number of words in utterances combined with subordinate clauses ('when we go downstairs') indicates syntactic competence and places them in the post-telegraphic stage.

■ Play and language acquisition

Lev Vygotsky, an early child development researcher, observed children's play and linked it to both cognitive and social development. Young children often use props as 'pivots' to support their play but, when older, use their imagination instead. Vygotsky also observed how children role-play adult behaviours as part of exploring their environment, which has interested more recent researchers.

Catherine Garvey's study of pairs of children playing found that children adopt roles and identities, acting out storylines and inventing objects and settings as required in a role-play scenario. This is termed pretend play and fulfils Halliday's imaginative language function. Children play together because it is enjoyable, but it also practises social interactions and negotiation skills, with players' roles and responsibilities often decided as they play. Sometimes called sociodramatic play, it involves both social and dramatic skills, with explicit rules and reflecting real-world behaviour.

Sociodramatic play usually begins when children are around 4 years old, possibly linking to their cognitive understanding as they understand the different roles people have and how these affect language. In their re-enactments they use field-specific lexis and structure them in some of the formulaic ways that adults use in precisely these situations, suggesting that they can observe and imitate adult behaviours. To illustrate children's real-world imitation, look at the transcription below of two children playing shops.

Transcription conventions are given on page v.

Context: two 4-year-olds, Hollie and Ewan, playing shops at Ewan's house, while their aunt, Laura, watches.

[*Till sounds*]
Hollie: I've got loads of scans one at the top
Ewan: I'm gonna put all of them on (1.0) me got real one
Hollie: this is a real one an' all (1.0) would you like cashback
Ewan: no but Laura does
Hollie: Laura can you play please
Ewan: it's two pounds then that
[*Till drawer opens*]
Hollie: and then you say would you like cash back
Ewan: do you like cash back
Hollie: no not yet

Laura Grimes, AQA June 2007

Classroom activity 7

Apply researchers' ideas about play, along with the gender and power debates you looked at in Unit 1 Section B of the AS book, to evaluate its function in language development in this interaction.

The lexis reflects a modern shop ('scans', 'cashback') and they are clearly undertaking the activity of putting objects through a till. Even the politeness is linked to the formulaic utterances made within customer transactions when Hollie gives Ewan the correct phrase to use ('would you like cash back') and the request for payment ('it's two pounds then').

Transcription conventions are given on page v.

Context: the children are dressed in fairy outfits and are playing in Keri's bedroom.

> **Anya:** here's a lovely thing (.) a lovely princess thing
> [*pointing at Keri dressed up in a fairy outfit*]
> **Anya:** I can be the (.) I can be the mother (.) right
> **Keri:** I can be a princess
> **Anya:** lie in your bed now princess (.) it's too late (1.0) right (.) straight to bed (.) mummy has to go to bed too
> [*Keri gets into bed*]
> **Keri:** your had to kiss me Anya
> **Anya:** right (.) you want me to read a story
> **Keri:** no (.) your had to kiss me
> **Anya:** okay then
> [*Anya kisses Keri on the forehead and Keri laughs*]
> **Anya:** go to sleep now
> [*Keri shuts her eyes for a few seconds then gets up*]
> **Anya:** not morning yet baby
> **Keri:** I not a baby
> **Anya:** it's still bedtime (.) go to sleep fairy (.) fairy
> **Keri:** I going to play in mummy's bedroom
> **Anya:** no (.) go back to sleep now fairy (.) go to sleep (.) what mum says (.) right (1.0) mums says (.) right (1.0) go to bed (.) let's go back to bed now (.) go to sleep (2.0) hum (.) this is my bed (.) I go to sleep (.) shh (.) shh

Amanda Coultas, AQA specimen paper

The role of parents

Although you will be evaluating language acquisition theories later, the role of parents cannot be overlooked. They are the main communicators with their children. The terms used to describe the non-standard form of language used by adults with young children have changed over time: baby talk (the traditional term used by non-linguists) became 'motherese', then changed to 'parentese'. The current preferred term used by linguists is **child-directed speech (CDS)** because it focuses on the child rather than the specific role of the adult.

What do you think these examples of English baby talk highlight?

beddy-byes	jim-jams	din-din	ickle	bic-bic
oopsie-daisie	wee-wee	yum-yum	pussy	doggie

Baby talk seems to rely on reduplication ('din-din', 'bic-bic'), deletion and substitution ('ickle') and addition ('doggie') with the adult speaker adopting child-like characteristics. When you learn about acquisition theories, evaluate what the linguistic theorists might think about the value of baby talk. Baby talk focuses on simple lexical features and exaggerated prosodic features, such as sing-song intonation.

Key terms

Child-directed speech (CDS): any of various speech patterns used by parents or care givers when communicating with young children, particularly infants, usually involving simplified vocabulary, melodic pitch, repetitive questioning, and a slow or deliberate tempo.

Features of child-directed speech (CDS)

Parents are likely to use some (or all) of the following:

- repetition and/or repeated sentence frames
- a higher pitch
- the child's name rather than pronouns
- the present tense
- one-word utterances and/or short elliptical sentences
- fewer verbs/modifiers
- concrete nouns
- **expansions** and/or **recasts**
- yes/no questioning
- exaggerated pauses giving turn-taking cues.

Child-directed speech has a far broader reach than baby talk. The benefits of CDS, some argue, are in teaching children the basic function and structure of language. Not all cultures use CDS, either not speaking to their children until they have reached a certain age (as in Samoa and Papua New Guinea), or not simplifying adult language for children.

Chomsky maintained that language structures cannot simply be acquired by repeating language from varieties such as CDS, because of its 'impoverished' and 'random' nature – using incomplete grammatical utterances. However, this now seems to be less valid, as studies of CDS features suggest that this register is more structured and regular than previously thought.

Some people have also looked at whether men use a different language register to their children. This has been dubbed fatherese. Men seem to use more direct questioning styles, seek more information and use a wider vocabulary than women.

Some of the evidence about the effects of CDS appears contradictory. In her 1970s research, Alison Clarke-Stewart found that children had a larger vocabulary if their mothers talked to them a lot. However, Roger Brown found that children were rarely corrected for grammatical mistakes, though they were for their lexical errors or for the content of their speech. So child-directed speech alone cannot explain children's acquisition of language, but may affect their linguistic competence.

Key terms

Expansion: the development of a child's utterance into a longer, more meaningful form.

Recast: the commenting on, extending and rephrasing of a child's utterance.

LASS (Language Acquisition Support System): this refers to the child's interaction with the adults around them and how this interaction supports language development.

Research point

Just as Chomsky thinks language occurs from an inbuilt processing device (LAD), others, like Jerome Bruner, think that there must also be a **Language Acquisition Support System (LASS)**. He particularly looked at ritualised activities that occur daily in young children's lives – mealtimes, bedtimes, reading books – and how carers make the rules and meanings of these interactions explicit and predictable so that children can learn.

Bruner cites the game of 'Peek-A-Boo' as an example of these educational rituals. In this game, parents hide their faces and then seem to reappear. As well as the non-verbal actions, this is accompanied by such phrases as 'bye bye', 'where am I?', 'here I am' and prosodic indicators such as pitch and intonation. So, for Bruner, this teaches children important linguistic aspects such as turn-taking, formulaic utterances and syntax.

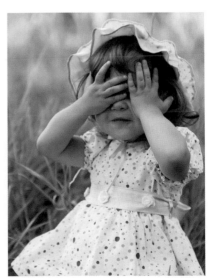

Fig. 15 *Games like Peek-A-Boo can teach a child many things*

■ Key terms

Object permanence: the awareness that objects continue to exist even when they are no longer visible.

Piaget would also use this game to test **object permanence**, where children understand that an object still exists even when it is no longer in sight. Some also link object permanence with the lexical growth from 36 months, as well as the emerging ability to use personal pronouns, distinguishing between 'I', 'me' and 'you'.

Thinking points

1. What might nursery rhymes and songs encourage children to learn about language (some suggestions are 'One, two, three, four, five, once I caught a fish alive' or 'Hickory, dickory, dock')?

2. Why is it important to understand the difference between 'I', 'you' and 'me'?

Classroom activity 8

What child-directed speech techniques do the parents use in the interactions in Texts A and B?

Transcription conventions are given on page v.

Text A

Michael:	[3 months; loud crying]
Mother:	[enters room] oh my word (.) what a noise (.) what a noise [picks up baby]
Michael:	[sobs]
Mother:	oh dear dear dear (.) didn't anybody come to see you Let's have a look at you [looks inside nappy] no (.) you're all right there aren't you
Michael:	[sputtering noises]
5 **Mother:**	well what is it then Are you hungry Is that it Is it a long time since dinner-time
Michael:	[gurgles]
Mother:	[nuzzles baby] oh yes it is a long time
Michael:	[cooing noise]
Mother:	yes I know (.) let's go and get some lovely grub then

David Crystal, Listen to Your Child: A Parent's Guide to Language, *1989*

Text B

Mother:	how many chickens are there
Tom:	(2.0) there's many chickens (.) one (.) two (.) three (.) four (.) five (.) six (.) seven (.) eight (.) nine (2.0)
Mother:	hmm (.) shall I count them now
5 **Tom:**	yeah
Mother:	one (.) two (.) three (.) four (.) five
Tom:	yep
Mother:	and we saw chickens this morning didn't we
Tom:	we did
10 **Mother:**	at Pascale's house (.) she's got some pet chickens
Tom:	has (.) have (.) has (.) has she I (.) stroke one chicken

Mother:	you did (.) didn't you You stroked it
Tom:	yeah
Mother:	Pascale had to hold it still and then you stroked the feathers didn't you 15

J.A. Darby, AQA January 2005

Research point

Interesting views have developed about the role of parents in providing linguistic support. Vygotsky, again, was influential in this area. His phrase 'zone of proximal development' describes how adults and children work together to move children towards independence, knowledge and competence. Jerome Bruner, with other researchers, introduced the concept of '**scaffolding**' to refer to the ways adults help children advance cognitively. He observed that adults withdraw support as children's skills develop.

The 'scaffolding' metaphor relates the support offered to children's language development with that offered by scaffolding around a building. Once the building or the child can support themselves independently, scaffolding is no longer required. Likewise, the carer plays an important role in early development, and the nature of their support changes with the child's needs and understanding.

Key terms

Scaffolding: the process of transferring a skill from adult to child and then withdrawing support once the skill has been mastered.

Thinking points

1. How might parents encourage children to reach 'the zone of proximal development' in activities such as completing jigsaws or with other practical toys?

2. What verbal support could adults withdraw as children's speech develops? (For example, think back to typical features of CDS.)

Extension activity 1

Using a style model from parenting magazines like *Practical Parenting*, write an informative article for parents, advising them about effective ways to speak to their children. If you are planning a child language investigation, this will help with the media task.

🔍 *i* 💡 Competing language acquisition debates

You have already read about many of the important theorists' views as you have studied children's linguistic development, and have seen how it applies to data of real children speaking and interacting with others. Knowing the theories is important as it makes up AO2, for which you will be awarded marks. But having an open mind and evaluating the diverse perspectives will help you in the examination as you interpret data that you have never seen before.

So, to summarise, the key debates are whether:

■ children learn language from imitation
■ language is inbuilt, with humans pre-programmed to acquire it
■ children need input from others to communicate effectively
■ children use cognitive skills to develop language by themselves.

Debates over language acquisition really started from a simple nature vs nurture perspective. These opposing stances were taken by two theorists, Noam Chomsky and B.F. Skinner, in the 1950s and 1960s. The nature view foregrounds the ability to use language as innate, whereas the nurture argument suggests that language acquisition is affected by others. Other linguists and psychologists challenged that either of these was capable of completely explaining language acquisition. Some, like Jean Piaget, took a cognitive approach, linking thought and language development, and others were interested in the role of other people and the social interaction needed to make children successful speakers. What has happened now is that many of these ideas have come together in order to explain the very complex process of acquisition and the factors needed to make it happen successfully.

Table 17 *Language acquisition theories*

Theory	Definition	Key theorist
Nativist	Humans have an inbuilt capacity to acquire language	Noam Chomsky, Eric Lenneburg
Behaviourist	Language is acquired through imitation and reinforcement	B.F. Skinner
Social interactionist	Child language is developed through interaction with adults	Jerome Bruner, Lev Vygotsky
Cognitive	Language acquisition is part of a wider development of understanding that develops	Lev Vygotsky, Jean Piaget

■ **Key terms**

Nativists: those who believe that humans have an inbuilt capacity to acquire language.

Noam Chomsky and nativist theory

Chomsky has changed his ideas over the years, although not from the core concept of children's innate ability to learn language (**nativism**). His focus is useful to explain grammatical development, but you can see that it does not go all the way to explaining other aspects of language.

Table 18 *Arguments for and against nativist theory*

For	Against
Children: ■ experience the same stages of development and at the same pace ■ resist correction ■ create forms of language that adults don't use (overgeneralisations) ■ make their own rules for language use that seem to understand that all languages have grammatical rules ■ produce correct language when surrounded by 'impoverished' faulty adult-speech, i.e. with false starts, incomplete utterances	**Children:** ■ stop overgeneralising and learn to use language correctly, as with irregular verbs ■ need input to give them more skills than grammar, for example pragmatic understanding ■ children who have been deprived of social contact can't achieve complete communicative competence
Relevant studies: ■ 'wug' test suggests children apply grammatical rules	**Relevant studies:** ■ studies of Genie (a girl deprived of social contact until she was 13 and then unable to learn speech beyond a very basic level) and feral children support the 'critical period' hypothesis that says that language needs to be acquired within a certain time frame. This challenges Chomsky's early argument that the ability to acquire language is simply innate within us as it shows that some interaction is needed for language completency.

Eric Lenneburg (1967) furthered the nativist argument by proposing that language has to be acquired within a critical period – really within the first five years. Case studies of feral ('wild') children, where human input has been limited, show that although some language processes can be acquired, full grammatical fluency is never achieved.

However, feral children who have grown up outside human society are not able to acquire language effectively when they return to live alongside others. Their individual stories, although sad, have allowed linguists and psychologists to test their theories about whether language is innate or if nurture is important too.

Extension activity 2

Find case studies of feral children, using www.feralchildren.com or sites such as Wikipedia. Read their stories, focusing on their language development. What does the children's development, or lack of it, suggest about the importance of human interaction to acquiring language? Do their experiences support any other theoretical views?

B.F. Skinner and behaviourist theory

Skinner's views have been largely discounted as a way of explaining language acquisition, although you might see that parents do use reinforcement when speaking to children and that children do copy language heard around them.

Table 19 *Arguments for and against behaviourist theory*

For	Against
Children: ■ imitate accent and dialect ■ learn politeness and pragmatic aspects of language ■ repeat language they have heard around them and incorporate it into theirs – lexical knowledge must be gained from being told the right labels	**Children:** ■ do more than just imitate language and can form sentences that they have never heard before ■ hear ungrammatical spoken language around them but can still learn correct language ■ do not seem to respond to correction ■ aren't negatively reinforced for language use ■ aren't always corrected by parents for incorrect grammar ■ corrections might actually slow down development ■ imitate but don't necessarily understand the meanings **Other limitations:** ■ 'fis' phenomenon suggests that children can hear and understand the correct pronunciation but simply can't produce it themselves at that stage ■ research was conducted on rats and pigeons, not on humans

Extension activity 3

Go to the Developing reading topic (page 36) and look at how parents use positive and negative reinforcement to help children read. Can you think of other literacy experiences where reinforcement by an adult might be useful?

Social interactionist theory

This is an appealing explanation for children's development in some key linguistic areas, foregrounding the roles of both carers and children. Clearly humans are sociable creatures and gain much from communicating with others. Increasingly, linguists have seen how important the help and 'scaffolding' given to children is, but it is still debated whether a greater adult linguistic input gives children an advantage.

Table 20 *Arguments for and against social interactionist theory*

For	Against
■ Routine/rituals seem to teach children about spoken discourse structure such as turn-taking ■ Pragmatic development suggests that children do learn politeness and verbally acceptable behaviour ■ Role-play and pretend play suggest that more interaction with carers can affect vocabulary	■ Children from cultures that do not promote interaction with children (e.g. Samoa) can still become articulate and fluent language users without adult input
Relevant studies: ■ Halliday's research into the functions of language supports the importance of social interaction ■ Vincent, a hearing child born to deaf parents, learned to communicate using sign language. As a hearing child he enjoyed watching televison, but he ignored the sounds. He did not start to speak until he went to school, where people talked to him.	

Extension activity 4

Look back at the extracts of children's and adults' speech in this topic. Can you find evidence of adults 'scaffolding' the children's language? How do the interactions help children's linguistic development?

Cognitive theories

Today cognitive theories go hand in hand with social interactionist theories, as people see how adult input helps children's understanding. Much of the research into children's developmental stages provides a convincing argument to explain the maturing of their language. These theories emphasise the active role of children themselves, seeing them not as passive beings in an adult-controlled linguistic world, but as humans who want to discover their surroundings and who use language to reflect this.

Table 21 *Arguments for and against cognitive theory*

For	Against
Children: ■ can't grasp aspects of language until they are ready; stages of development support this ■ produce utterances which increase in complexity as they work towards mastering a rule	**Children:** ■ with cognitive difficulties can still manage to use language beyond their understanding ■ acquire language without having an understanding of it, especially in the early stages of development
Relevant studies: ■ Brown's morphemes ■ Bellugi's stages for pronoun and question formation	■ 'fis' phenomenon suggests children's cognitive understanding can be present but their physical development still impacts their ability to use language

On a final note, there are many arguments and researchers' case studies apart from the ones cited here, offering evidence for and against aspects of all theories, especially the earlier ones – Skinner and Chomsky. Recent linguists have focused on the whole picture and concluded that:

■ the ability to produce language is within all humans

■ cognitive skills develop and link to language development

■ all children exposed to language acquire it naturally, without deliberate teaching but social input is needed and sought by children to help them communicate effectively and explore their environment.

Developing reading

When does reading start?

Literacy differs from oracy in that reading and writing skills are explicitly taught to young children, as an established part of formal schooling (from age 4). However, for young children, as for adults, reading books is just one literacy experience as they encounter the written word in other aspects of daily routines and cultural experiences. All around are words and symbols to interpret, not always written in strings of words or in the narrative structure of story books: PUSH and PULL on the doors of buildings provide information about how to use them, as does the word STOP alongside a picture on a pedestrian crossing. Even company logos and names of shops become a way to interpret their environment. Children also absorb information from television and computer sources (including games), and these have become part of the young learner's literacy environment.

Research point

S.B. Heath, in the 1980s, studied three different American communities' use of both spoken language and writing/reading practices within the home. Comparing two working-class areas – one predominantly black, the other white – with a middle-class suburb, she found that early school literacy experiences reflected middle-class values, with activities based around shared books/reading and creative writing.

The other communities' cultural activities were more oral. Storytelling, singing and rhymes were part of daily experiences. Actions, gestures and visual images played a more active part, perhaps resulting from community gatherings. She argued that, because early literacy is shaped by the community and the home, schools should recognise children's literacy experiences instead of imposing their own.

Thinking points

1. Did your own pre-school or family experiences shape your attitudes to reading and writing and your confidence at school?

2. Technologies (interactive television, the internet and video games) offer a new kind of literacy. What literacy skills do you need to use these?

3. Should other cultural practices (such as video games) be valued within schools?

Different types of reading books

First, recognising the variety in the types of books written for young children highlights their different functions. Many baby and toddler books aim to help with speech development by providing pictures for children to label and package/network build. These are often based around themes or topics using hypernyms (weather, clothes, animals) to provide children with relevant hyponyms (rain, socks, dogs). Nouns and adjectives are the most common word classes in early books that contain only a few words. These link children's literacy experiences with the equivalent stage of speech acquisition, by giving labels for objects and increasing children's knowledge of their immediate environment.

Early story books are designed to be read to children, not by them. They contain complicated words and grammatical structures that children can understand, even though they cannot read them or use them in their own speech. Children's understanding of words and structures is ahead of their ability to use them.

Books for young children aim to be enjoyable and act as a shared experience; such books introduce children to stories and storytelling, as well as often being instructional. Reading schemes for school-age children are slightly different in that, although entertaining, they have been created to help in the formal learning process, being graded to assist children in acquiring fluency skills.

And then what? Well, children become independent readers around the age of 8. Books for older children are still entertaining, informative and instructive, but are centred on them as active, solo readers.

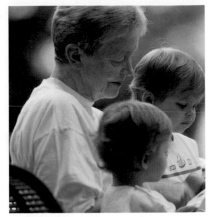

Fig. 16 *Early story books are designed to be read to children*

■ Research point

Jerome Bruner's LASS (Language Acquisition Support System) theory explains how adults encourage children's speech by using books to interact with babies and young children.

He saw parent–child interactions with books as four-phased:

1. **gaining attention**: getting the baby's attention on a picture
2. **query**: asking the baby what the object in the picture is
3. **label**: telling the baby what the object in the picture is
4. **feedback**: responding to the baby's utterance.

Bruner was inspired by Vygotsky, who believed that children learn not by being told how to do something but by being helped to do it when they are ready – and part of the 'scaffolding' process (see page 31). Both Bruner and Vygotsky see children as active learners and believe that the social contexts of their experiences are very important.

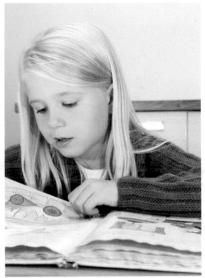

Fig. 17 *Children become independent readers around the age of eight*

Thinking points

1. How might early exposure to books help children's language skills?
2. In what ways do children use books to become active learners?
3. Apart from books, what other toys might help their speech development?

Classroom activity 9

Collect a selection of children's first books. Categorise them: for example, lift-the-flap, touch/feel, press/sounds, characters (Spot the dog) etc. Investigate key linguistic features and their effects. Think about how the texts:

- interact with their audience
- suggest values (e.g. behaviour/politeness/morals)
- use rhyme and other phonological devices
- depict characters (animal or human)
- use spoken language features
- proportion the amount of text to pictures; use pictures; use colour
- use hypernyms/hyponyms and semantic fields (what typical word classes are there?)
- use rhetorical devices (repetition, parallel sentence structures etc.)
- create textual **cohesion** (lexical repetition, syntactical repetition, connectives)
- vary sentence moods (declarative, exclamatory, interrogative or imperative).

What do young readers need to know?

Children need to understand that written texts:

- reflect the relationship between written symbols (**graphemes**) and sounds (phonemes)
- have cohesion, with different parts interconnecting
- are organised in particular ways, with chapter headings, page numbers, etc.
- differ in their organisation according to genre (e.g. fiction and non-fiction books are organised in different ways)
- represent the original culture, following its rules and conventions (e.g. English is read from left to right; narratives are organised in particular ways; certain 'characters' are well known in English-speaking cultures, etc.).

🔍 Analysing early books

An interesting feature of books written for young children is the use of animals, rather than human characters, as the central focus of fictional narratives in English-speaking cultures. *The Gruffalo*, by Julia Donaldson and Axel Scheffler, a popular and well-known story, exemplifies typical features of the genre.

Focusing on these four aspects of the text will show you how effective writing for children can be:

1 the significance of the characters of a mouse and a fox
2 the kinds of phonological devices
3 the use of direct speech
4 the types of pictures and layout chosen.

Choosing a mouse (usually the prey) as the hero of the tale and a fox (usually the predator) is significant, with breaking of stereotypes suggesting a moral or implied meaning for children to absorb. Here the mouse is the bravest animal, outmanoeuvring other animals, revealing their cowardly natures when confronted with the idea of a fierce-sounding

■ Key terms

Cohesion: the way in which a text appears logical and well constructed.

Grapheme: a written symbol, letter or combination of letters that is used to represent a phoneme.

AQA Examiner's tip

Look for patterns in texts and cluster your comments in your written responses. This helps to avoid the pitfalls of either analysing data chronologically, repeating ideas, or simply describing what you can see in front of you.

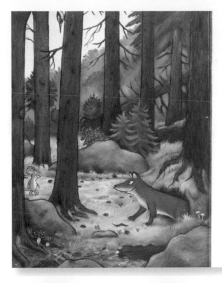

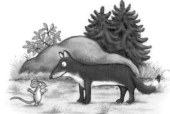

A mouse took a stroll through the deep dark wood.
A fox saw the mouse and the mouse looked good.
"Where are you going to, little brown mouse?
Come and have lunch in my underground house."
"It's terribly kind of you, Fox, but no —
I'm going to have lunch with a gruffalo."

"A gruffalo? What's a gruffalo?"
"A gruffalo! Why, didn't you know?"

"He has terrible tusks   and terrible claws,

And terrible teeth in his terrible jaws."

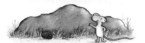

"Where are you meeting him?"
"Here, by these rocks,
And his favourite food is roasted fox."

"Roasted fox! I'm off!" Fox said.
"Goodbye, little mouse," and away he sped.

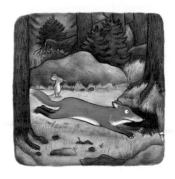

"Silly old Fox! Doesn't he know,
There's no such thing as a gruffalo?"

Julia Donaldson and Axel Scheffler, The Gruffalo, 1999

unknown animal, the Gruffalo. These stereotypes are probably already recognisable to children, from fairy tales or television cartoons. Even the monster's name ('Gruffalo') is interesting, with hints of the invented terms and names used in Lewis Carroll's 'Jabberwocky'. It echoes a real animal name (buffalo), and the adjective (gruff) has semantic connotations of grumpiness or badness.

Poetic phonological devices are used, as in the line-end rhymes ('wood'/'good'). This typical characteristic helps young children to remember words when hearing the text read aloud. Young children enjoy having the same book read to them repeatedly, responding to the repetitive nature and familiarity in a very different way from adult readers, who are more likely to search for new reading matter. Aside from predictability, rhyme is a common feature of nursery rhymes and songs, where the emphasis is on the interactive and multimodal nature of the experience (actions and words) and on sharing these. The rhythmic pattern is another poetic feature, linking the written word with oral storytelling; the sound effects in the plosive alliterative choices ('terrible tusks', 'terrible teeth') are reminiscent of poetry or descriptive literature. Repeated structures emphasise phrase structure, helping to extend vocabulary; the placing of a new word ('tusk') makes sense in the parallel structure to a near **synonym** ('teeth').

Key terms

Synonyms: words with very similar semantic value.

39

Most of the text is a dialogue. Direct speech, as a narrative feature, creates interesting variations of animal voices, but also becomes a grammatical and rhetorical patterning device. Syntactical structures used by the fox, and the other would-be eaters of the mouse, are repeated; only different lexical choices signal the places where the mouse might be enticed to be the predators' next meal. For example, the next creature to suggest to the mouse that they have a meal together, the owl, replaces 'underground house' with 'treetop house'.

Graphologically, placing the picture on the left of the page draws the child's attention to the images of the animals and the woodland context, before attention shifts to the text on the right. Already the child is encouraged to 'read' from left to right. Facial expressions can be interpreted – the mouse's innocence and naivety decoded from its smiling face, contrasting with the rather evil smile of the fox. Another recurrent feature is the placing of pictures both within the page and between passages of text, providing text–image cohesion. The pictures either link to the action, giving context to the dialogue, or help children understand the meanings of words – as where the adjectival material ('terrible claws') is pictured to give a visual impression. The **typographical** device of italics to present the speech of the fox is aimed at the adult reader of the text, who can create a different voice for the animal speaker.

Extension activity 5

Conduct a small-scale linguistic investigation of children's story books. You could focus on books aimed at specific ages, or particular genres. Look for some of the stylistic devices used to engage children's interest. Which linguistic methods do you think are used most to appeal to the child audience?

i How are children taught to read?

All this may have triggered memories of your first school reading books. Can you remember how you were taught to read words and produce the sounds that they represent? Changes in literacy strategies have changed some teaching methods within the classroom, but the main teaching approaches haven't altered significantly. Recently, debate has been fierce about the most effective methods for teaching reading. While you won't be asked in an examination to evaluate the different approaches, it is helpful to be aware of the strategies children apply and the support parents and teachers offer to advance their skills.

The 'look and say' and **phonics** methods are the two used in British classrooms.

'Look and say' or whole-word approach

Children learn the shape of words, not breaking them down phonologically. With the 'look and say' method, children learn to recognise whole words or sentences rather than individual phonemes. Flashcards with individual words written on them are used for this method, often accompanied with a related picture so that children can link the object and the referent.

Phonics

Children learn the different sounds made by different letters and letter blends and some rules of putting them together. Emphasis is on developing phonological awareness and on hearing, differentiating and replicating sounds in spoken words. The two main approaches to teaching phonics are analytic and synthetic (Table 22).

Table 22 *The key features of the analytic and synthetic phonics approaches*

Analytic phonics	Synthetic phonics

Children learn:
■ to break down whole words into phonemes and graphemes, looking for phonetic or orthographic patterns.
■ to decode words by separating them into smaller units:
  – *onset* (the vowel or syllable at the start of a word)
  – *rime* (the rest of the word, always beginning with a vowel)
■ to use rhyme or analogy to learn other words with similar patterns, e.g. c-at, m-at, p-at
■ to recognise one letter sound at a time, seeing pictures showing words beginning with the same letter sound
 	
Children learn initial letter sounds first, then middle sounds, followed by the final sounds of words and consonant blends.
 	
Children are competent readers within three years, breaking down and sounding out unfamiliar words. This phonics method runs alongside whole-word approaches and reading-scheme books.
	Children learn:
	■ to remember up to 44 phonemes and their related graphemes (one phoneme can be represented by different graphemes, for example 'ough', 'ow' and 'oa')
	■ to recognise each grapheme, sound out each phoneme in a word, blending the sounds together to pronounce the word phonetically
	■ to memorise phonemes quickly (up to five or six sounds a week)
	■ often through a multi-sensory approach whereby they:
	1) see the symbol
	2) listen to the sound
	3) use an action (such as counting phonemes on fingers or using magnetic letters to correspond to the phonemes)
	Children learn in whole-class teaching groups. Reading schemes are not used in the early stages of learning synthetic phonics, as the method can be taught in a few months.

Phonics is currently viewed as the most effective teaching method, but encouraging and motivating children to read independently outside school also ensures confident readers. This extract from a seven-year old's reading shows how parents support school literacy programmes.

Transcription conventions are given on page v.

Context: Oliver is reading his school book to his mother at home.

> **C:** the horse needs a new shoe (.) got any jobs mister (.) asked Vicky I'll give you a penny to jump
>
> **M:** not jump
>
> **C:** pump
>
> 5 **M:** yeah
>
> **C:** the pi b-billows
>
> **M:** not (.) not (.) billows what does that say what does that part of the word say [*mother covers up the end of the word to leave 'bell'*]
>
> **C:** bell [*mother takes hand off word*] ows
>
> 10 **M:** yes bellows

Author's own data

Already a confident reader, the child reads most words easily. The mother helps him to read an unfamiliar word ('bellows') by separating the syllables visually. Here phonics seems to help him decode syllables as, even prior to his mother's help, he uses his knowledge of rhyme to guess the word ('pi b-billows'). She also confirms he is reading accurately ('yeah', 'yes bellows'), repeating words for reinforcement.

Research point

Skinner's ideas about reinforcement could be useful to link to literacy acquisition. His view that learning takes place through positive reinforcement is perhaps evident in the way parents and teachers correct children's reading. The mother here limits her positive reinforcement to affirming the child's' correct reading of words ('yeah') but you could equally see an adult using praise words, such as 'well done' or 'good boy/girl', congratulating children's successful pronunciation or interpretation of words. Negative reinforcement in this interaction is limited to the mother telling the child when they have read a word wrongly ('not billows').

Thinking points

1. What other kinds of positive reinforcement are teachers/parents likely to offer to children learning to read?

2. Do you think negative reinforcement would be effective as a teaching method?

Classroom activity 10

Using the information provided on the previous couple of pages about the various methods of teaching children to read (whole-word, phonics, analytic and synthetic phonics), list some of their advantages and disadvantages.

Extension activity 6

Write an article evaluating the different teaching strategies, to appear in a magazine for parents.

🔍 The cues children use

So far we have concentrated mainly on phonological methods, but an early reader acquires many tools to interpret the written word, using **cues** to decode words and meanings within texts. Writers of children's reading books build cues into their texts. You will see this when you look at reading schemes.

Key terms

Cueing: the strategies used to help decode written texts successfully.

Table 23 *Types of reading cues*

Cue	Activity
Graphophonic	Looking at the shape of words, linking these to familiar graphemes/words to interpret them
Semantic	Understanding the meanings of words and making connections between words in order to decode new ones
Visual	Looking at the pictures and using the visual narrative to interpret unfamiliar words or ideas
Syntactic	Applying knowledge of word order and word classes to work out if a word seems right in the context
Contextual	Searching for understanding in the situation of the story – comparing it to their own experience or their pragmatic understanding of social conventions
Miscue	Making errors when reading: a child might miss a word or substitute another that looks similar, or guess a word from accompanying pictures

Text A is an extract from the opening of *Victorian Adventure*. Text B is a transcript of Oliver, aged 7, reading from the book. These texts show Oliver's use of cueing to read accurately.

Transcription conventions are given on page v.

Text A

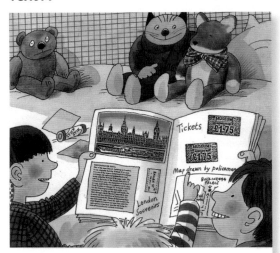

Biff and Chip had been to
   London with Gran.
They had some pictures which
   they put into a scrapbook.
They wanted to take the book to school.

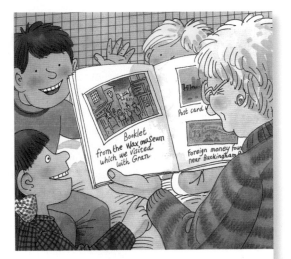

Gran came into Biff's room to
   look at the children's scrapbook.
'We had a great time in London,' said Biff.
'Thank you, Gran.'
Gran was pleased.

Roderick Hunt and Alex Brychta, Victorian Adventure, *1990*

Text B

M: okay are you going to read your book to me Ollie (2.0) what's it called

O: Victorian Adventure

M: yes

5   *O:* Biff and Chip had been to (.) London (1.0) with Gran (,) they had some pictures which (.) they put into a scrapbook (.) they wanted to take the book to school

M: it's like when we went to London isn't it

O: Gran came into Biff's room to look at the children's
10   scrapbook(.) We had a great time in London said Biff (1.0) thank you Gran (.) Gran was pleased (2.0) suddenly the magic (.) key glowed it was time for an adventure (.) the magic took the children into the (.) little house (.) but didn't it take Gran

M: no no what does it say

15 *O:* but did it take Gran

M: that's right good boy [*sound of pages turning*]

O: the magic took them back in time to a street on a foggy day (1) a boy was standing under a (.) gas lamp (.) he looked at the children in surprise (.) excuse me (.) said Biff do you know
20   where we are (.) don't you know said the boy (.) this is London (.) he took his cap off it wasn't a boy it was a girl

M: [*laughs*]

Author's own data

Oliver appears to have little difficulty using graphophonic cues; he reads the words in this opening section accurately with his only error being a **miscue** ('didn't' for 'did'). This 'virtuous' error reveals his understanding of syntax, although the two words have opposite meanings. His pauses before the nouns ('gran', 'gas lamp') suggest that his semantic understanding is not as confident; perhaps Oliver does not usually use the word 'Gran' to address his grandmother, needing the visual clue on page two to connect the white-haired woman with the word 'gran'. Regular pauses vary in length from a micro-pause to two seconds. In some instances these show his uncertainty with a word. The pauses before the proper noun ('London') suggest it is unfamiliar and he looks for prompts from picture clues. The pictures of Big Ben and Buckingham Palace in the text provide him with a cultural context.

The prosodic features, with stresses on words ('great', 'know' and 'girl'), show that Oliver has semantic awareness. By stressing what he thinks are key elements of the story ('it was a girl'), rather than particular word classes, he engages with the listener's needs. When reading to his mother, he seems to understand that dialogue creates a character's voice. He tries to inject emphasis and stress into key words when reading aloud ('Don't you know, said the boy').

Oliver's use of syntactical cueing is influenced more by the line breaks than the grammatical sense of sentences, as in the pauses after 'to' and 'which' on the first page of the book. More sophisticated grammatical awareness is apparent when he uses pauses to show a completed clause ('he looked at the children in surprise'). Although inconsistent throughout the transcript, this confirms that his reading ability is developing.

His awareness of context is not really tested here. Despite the unfamiliarity of the 'Victorian' context, the book actually focuses on a London trip. That he can relate to this experience is reinforced by his mother's unacknowledged interrogative ('it's like when we went to London isn't it'). Because this is a staged reading scheme, he has encountered the 'magic key' before and does not question this narrative device ('the magic took the children into the little house').

The stages of reading development

Jeanne Chall identified six stages from her studies with children (Table 24). Although your focus is on children reading from toddlerhood to age 11, it is interesting to see how our reading motivations change, and the types of texts we choose alter, as we become accomplished readers. As with all stages, remember that these offer simplified guides and not definitive judgments about all children's development at these ages.

Returning to Oliver, you can see that he is in the 'confirmation and fluency' stage; he reads quickly with few pauses or inaccuracies. Confident with high-frequency words, he struggles only with unfamiliar ones. Each book he reads adds to his word bank, in both lexical and semantic terms. But he is still reading to learn that skill rather than for the content of a text, i.e. reading for knowledge and enjoyment.

Extension activity 7

Record and transcribe children of different ages reading. (You could use younger siblings, friends' families or through school/nursery visits.) Focus on specific aspects of the data that you find interesting. For example, you could look at the interactional nature of reading and social development, or compare a child's reading development over time.

Table 24 *Chall's stages of children's reading development*

Stage	Description	Age (years)	Key characteristics
0	Pre-reading and pseudo-reading	Up to 6	'Pretend' reading (turning pages and repeating stories perhaps previously read to them)
			Some letter and word recognition, especially letters in own name
			Predicting single words or the next stage of a story
1	Initial reading and decoding	6–7	Reading simple texts containing high-frequency lexis (this happens when children start to learn the relationship between phonemes and graphemes)
			How many written words understood? Chall estimated around 600
2	Confirmation and fluency	7–8	Reading texts more quickly, accurately and fluently, paying more attention to the meanings of words and texts
			How many written words understood? Chall estimated around 3,000
3	Reading for learning	9–14	Reading for knowledge and information becomes the motivation
4	Multiplicity and complexity	14–17	Responding critically to what they read and analysing texts
5	Construction and reconstruction	18+	Reading selectively and forming opinions about what they have read

■ Reading schemes

References have already been made to graded reading schemes designed to help children's development. You might recall characters from your school reading-scheme books and the types of narratives they involved, such as Biff and Chip and the 'magic key' genre. This genre is used in the Oxford Reading Tree scheme and uses the narrative structure of a magic key that begins to glow and transports children back to the past for an adventure. Reading schemes are deliberately staged in difficulty to help children acquire and extend lexical and semantic knowledge, as well as developing grammatical understanding. Familiarity is established through character-based and narrative approaches as the aim is to build confidence through the stages. Like early reading books, texts designed for teaching purposes often offer opportunities for developing pragmatic understanding through modelling good behaviour and politeness conventions, and by using multicultural and gender representations to negate stereotyping. Recently the value of non-fiction books has been recognised, especially to motivate and encourage boys to read.

Reading-scheme books use different linguistic choices from the kinds in *The Gruffalo*, because their primary purpose is to teach reading skills rather than to entertain.

Key features of reading schemes are:

■ **lexical repetition**: especially the new lexis introduced in each book but also proper nouns

- **syntactical repetition of structures**: usually subject-verb-object order and simple sentences containing one clause (in early books)
- **simple verbs**: single verbs used (i.e. is) rather than verb phrases
- **one sentence per line**: helping children to say complete phrases
- **anaphoric referencing**: pronouns (she/he) refer to the names of characters already used
- **limited use of modifiers**: this makes graded reading schemes different from imaginative stories where adjectives add detail and description
- **text-image cohesion**: the picture tells the story of the text on the page.

Classroom activity 11

1. Below is an extract from *Going for Gold*, part of the Wellington Square reading scheme.

2. Using the list of key features of reading schemes above, identify the language devices chosen by the writer to help develop children's reading skills.

Training for the race

It was Sports Day at Waterloo School.
Ben's Dad had come to see him run.
Ben was a good runner.
He was in the 200 metres and
he wanted to win.
Kevin was also in that race.
He was a good runner and
he wanted to win the race too.
Kevin and Ben lined up with
the other runners.
'Ready, steady, go!' shouted Mr March.
Everyone ran very quickly but
Kevin and Ben finished first.
They finished the race together.
'Well done!' shouted Mr Belter.
'Well done!' shouted Mr March.
Ben's Dad was very pleased.

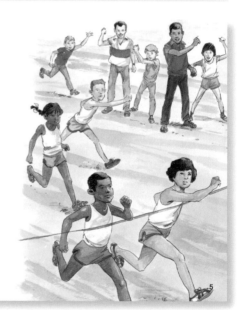

Tessa Krailing, Keith Gaines, Wendy Wren, Shirley Tully, Going for Gold, *1993*

Extension activity 8

Look back at the data extracts in this topic and evaluate how they link to these acquisition debates:

1. Can you apply the nature versus nurture debate to literacy acquisition? Is learning to read an innate skill (Chomsky) or does it have to be acquired through imitation (Skinner)?

2. Is there evidence that the methods used to teach children reading support the interactionist viewpoint?

3. How far to you think cognitive acquisition theories relate to reading development? Do children have to understand concepts before they can read words, or is reading different from spoken acquisition?

Developing writing

Key terms

Cursive handwriting: handwriting in which the characters are joined in rounded and flowing strokes.

Convergence: a process of linguistic change in which people adjust their dialect, accent or speech style to those of others, often occurring to express solidarity and understanding.

Sociolect: a defined use of language as a result of membership of a social group.

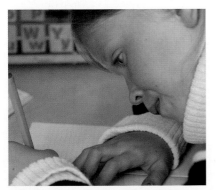

Fig. 18 *Writing can be used to communicate, to record and to express yourself*

What is writing and why do we need it?

A useful starting point is to remind yourself of the main differences between speech and writing modes (a key part of your AS study). Other questions to ask yourself are:

- Why do we write? What are the functions and purposes of writing?

- How do our writing skills develop and how do we personalise these?

- How do we adapt our style of writing for different genres and in different registers?

You may believe that writing can be used:

- to communicate with others for social, interactional and phatic purposes (text messages, letters, birthday cards)

- referentially to record information (notes, lists, reminders, official forms)

- expressively (diaries, creative writing).

Writing often supports or replaces oral communication; for example, you can text a message to a friend to arrange a meeting, or give bad news that you would rather not deliver in person.

Before looking at children's writing development, think back to your own. How did your writing style and skills develop? Were you excited when you were allowed to use a pen in your schoolwork instead of a pencil, as this meant that you were now a competent writer? Another milestone may have been when you joined up your **handwriting cursively** and made decisions about your writing style (sloped, upright), letting you personalise your work and define your identity.

You might also remember your pride at having your work displayed on the classroom walls. If you find your old exercise books, your spellings might make you laugh, as might your phrasing of ideas. These sound odd to you now because of your knowledge of grammatical structures and spelling rules. What might surprise you is how creative with language you were as a child.

As an adult writer, you have learnt to manipulate register. In text messaging you probably adapt standard spelling, punctuation and grammatical rules to conform to text conventions, and to **converge** to the **sociolect** of your audience. By doing this you can also display your idiolect, creating a style that others recognise as yours (a little like your handwriting). You do this because you know the 'rules' of written language and choose to break them.

So you can see that children have much to learn. It's not just about mechanical and physical control of the pen or pencil, it is as much about:

- combining words and sentences to convey ideas

- recognising that writing generally has an audience

- using recognisable discourse and genre conventions

- manipulating language to achieve specific purposes.

It's also about being an active learner, discovering that writing can do all these things.

Recent research into children's literacy emphasises the effects of home cultural and social practices on their reading and writing development. But children don't just experience the written word in books, they also find it through computers and television.

Writing is one of the key communication modes, acquired after speech and having its own separate system. In any language, writing uses a common and agreed code of symbols. Individual graphemes combine to make words that a language user can recognise. But writing is only effective when the order is right; this order can be syntactical and in the spelling and **orthography** of words.

To summarise, writing means being able to use:

- the vocabulary system and associated meanings of words and phrases (lexis)
- sentences to create meaning (grammar)
- graphemes that relate to phonemes, and other devices to create prosodic effects, for example in punctuation choices (phonology)
- social conventions within certain types of written texts (pragmatics)
- cohesive structures (discourse)
- the layout of texts, the use of graphemes and images to create semiotic meaning (graphology)
- variations in language to suit audience, purpose and context (register).

Orthography too is important. It's the part of language study to do with spelling and the graphemes used. For some linguists, orthography also includes the use of capital letters.

The list above should remind you how complex writing is. Written texts are often constructed far more deliberately than speech. As children have so much to learn, it is unsurprising that it takes a long time to learn to write effectively in all areas. As you know from your own experience, writing is far more prescriptive than speech and follows established rules. Schooling, too, places emphasis on children becoming literate, with national literacy strategies and initiatives like the 'literacy hour' encouraging a focus on successful reading and writing development.

A major difference between reading and writing is that the latter requires motor and mechanical skills; children have to hold pencils and pens, controlling them in order to transfer their thoughts and ideas onto paper. Increasingly, access to computers means that children can combine the letters and symbols on a keyboard to make words and sentences into meaningful texts. Using computers also introduces graphological and typographical choices that are unavailable when writing by hand.

🔍 Stages of writing

To introduce writing development, the list below outlines the stages:

- drawing
- letter-like forms
- copied letters
- child's name and strings of letters
- words
- sentences
- text.

Children's skills start with putting a writing instrument on paper (usually crayons and paints). Images and shapes become words, sentences and whole texts. Put like this it seems rather mechanical, but, of course, writing is also about conveying ideas and meanings and so both thought and planning have to apply to any written text.

Early writing

The term **emergent writing** is used to describe children's early scribbles or representations of the written word. Below is Oliver's early attempt, aged 3, at writing his thoughts down on paper. This accompanied a picture he had drawn at nursery school.

Oliver's message would have been impossible for others to interpret without the teacher asking what he had written, and recording this message using recognisable words. He clearly has meaning for his scribbles, indicating semiotic understanding. But he needs to learn mechanical skills to make his graphemes recognisable.

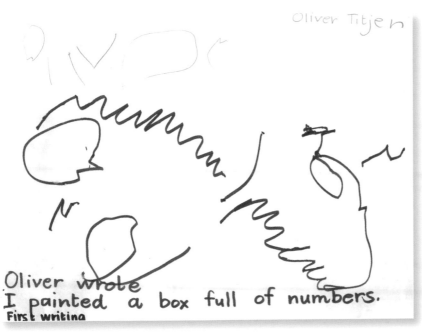

Author's own data

Typically for a 3-year-old, the letters in his name are written clearly. The rest resemble scribbles, but Oliver is aware of directionality (working from left to right) and that English is written from top to bottom of a page. A sense of authorship is already present in the placing of his name at the top left of the text. The teacher reinforces this by writing Oliver's full name. Spaces between the scribbles show that Oliver is aware that individual words have discrete meanings. Letter shapes resemble some of the alphabet ('w', 'm') and **ascender/descender** graphemes ('p') suggest an emerging orthographical awareness. For Oliver, however, there seems to be no separation yet between words and pictures. The text is multimodal, conveying his message in both the picture and the scribble writing.

From this early writing, you can see that Oliver has achieved the first four stages of writing development. His writing still resembles a drawing, yet within it are letter-like forms, written in strings, and his name is clearly evident. Oliver's next stage is to create words, sentences and texts. This will be encouraged during his school experiences within a more formal framework of literacy teaching.

Classroom activity 12

Look at this story by Cameron, aged 5.

■ How has he developed from Oliver's stage?

■ What does Cameron understand about constructing texts?

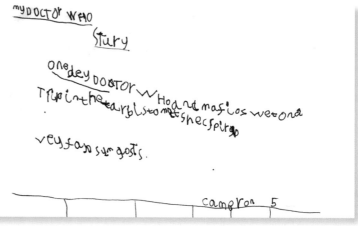

Transliteration:

My Doctor Who story

One day Dr Who and Martha Jones went on a trip in the Tardis to meet Shakespeare and they found some ghosts.

Cameron 5

Author's own data

■ Extension activity 9

Gather examples from emergent writing onwards. This could be from young family members, or through visits to local primary schools or, if you have kept your books, you could chart your own writing development through junior school.

Kroll's four phases/stages of development

Barry Kroll (1981) identified four phases of children's development, and further work by other researchers, such as Katherine Perera, added suggested age ranges for these stages (Table 25).

Table 25 *Kroll's stages of development*

Stage	Age (years)	Characteristics
Preparation	Up to 6	Basic motor skills are acquired alongside some principles of spelling.
Consolidation	7/8	Writing is similar to spoken language (including a more casual, colloquial register, unfinished sentences and strings of clauses joined by the conjunction 'and').
Differentiation	9/10	Awareness of writing as separate from speech emerges. A stronger understanding of writing for different audiences and purposes is evident and becomes more automatic.
Integration	Mid-teens	This stage heralds the 'personal voice' in writing and is characterised by evidence of controlled writing, with appropriate linguistic choices being made consistently.

Looking at Oliver's 'I painted a box full of numbers' (see page 49) and Cameron's 'Dr Who story' (see page 50), which stage would you place them in? What support would you give for your decisions?

Later you will see evidence of children's writing in later stages; compare their development with Kroll's stages.

Understanding genre

From an early age children see specific writing genres, usually ones related to their own experience. Think of key events when you were younger, such as parties, and recall the invitations sent out on your behalf and the birthday cards that you first signed and then wrote using genre conventions (dear Emily, happy birthday, love Jenny). Other early home writing experiences might have been writing a list for Father Christmas or a note for the Tooth Fairy.

Understanding register is important in order to meet genre conventions, and children have to learn that vocabulary choices and grammatical constructions contribute to the overall tone. Also significant is the purpose of the text as well as the audience and the relationship between reader and writer. As writing matures, pragmatic awareness becomes more sophisticated, with references to shared experiences and the use of either a humorous or serious tone reflecting the personality of the writer. These pragmatic skills make writing less mechanical and more engaging.

Here are some pieces of writing in specific genres. The first text is a 7-year-old boy's letter to Santa. The second is a 4-year-old girl's invitation for her teddy to attend a tea party celebrating the end of her Reception year.

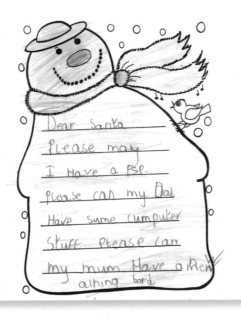

Transliteration:

Dear Santa

Please may I have a PSP. Please can my dad have some computer stuff. Please can my mum have a new ironing board.

Author's own data

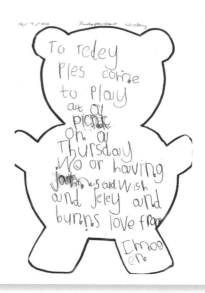

Transliteration:

To Teddy

Please come to play at a picnic on Thursday. We are having jam sandwiches and jelly and buns

Love from Imogen

Author's own data

Both children show the pragmatic understanding that politeness is needed in invitations and certain types of letters, notably those in which you make a request. In the letter to Santa, the child repeats words ('please'), foregrounding this at the beginning of each sentence, as well as using modal auxiliary verbs ('can', may') to reinforce the polite tone. This repetition of sentence structure also makes the text cohesive. Although careful to put his own wish first, the child also refers to his parents and identifies items that they may (or may not in the mother's case) be grateful to receive. You might perceive some gender-stereotype issues here! His use of the possessive pronoun ('my') could be an acknowledgement that Santa needs to know the recipients of the presents.

Within the letter to Santa, the child understands letter conventions, choosing 'Dear' to address Santa formally. In the tea invitation the child also demonstrates strong awareness of generic conventions with the address ('To Teddy') and the sign-off ('love from Imogen'). Imogen is also aware of certain conventions associated with invitations in her request for 'Teddy' to join her at an event (a picnic), offering a time, but not a venue, which shows that she has still to learn all the information that Teddy logically would need to know in order to attend. Not only does she show an awareness of genre conventions, she also demonstrates an understanding of the persuasive nature of an invitation, tempting Teddy with promises of jelly and buns. Both texts display an understanding of the correct register, and both have a formal tone.

How are genres used in children's early writing at school?

A useful way to help you evaluate children's writing is to use Joan Rothery's categories, identified from investigating young children's writing in Australian schools (Table 26). She found that early writing within school fell into some distinctive groupings: observation/comment, recount, report and narrative.

Table 26 *Rothery's categories for evaluating children's writing*

Category	Features
Observation/ comment	The writer makes an observation ('I saw a tiger') and follows this with either an evaluative comment ('it was very large') or mixes these in with the observation ('I saw a very large tiger').
Recount	Usually a chronological sequence of events. A typical example would be a recount of a school trip, which children are often asked to do as a follow-up activity. It is written subjectively ('I'). The structure of a recount usually follows a set pattern: Orientation – Event – Reorientation. The orientation sets the scene, perhaps the journey to the place or the name of the place visited. The reorientation at the end of the recount completes the writing.
Report	A factual and objective description of events or things; it tends not to be chronological.
Narrative	A story genre where the scene is set for events to occur and be resolved at the end. It also has a set pattern: Orientation – Complication – Resolution – Coda. The coda, which identifies the point of the story, is not always added. Because of the structural complexity few children will achieve the whole structure early on, despite their experience of reading stories that follow this narrative structure.

Classroom activity 13

Apply Rothery's categories to the following three texts.

- Which text exemplifies each category?
- What evidence is there in the texts to support your choices?

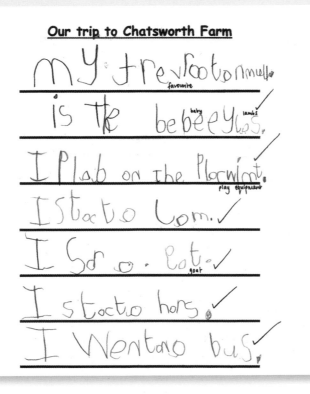

Our trip to Chatsworth Farm

Transliteration:

My favourite animal is the baby lambs. I played on the play equipment. I stroked a lamb. I saw a goat. I stroked a horse. I went on a bus.

Author's own data

> Thursday 10th April
>
> <u>My favourite place</u>
>
> <u>where is it.</u>
> Portugal is a warm place. in ~~summer~~
> summer. It has lovely restaurants
> and ~~delys~~ delicious food. I
> like to go there with my family
> It is a cheerful place.
> <u>what is it like.</u>
>
> Portugal has delightful beaches
> and in some beaches there are
> Rock Pools. It has the most
> wonderful villa's with good pools.
> <u>what happens there.</u>

Transliteration:

My favourite place

Where is it

Portugal is a warm place in summer. It has lovely restaurants and delicious food. I like to go there with my family. It is a cheerful place.

What is it like

Portugal has delightful beaches and in some beaches there are rock pools. It has the most wonderful villas with good pools.

What happens there.

Author's own data

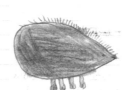

> wednesday 10th Seblember
>
> <u>Hedgehogs</u>
>
> ~~I did a~~ I am doing a rePort
> on hedgehogs ~~Because I like them~~.
>
> Hedgehogs have Short SPines. often on
> there back and they can Prick you
> when you touch them. Hedgehogs will
> curl uP into balls when they smell
> danger.
>
> Most hedgehogs live under leaves
> and Some live in PeoPles gardens.
>
> Some hedgehogs eat foul things
> like dead toads but Some Just eat
> Snails and worms.
>
> Most hedgehogs wander around and
> Some just Stay in thier nests.
>
> I wrote this rePort on hedgehogs because
> i like them

Transliteration:

Wednesday 10th September

Hedgehogs

I am doing a report on hedgehogs.

Hedgehogs have sharp spines on their back and they can prick you when you touch them. Hedgehogs will curl up into balls when they smell danger.

Most hedgehogs live under leaves and some live in people's gardens.

Some hedgehogs eat foul things like dead toads but some just eat snails and worms.

Most hedgehogs wander around and some just stay in their nests.

I wrote this report on hedgehogs because I like them.

Author's own data

Other genre perspectives

Britton proposed three modes of writing used by schoolchildren: expressive, poetic and transactional (Table 27). These modes focus more on stylistic choices than on the content of the writing, as with Rothery's categories.

Table 27 *Britton's three modes of children's writing*

Mode	Features
Expressive	The first mode to develop because it resembles speech.
	Uses the first person perspective and the content is usually based on personal preferences.
Poetic	Develops gradually, requiring skills in crafting and shaping language, but is encouraged early on because of its creativity.
	Phonological features such as rhyme, rhythm and alliteration, as well as descriptive devices such as adjectives and similes, are common.
Transactional	Develops last, around secondary school age, once children have finally dissociated speech from writing. It is the style of academic essays, as it is more impersonal in style and tone. The third person is used to create a detached tone. Formal sentence structures and graphological features are used to signpost sections and ideas and structures tend to be chronological.

■ Research point

Katherine Perera suggested an alternative framework for classifying texts: chronological and non-chronological. Chronological texts rely on action words (verbs) and on linking ideas using connectives. Non-chronological texts are considered harder to write because they rely on logical connections between ideas.

This framework complements Rothery's genre categories, focusing also on the importance of the discourse structure of the writing task as a way of assisting children to become competent and confident writers. It is interesting that non-chronological texts are considered harder to write, but Britton suggests that children are encouraged to tackle these early on because of their creative aspect; for example, poetry is a writing activity that children accomplish early in school.

Looking at Imogen's 'leaves' poem (written at age 4) and Oliver's 'animal' poem (written at age 7) will help you with the Thinking points.

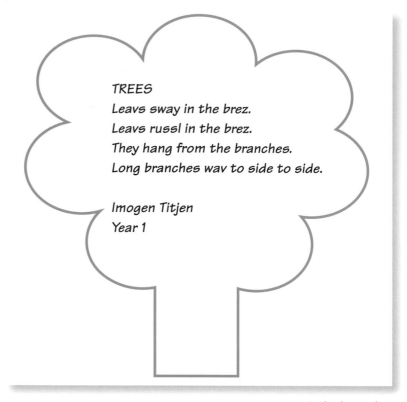

TREES
Leavs sway in the brez.
Leavs russl in the brez.
They hang from the branches.
Long branches wav to side to side.

Imogen Titjen
Year 1

Author's own data

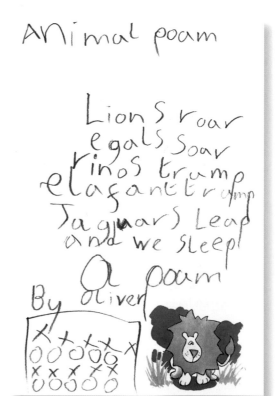

Author's own data

Transliteration:

Animal poem

Lions roar
Eagles soar
Rhinos tramp
Elephants trump
Jaguars leap
And we sleep

A poem by Oliver

1. Why might children write chronological texts first?

2. What kind of genres fit with chronological approaches?

3. What genres might encourage children to practise non-chronological text skills?

Extension activity 10

Return to the texts used in Classroom activity 13. Apply Britton's writing modes to these texts. To what extent can you classify each text as expressive, poetic or transactional? Evaluate the differences you can find when you apply Rothery, Perera and Britton's classifications.

Spelling

How do you spell a word you haven't heard before? We all use various strategies to help us spell accurately, including many we learned as children. The main ones are:

■ sound clues, sounding out words to stress the sounds and separate syllables

■ clues from the word's meaning to make links with similar words

■ writing it down until it 'looks' right

■ using grammatical knowledge to predict spelling (such as patterns in affixing to change word class and the common inflections/morphemes that are added to English words)

■ a dictionary or a computer spell-checker.

Children become like detectives looking for clues and making guesses but, as they become more experienced, they rely less on guesswork and more on their knowledge of spelling patterns.

Difficulties arise with spelling despite the alphabetic principle (in which a symbol represents a sound or unit of sounds) because there is not a one-to-one correspondence between sound and symbol; in English, 26 letters represent 44 phonemes. Decisions need to be made about whether individual graphemes represent the sound or whether a **digraph** (two letters produced as a single sound, for example 'sh') is needed to create a single sound. The sounds of letters are often affected by their position in the word or by the surrounding letters, so phonetic strategies are insufficient for accurate spelling. To demonstrate the potential pitfalls of spelling, say the following words out loud:

careful   rat   favour   ball   was

Possible problems also occur because of the number of **homophones** in English. Here are some examples of homophones beginning with the letter 's':

sea/see   sale/sail   stare/stair   son/sun   some/sum   steak/stake

Children have to learn and practise homophones so that they can use the right one in their written work. Another difficulty is created by the addition of inflections, which can affect the phonology of a word, as in 'house' and 'houses'.

Key terms

Digraph: a graphic unit in which two symbols combine, or any sequence of two letters produced as a single sound, e.g. 'sh'.

Homophone: a lexical item that has the same pronunciation as another.

The five spelling stages

Research has pinpointed five spelling stages (Table 28) but, again, remember that individual children can reach these at different ages.

Table 28 *Spelling stages*

Stage	What can a child do at this stage?
Pre-phonemic	Imitate writing, mainly scribbling and using pretend writing; some letter shapes are decipherable
Semi-phonetic	Link letter shapes and sounds, using this to write words
Phonetic	Understand that all phonemes can be represented by graphemes; words become more complete
Transitional	Combine phonic knowledge with visual memory; an awareness of combinations of letters and letter patterns, including the 'magic e' rule
Conventional	Spell most words correctly

💡 Categories of spelling error

Table 29 shows the main types of spelling error. It is often interesting to consider the errors made and how many or few there are within a text. This could link with analyses of other linguistic competencies, building a picture of a child's overall understanding of writing. Remember that children might overgeneralise rules in the same way they do when acquiring speech, which is not always helpful with irregular spelling patterns. Another factor to consider is the effect of accent on some phonetic choices and that some spelling choices might vary according to where children live.

Table 29 *The main types of spelling error made by children*

Term	Definition
Insertion	Adding extra letters
Omission	Leaving out letters
Substitution	Substituting one letter for another
Transposition	Reversing the correct order of letters in words
Phonetic spelling	Using sound awareness to guess letters and combinations of letters
Over/undergeneralisation of spelling rules	Overgeneralising of a rule where it is not appropriate to apply it, or undergeneralising it by only applying it in one specific context
Salient (key) sounds	Writing only the key sounds

AQA Examiner's tip

Remember the phrase 'virtuous error', as this will help you take a positive approach to describing what children can do and the logical reasons for their choices, rather than adopting a deficit model and focusing judgementally on their mistakes.

Classroom activity 14

The table below shows a selection of spelling errors made by children aged 7 and 8. Copy and complete the table, identifying:

■ what the actual spelling is

■ what types of errors the children have made.

You might put some words into more than one category.

You can then go on to consider:

■ why these might have occurred

■ what effect accent might have on spelling.

Child's spelling	Actual spelling	Type of spelling error(s)
suddnly		
peculier/perculiar		
cloke		
kitchin		
discusting		
(golf) corse		
shale (shall)		
exspensis		
twincling		
butifull		
kitins		
fraindly		
becuase		
correg (meaning bravery)		
bissnis		
chearful		
intelgent		

Extension activity 11

When you looked at the ways in which children acquire speech, you evaluated arguments of nature (language as innate within us) and nurture (as supported by teaching and environmental factors). Which acquisition arguments apply most relevantly to writing acquisition?

■ Punctuation and grammatical development

What is punctuation and why is it important? It marks boundaries between units of language: words, phrases, clauses and sentences. These boundaries are marked by spaces, capital letters, full stops and commas. Certain sentence moods, specifically exclamatory and interrogative moods, are indicated by exclamation and question marks. Punctuation also makes meaning clear to a reader.

These typed extracts written by the same child were produced two years apart. Although not in the child's handwriting, the texts have been reproduced using the original spelling and punctuation. Note the differences between the punctuation of each text and the effect this has on the overall success of the narrative for an audience.

A terrible day (child, aged 8)

It all started one morning when the alarm clock rang very loud and I fell out of bed and bumbed my head. I got dressed and had breakfast my sister got a toy in her breakfast and I got nothing. and I lost my toothbrush so my Mum told me of. when I was brushing my hair my brush broke. when I was on my way to school my car broke down and I had to walk to school. Then I dropped my bag and its strap broke in half. when I got into school I had to do a hard test and I got all my spellings wrong. in the playground I had a fall out with my best fraind, and I fell over and hurt my knee.

Author's own data

A Space Adventure (child, aged 10)

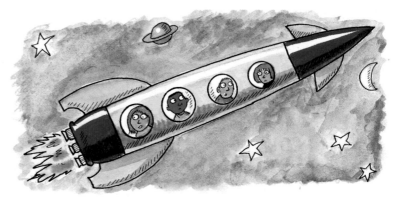

Fig. 19 *'Suddenly the ship made a sudden jolt …'*

Somewhere in deepest, darkest space travelled a team of explorers on board. No one could of predicted the mayhem and misfortunate happenings lying ahead. This was only the beginning…

The crew inside the spaceship wasn't a big crew, there was only 4, but they were always arguing; they could never agree on anything! They were called Katie, Jessica, Tom and James and all they thought about was themselves. Nevertheless, they were stuck together.

Suddenly the ship made a sudden jolt and everyone was thrown of their feet and fell with a bump to the floor.

'What was that?' asked Katie

'It wasn't me!' replied Tom

Author's own data

The 'terrible day' writing contains full stops to show the end of ideas, but some are non-standard, such as the full stop before the conjunction ('and I lost my toothbrush'). As stylistic awareness develops, writers learn to break rules for effect. Yet here the child is trying to think of another terrible event to describe, so the connective ('and') simply acts as a continuation, rather than trying to make this sentence stand out to a reader. This is typical of Kroll's consolidation stage (see page 50), where writing is similar to speech; look at the number of times 'and' is used as a connective. The child still uses capital letters inconsistently after full stops and, interestingly, tends to not capitalise sentences starting with the subordinating conjunction ('when') and coordinating conjunction ('and'), perhaps because of their roles as conjunctions. The one comma in the passage suggests the addition of another terrible event ('I had a fall out with my best fraind, and I fell over') showing some development in punctuation.

When reading this story, or imagined account, of a bad day you might have noticed some sophistication emerging in the grammatical structure; the child is using subordinate clauses to create complex sentences, and uses the subordinating conjunction at the start of a sentence to create clarity and interest for a reader. Adverbial phrases ('in the playground') are important, rather than description, and lexical choices are mainly limited to nouns ('alarm clock', 'toothbrush').

Two years later the same child has advanced to Kroll's differentiation stage. There is a strong narrative, and stylistic choices are used deliberately to entertain an audience and sustain their interest. A range of punctuation is used for effect: ellipsis creates tension (…); commas provide parenthesis, showing grammatical understanding that the ideas contained within the commas provide additional information to the main clause; and semicolons add further information. Direct speech is now punctuated (' ') and separated, so the child distinguishes between represented speech and continuous prose. Question marks and exclamation marks add prosodic effects, illustrating the writer's desire to craft an interesting story. Although complex sentences were used when the child was 8, here the same child uses simple sentences for dramatic effect. More sophisticated adverbs ('suddenly') make cohesive links or change direction in the narrative. Another significant development is the use of paragraphs to structure the narrative, again highlighting greater control of discourse structure and graphological understanding of the right layout of a text. Superlatives ('deepest', 'darkest') and other descriptive adjectives set the scene, with elision used to create a casual register.

As children grow older they also develop skills in checking, editing and correcting their work. If writing is considered a process, this might be separated into thinking and reflecting about their ideas, planning and composing how best to convey them, then writing down, revising and editing them. You can see in children's writing from different stages how the latter skills begin to appear.

Extension activity 12

Collect a range of writing by children of different ages and undertake a detailed investigation as to how it develops in all the linguistic areas. You could compare by genre, such as story writing, or just look for patterns in development.

Examination preparation and practice

Assessment

As part of the $2\frac{1}{2}$ hour examination you will spend half of the time allowed on Section A: Language acquisition and half the time allowed on Section B: Language change. You need to answer one question from each section, so this will give you 1 hour and 15 minutes for each.

You will have the choice of two questions for Section A: Language acquisition. The usual pattern is one spoken and one literacy option. However, there can be some mix/matching between the topics, for example a spoken transcript accompanied by written texts, so make sure you revise all topics. All questions are data-based, meaning that you will have to analyse transcripts of real interactions or facsimiles of written material produced for, or by, children.

Assessment objectives

AO1: Select and apply a range of linguistic methods, to communicate relevant knowledge using appropriate terminology and coherent, accurate written expression (7.5%).

AO1 is worth up to 24 marks. You are credited at the highest level for being systematic in your approach to the data in front of you. Read the question carefully, note the main parts of it and annotate the exam paper before you start writing. Focus particularly on identifying relevant linguistic features, using the linguistic methods you are familiar with from your English language study (grammar, phonology etc.). Make sure you write clearly and accurately in the exam, as this shows the examiner that you are able to use English language yourself effectively.

AO2: Demonstrate critical understanding of a range of concepts and issues relating to the construction and analysis of meanings in spoken and written language, using knowledge of linguistic approaches (5%).

This is worth 16 marks. It is testing what you know about the theories and concepts you have studied in English language, from both AS and A2. Getting high marks for this assessment objective is about being selective in your choice of theories and theorists to discuss. Making them relevant to the data in front of you and integrated into these examples will avoid huge chunks of 'all I know about Chomsky', which is not what the examiner wants to know. Don't forget that using your own observations of younger family members' language use, or your Unit 4 child language investigation findings, might be just as pertinent to the data as recognised theorists.

AO3: Analyse and evaluate the influence of contextual factors on the production and reception of spoken and written language, showing knowledge of the key constituents of language (2.5%).

This is worth 8 marks. Read both the question and the data carefully, noting down the significant features of context you can see. Such information could include that the setting of the children's conversations was a home context, or that the written texts were produced in school. Look also for who the participants are and their relationship to each other. Context on its own is not enough to discuss. To get the highest possible mark for context, the examiner is looking for you to link the contextual points to your interpretation of features within the data. So consider how the context affects the language used and don't make a discussion of context separate from your analysis of the data.

■ Practising for the exam

In this section you have the opportunity to practise some of the types of questions that you could see in the Unit 3 examination. Practising small tasks, as you have done throughout the topics, was important to ensure your understanding of all the different linguistic areas and methods you can use in your analysis. However, practising extended writing tasks is the most useful thing you can do, as it tests your ability to look at data in a detailed manner, and assesses your ability to apply what you know about language acquisition.

Write your answers to the questions below, keeping the assessment objectives and mark scheme in mind. Check your answers against the sample responses that follow and read the examiner's comments, matching these to the Mark Scheme extracts provided. Add these to your own ideas to see what a comprehensive answer for each question could have contained. Evaluate your own answers to identify what you could have done differently to maximise your marks.

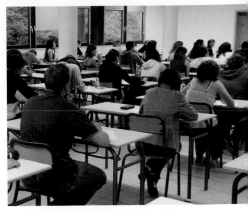

Fig. 20 *A thorough knowledge of the topic area will be the biggest help to you in the exam*

You have one spoken acquisition question and one literacy-style question to practise.

Preparing wisely

Knowing the topic area thoroughly will be the biggest help to you, giving you confidence when you face previously unseen data. You know what revision methods work best for you but remember the assessment objectives, and their weightings, when you are revising and, in the examination, when you are constructing your answer:

Transcription conventions are given on page v.

▶ Examination question: spoken

Q1) **Texts A** and **B** are transcripts of a child, Tom, aged 2 years and 7 months, talking with his parents. **Text A** is a transcript of the conversation which occurred as he helped mend bikes with his mother and father. **Text B** is a transcript of a conversation while he did a jigsaw with his mother.

Referring in detail to the transcripts, and to relevant ideas from language study, explore the language used by Tom and his mother.

You may wish to comment on **some** of the following: the initiation and development of topics; the lexical and grammatical choices made; interactions with caregivers.

AQA January 2005

Text A

[Tom is sitting on his bike outside in the garden]

Tom: oh please

Mother: so what are you doing Tom

Tom: I sitting on the bike (.) it make noises

Mother: it makes noises

5 **Tom:** yeah

Mother: what sort of noises

Tom: the bike (.) the dad bike

Mother: dad's bike

Tom: yeah (.) the dad (.) dad's bike (.) dad's bike mum (.) dad's bike

10	*Mother:*	you're not on dad's bike (.) you're on your bike
	Tom:	I am on dad's bike but I not on dad's bike
		[Tom notices tape recorder]
	Mother:	don't touch (.) don't touch
	Tom:	no (.) can I put it on
	Mother:	in a minute
15	*Tom:*	please
	Mother:	please (.) where are you gonna go are you going for a ride
	Tom:	*[giggles]*
	Mother:	you
		[Tom moves over to father's bike and sticks screwdriver down the handlebar]
	Tom:	me (.) I need to fix dad's bike OK
20	*Mother:*	you need to fix dad's bike
	Tom:	I need to fix dad's bike (.) go (.) on (.) oh (.) I need to fix dad's bike again
	Father:	my bike
	Tom:	yeah
25	*Father:*	really
	Tom:	an
	Mother:	oops
	Tom:	I just get the bits out OK

J.A. Darby

Student answer

Tom appears to be in the telegraphic stage as he can create a complete sentence consisting of a subject, verb and complement 'it make noises', although he hasn't acquired the third person singular inflection.

The mother uses an interrogative, 'so what are you doing Tom?' to begin the conversation and Tom has learnt that in conversation if you are asked a question it is polite to answer and he can take his turn in an adjacency pair. Tom's mother is using child-directed speech (CDS) as interrogatives are a feature of this and CDS is often used by parents to aid their child in their language acquisition. The mother begins the conversation with a question, illustrating that she has the power in the conversation.

Tom's mother attempts to correct Tom's grammar, 'dad's bike', which provides support for Piaget's cognitive theory as Tom needs to understand possession. By the end of the transcript, however, Tom does understand this and has grasped the concept of dad's bike.

As he is in the telegraphic stage, Tom has acquired some use of auxiliary verbs and can use these to construct interrogatives, 'can I put it on?'. However, when constructing an utterance in the progressive aspect he doesn't use the auxiliary verb 'am', but says 'I sitting'. This virtuous error shows that although Tom is at Stage 4 in his auxiliary verb usage he is still struggling with the progressive, which is often acquired later in the telegraphic stage.

Tom knows what to do with a screwdriver '[*sticks screwdriver down the handlebar*]', which suggests he has used one before. This is a stereotypical game which fathers play with their sons. There is a semantic field of DIY which reflects the male gender.

Response starts with focus on the data, selecting an appropriate linguistic method of analysis (grammar) and using relevant and precise terminology (AO1). As AO1 secures the most marks, this approach is likely to be successful.

Here the grammatical exploration of the data is continued in a systematic manner, along with development into discourse analysis.

AO1 is linked to ideas about language development (AO2) with some development of points.

Again clear connections are being made between the data and concepts surrounding language development, showing evident AO1 and AO2 strengths.

References to theory are implicit and bedded into the detailed analysis.

Tom uses tag questions, 'I just get the bits out OK?' in his speech. This is typically a feature of female speech, suggesting he is imitating his mother's speech, which supports Skinner's behaviourist view that children learn through imitation.

Text B

	Mother:	where do they go
	Tom:	it goes (2.0) here
	Mother:	pop it in (.) fantastic (.)
	Tom:	ha (.) ha *[laughs]* I put (.) I put (2.0)
5	*Mother:*	what animal's that
	Tom:	*[looking at the logo on mother's coffee cup]* is these drawing Cartoon Network cup of tea mum
	Mother:	um (.) no (.) it's a moving shadow mug (.) it looks like the Cartoon Network logo (.) but it's actually something else
10	*Tom:*	it is [i:s]
	Mother:	OK (1.0) and another piece
	Tom:	is (.) is dat your talker
	Mother:	my talker? yeah (.) that's a tape recorder
	Tom:	hello
15	*Mother:*	hello (.) I'm recording you
		[Tom laughs]
	Mother:	you stood on my fingers (.) *[Tom pushes the piece in the puzzle quite forcefully]* well done (.) can you find the other bit
	Tom:	I (.) I killed it (.) I (.) killed the sh (.) sheep (.) mum (.)
20		yeah
	Mother:	did you? what you squashed it
	Tom:	yeah (.) I squashed it
	Mother:	poor little sheep (.) oh (.) oh (.) oh
	Tom:	did I kill [ki:l] you
25	*Mother:*	um (.) did you kill me
	Tom:	I didn't
	Mother:	how many chickens are there
	Tom:	(2.0) there's many chickens (.) one (.) two (.) three (.) four (.) one (.) two (.) three (.) four (.) five (.) six (.) seven (.)
30		eight (.) nine (2.0)
	Mother:	hmm (.) shall I count them now
	Tom:	yeah
	Mother:	one (.) two (.) three (.) four (.) five

J.A. Darby

Student answer

In Text B Tom uses substitution, 'is dat your talker'. As Tom is in the telegraphic stage it is surprising to find substitution in his speech as it typically occurs in early phonological development. This shows that language acquisition is an ongoing process. However, this utterance does reveal that Tom is using language to explore his environment, which fulfils Halliday's heuristic function of the pragmatics of language.

Tom's mother is using CDS in this extract also, as when Tom asks if it's a 'talker' she corrects his lexical choice calling it a 'tape recorder'. Like many parents she corrects his lexical choices rather than errors in grammar, as previously Tom made a virtuous error using the plural rather than the singular 'is these drawing'. The fact that children learn the correct grammatical rules without being corrected indicates that language is innate within us, as Chomsky believed.

In this text the jigsaw is being used as a tool for learning. Many children's toys have an educational purpose and in this case the purpose is counting, 'there's many chickens one two three four five'. Tom's mother directs the educational part of the conversation asking 'how many chickens are there?' After her interrogative there is an extended pause until Tom realises that it's his turn to speak. Extended pauses are a feature of CDS as parents teach their children the pragmatics of conversation and turn-taking.

As Tom is in the telegraphic stage he has learnt the '–ed' rule to create the past tense, 'I killed the sh (.) sheep (.) mum (.) yeah'. He is able to create a grammatically accurate correct sentence using a subject, verb and object.

Examiner's overall comments

The student takes a very systematic approach to the data and shows accurate linguistic knowledge, especially when discussing grammar (AO1). A range of theoretical perspectives are discussed (AO2) and challenged in the response to the data. Above all the examples chosen are judicious and discussed thoroughly (AO2). More could have been made perhaps of the different roles taken by each parent (seen later in the data for Text A) but a perceptive and thoughtful engagement with the data is in evidence throughout. This response would be placed in the top band for AO1 (22–24 marks) as the comments are completely led by the data in front of the candidate and for AO2 (15–16) all the references to theories are relevant, including some synopticity with the discussion of gender. Context (AO3) is integrated insightfully into the essay, especially with the comments on how toys are used, the roles taken by parents encouraging their children's speech and the understanding of the key developmental stages. This would be awarded at the highest level (8).

◤ Examination question: reading

Q2)   **Text C** is a transcript of George, aged just 7 years, reading his school reading book to his mother. **Text D** shows the pages that George is reading.

By reference to the texts and to ideas from language study, explore how George is being helped in his reading development.

AQA specimen paper

Text C

George:	in (2.0) the street it was (.) [lə] loaded
Mother:	that's it
George:	with (2.0)
Mother:	sound it out
George:	[sə] (.) [æ] (.) [nə]
Mother:	[də]

	George:	sandbags
	Mother:	well done
	George:	people were taking the s (.) sanbags
10	Mother:	sand
	George:	sand
	Mother:	bags
	George:	bags
	Mother:	good boy
15	George:	to their house
	Mother:	[e] [z] (2.0) watch the endings (3.0)
	George:	we never
	Mother:	nooo
	George:	no we need
20	Mother:	that's it
	George:	all to help said Mum (.)
	Mother:	what's happening (.) what do you think's happening (2.0)
	George:	look at that flood (.) you'll have to get loads there and one there (.) and one there and one there
25	Mother:	what are they doing with the sandbags
	George:	pile them up (.) so it can't get in (.) but it can get up to here but it isn't here (.) but he's letting them get inside is he
	Mother:	no
30	George:	Biff and Chip (.) helped to carry (.) the sandbags (.) they were very heavy (.) Dad put them in (.) front of the doors (.) I just hope the water doesn't come up (.) this (2.0) far said Dad
	Mother:	well done
35	George:	(3.0) Mum looked upstairs
	Mother:	no (.) it looks like upstairs doesn't it (.) but look at the word
	George:	up [sə] (.) [et] (.) upset
	Mother:	that's it
40	George:	the floods made
	Mother:	may
	George:	may get worse she said so there's (2.) only one thing to do (.) she picked up a chair (.) we'll have to take things 45 upstairs said Mum (4) now where they going

Text D

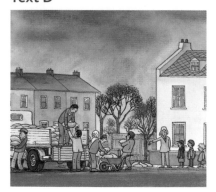

When the children got home, they saw a lorry in the street. It was loaded with sandbags. People were taking the sandbags to their houses.

"We need you all to help," said Mum.

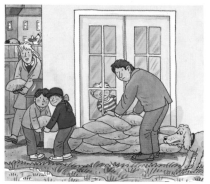

Biff and Chip helped to carry the sandbags. They were very heavy. Dad put them in front of the doors.

"I just hope the water doesn't come up this far," said Dad.

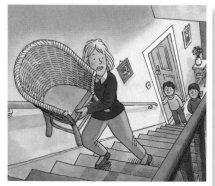

Mum looked upset.

"The floods may get worse," she said. "So there's only one thing to do."

She picked up a chair.

"We'll have to take things upstairs," said Mum.

Rod Hunt and *Alex Brychta*, Flood!, 2003

Student answer

Response is immediately grounded in the contextual factors of teaching methods (AO3) and references to concepts and issues from language development study (AO2).

Perceptive and critically aware comments show an engagement with the topic of reading development.

George is being helped to learn reading by an array of techniques, including the mother's use of feedback, correction and positive reinforcement. There is also evidence of the synthetic phonics teaching method which has been used to teach the child. There has been much recent debate regarding the correct methods to teach young children to read. This is mainly due to a strong emphasis on synthetic phonics and there is evidence supporting this style of teaching showing children's reading ability to be far greater than children taught reading by other methods.

General observations about phonics are now firmly rooted in examples from the data, linking AO1 and AO2 effectively.

Again AO2 strengths are evident, with the issues around children's reading development linked to salient examples from the data.

Within the text it appears the child uses phonics. This method is also taught to George by his mother who, when he is unsure of a word, tells him to 'sound it out', which George does based on the individual phonemes of the word 'sandbag': [sə] (.) [æ] (.) [nə]. George omits the phoneme [də] which is corrected by his mother. This error, which is clearly virtuous as it will later aid his learning, occurs later in the text in which he reads 'sanbags'. With his mother's emphasis (through her intonation) on 'sand', George corrects his error. However, it is arguable that through use of the 'look and say' method this mistake may not have been made as he would have seen the letter 'd'.

Examples from the data are clustered together from the data, demonstrating close reading and annotation before writing the response; this helps to meet the 'systematic and evaluative' aspect of AO1.

Another virtuous error occurs in line 17 in which George omits the plural for 'houses' and merely says 'house'. This is corrected by the mother saying 'watch the endings'. This error could have been caused by two things, either that George is trying to read on from one line to the next too quickly and therefore fails to notice the plural, or that George is not yet fully aware how words are plural and needs to learn the rule. The speed he is reading seems to be the most likely explanation as he makes a further three errors in a similar way. These include 'never' rather than 'need', 'upstairs' rather than 'upset' and 'made' rather than 'may'. These errors are made by George seeing the first two letters of the word and pronouncing words he knows which begin with the same letters and may fit syntactically into the sentence. This basis for predicting words is shown by his mother's statement 'it looks like upstairs, doesn't it'. However, this may also be a reference to the 'look and say' method in which George has registered that the word resembles 'upstairs'. George's error with 'upstairs' may also suggest that George is reading for reading's sake rather than for actual meaning.

The mother's role in the process is vital in aiding her child's development. This is not just in the form of correcting any mistakes, but in the form of positive and negative reinforcement, a behaviourist approach proposed by Skinner. George's mother uses positive reinforcement in abundance through the use of praise words, 'well done' and 'good boy'. Such statements encourage George to keep reading and to do so using the techniques he is already employing. Even corrections are done in a friendly and positive way, shown by the elongated vowel cluster in 'nooo'; it is likely her intonation would rise at this cluster making the reinforcement friendly whilst simultaneously aiding development. Any corrections are followed with more positive reinforcement, 'that's it', to avoid discouraging him. The mother also invites George to interact with the book by the use of interrogatives 'what do you think's happening'. This enables her to check that George understands the plot and what he has just read.

The book George is reading also aids his development. Such books contain pictures for visual input into the plot. An action in a picture can help a child decode the text underneath and this might be why George said 'upstairs' rather than 'upset'. The language of such texts also aids reading development. The sentences are short and simple, often only containing one clause. Speech is minimal so that the child can keep track of who is speaking and at what point. The lexis is often monosyllabic, making phonetic decoding easier. Full stops are used to teach children when to pause. This is effective in George's reading but is sometimes ignored, showing he still needs to learn the function of punctuation.

> Coverage of the data is full, looking at the language of the mother and the child, as well as the book itself.
>
> The range of linguistic methods (AO1) applied to the data is impressive here with lexical choices linked to discourse features and phonology.

> Here sensible observations are made evaluating the influence of context on George's language choices (AO3).

Examiner's overall comments

This is a fluent answer with a clear focus on the question. It meets AO1 criteria at a high level because of the controlled and accurate expression. Evidence of secure linguistic knowledge is demonstrated in the terminology used. The approach to the data is systematic, and there is evidence of a linguistic methodology applied. Critical understanding (AO2) is apparent in the discussion of the different reading methods. Exploration of the concepts and issues surrounding teaching methods is developed and perceptive; examples provided from the data show that this student has not only engaged with the debates but can apply them successfully to unseen texts. There is some consideration of context (AO3) integrated into the essay, although further consideration of context could have included the influence of home literacy practices. Contextual awareness is implicit in the discussion of attitudes to the phonics debate but more explicit links need to be made to specific language features in the data to achieve a high mark.

■ Further reading

Crystal, D. *Listen To Your Child*, Penguin, 1982

Crystal, D. *The Cambridge Encyclopaedia of the English Language*, CUP, 1995

Gee, J.P. *Language, Literacy and Learning*, Routledge, 2004

Gillen, J. *The Language of Children*, Routledge, 2003

Heath, S. *Ways with Words: Language, Life and Work in Communities and Classroom*, CUP, 1983

Myszor, F. *Language Acquisition*, Hodder Education, 1999

O'Grady, W. *How Children Learn Language*, CUP, 2005

Peccei, J.S. *Child Language: A Resource Book for Students*, Routledge, 2005

Perera, C. *Children's Reading and Writing*, Blackwell, 1984

Pinker, S. *Words and Rules*, Basic Books, 1999

B Language change

Introduction

In this section you will:

- identify the main linguistic changes to English from 1700

- learn about the main contextual factors affecting changes to the English language

- understand and evaluate the process of standardisation from the 18th century to the present day, and people's attitudes to changes to spoken and written English since 1700

- apply and select appropriate linguistic methods, key concepts and relevant contextual factors to spoken and written texts since 1700.

Key terms

Standardisation: making all variations of language conform to the standard language.

Mixed-mode: features of printed text combined with features expected in conversation.

Diachronic change: referes to the study of historical language change occuring over a span of time.

Synchronic change: refers to an approach that studies language at a theoretical point in time without considering the historical context.

Section B of Unit 3 focuses your language study on the historical and contemporary changes that have taken place in the English language from 1700 to the present day (Late Modern English). It covers two main areas:

- the main linguistic changes occurring since 1700 and some contextual influences on these

- the **standardisation** of English, the reasons for this and various attitudes to the changes in English usage.

So, what is language change and why is it important to study it? If you have already studied acquisition, you have learnt about the beginnings of spoken language in children – acquiring lexical and grammatical skills, along with the social pragmatics of communication. Focusing on language change will demonstrate how English has been shaped over time, but will also show that a language doesn't simply stand still. English, as a rich mixture of different language influences, fascinates linguists who both chart its development and discuss its contemporary use, theorising about its spoken and written forms. You won't be tested on a detailed historical knowledge, but an awareness of some of the key factors and attitudes affecting speakers' and writers' language choices in a given period of history is important to interpreting texts perceptively.

What debates surround language change? Well, you might have been corrected for 'improper' use of spoken language, and no doubt your written literacy has been assessed and corrected throughout your schooling. The reason for this lies in the prescriptive attitudes to language use that emerged as the English language was standardised. Society's views of English have always been as important in shaping English as the linguists who note the changes and consider their impact. These sometimes conflict because linguists seek to describe, rather than prescribe, language use; society is often more judgemental than the 'experts' and sees these changes as evidence of declining standards. In your lifetime, you have probably been part of a very significant change in English. Text messaging and instant messaging have affected writing styles, spelling and punctuation, greatly influenced by the spoken word. The boundaries between speech and writing seem to be blurring as **mixed-mode** styles become popular and the ways we use language transform.

Don't forget that Language change is a synoptic topic, so exploring again the social contexts of AS (power, gender and technology) relevant to texts from 1700, as well as investigating different text varieties and applying concepts of language study (such as register) are all still important. But added at A2 is a focus on major changes to English in the linguistic areas you have already studied, and the learning of new terminology to describe your knowledge.

Two linguistic approaches are a good starting point for language change. These are the **diachronic** approach – the study of the history and evolution of a language – and the **synchronic** approach – the study of language at a particular point in time.

■ Research point

Ferdinand de Saussure, a French linguist and semiologist of the early 20th century, became interested in synchronic change and looking at language in general, rather than his earlier preoccupation with diachronic change and looking at languages in history. He saw change occurring because of the way that language is continually being rearranged and reinterpreted by people. Taking the semiotic approach to linguistics, he saw language as a structured series of signs with meanings: one side of the sign he called the signifier, and the meanings and mental associations drawn from it the signified.

For example, the signifier 'cat' is made up from three verbal signifiers /c/, /a/, /t/. The signified are all the associations with the signifier. So for 'cat' these might be as follows:

Signifier	Signified
	furry, purring, independent, cunning, hunter, playful, etc.

All words have signifiers, or connotations. Moving from a tangible creature such as a cat, what associations would you have for the adjective 'wicked'? In 21st-century youth sociolect this might connote that something is really cool, good, excellent. But to an 18th-century audience they would have thought evil, bad, sinful, lacking in morals, mean, nasty and so on.

Thinking points

1. What can studying contemporary language tell us about how people's attitudes have changed, for example in using taboo language or dropping sounds from the ends of words as in goin'?

2. Do you think words can change their signified aspects and alter their meanings? For example what slang words have changed their meanings apart from wicked?

Within Unit 3 you have the opportunity to consider both approaches. Your attention is concentrated on texts from the Late Modern English period, which most agree is a period of more settled forms of English – for reasons you will encounter later. However, it is impossible to look at texts from the 18th century without feeling that the language used, the formality and the writers' styles differ greatly from our own. Even looking at early 20th-century writing, or hearing old sound recordings, shows a society with distinctive attitudes towards what it was to be polite, how to speak about different social groups and, to our ears, curious lexical choices.

Analysing and examining similar types of texts from across 300 years of the Late Modern English period (as in the recipes on page 84) will help you look at diachronic change; seeing how English has changed lexically, grammatically and graphologically should encourage an interest in discovering the reasons for the change.

Looking at different contemporary texts and data will reveal how language is used by English speakers and writers synchronically in a variety of ways.

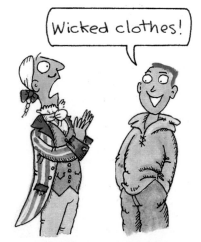

Fig. 1 *Language is constantly being rearranged and reinterpreted by the people who use it*

Changes in context, lexis and semantics

Key terms

Lexicon: the vocabulary of a language.

Understanding language change

As you study the individual linguistic areas of language change, you might reflect on some of the wider issues of why English, or any language, changes. This topic introduces concepts and terms that you may have touched on in AS, for example, when you looked at how words have been introduced to English – or changed their meaning – because of technology. Although understanding the **lexicon** is important, so too is an understanding of changes to word order, the written presentation of letters and texts and the structuring and ordering of ideas. The sounds of English have also altered and you can engage with some debates surrounding these, too.

You should, as ever, apply a range of linguistic methods to analysing texts. Key areas of change are in the:

■ English lexicon as words enter and leave the language or change meanings

■ syntax between earlier and later forms of English

■ phonology of spoken English and its representation in written texts

■ graphology (including typography and orthography): how texts are arranged on a page, font styles and their punctuation and spelling

■ discourse structure and the organisation of texts.

As you go through the linguistic areas, don't lose sight of what you should be aiming for with all the texts you encounter; bring your understanding of the separate ideas about lexical, grammatical, phonological and graphological change together effectively and systematically along with an understanding of changing audiences, writers' intentions and the conventions of the genre they are working in.

Changing contexts, changing words and meanings

Throughout your English language study you are encouraged to reflect on the social contexts of language use and now you have the opportunity to expand this to include historical perspectives. Simply identifying the linguistic features of texts is never enough; an overview of the effect of key factors on language change will increase your linguistic understanding as you can explain features, for example of lexis and grammar, by linking them to how people used them at a particular time.

Why does any language change over time? Of course, it's all to do with people as they:

■ invent things and need words to describe them

■ change attitudes because of changes in society, or are influenced by others such as politicians or the media

■ travel to, move to, trade with or invade other countries.

Research point

Linguists and historians have divided English into key dates and periods as a way to chart the main developments. Changes happened gradually and modern English has evolved over centuries. These divisions suggest that significant changes occurred between certain dates, enough to justify a change of name. Some disagree over the exact transition dates, especially from Middle English to Early Modern English.

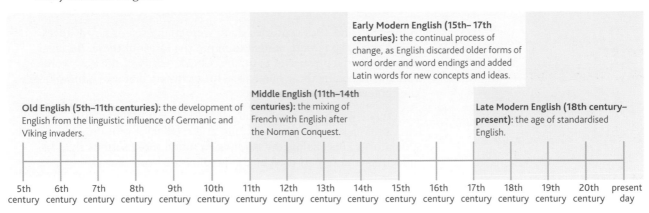

Early Modern English (15th– 17th centuries): the continual process of change, as English discarded older forms of word order and word endings and added Latin words for new concepts and ideas.

Old English (5th–11th centuries): the development of English from the linguistic influence of Germanic and Viking invaders.

Middle English (11th–14th centuries): the mixing of French with English after the Norman Conquest.

Late Modern English (18th century–present): the age of standardised English.

| 5th century | 6th century | 7th century | 8th century | 9th century | 10th century | 11th century | 12th century | 13th century | 14th century | 15th century | 16th century | 17th century | 18th century | 19th century | 20th century | present day |

Fig. 2 *Timeline showing the development of the English language*

Thinking points

Using the brief outline of English shown in Figure 3, think about the influences that can make a language change.

Migration, travel, the British Empire and globalisation

People have always moved to different parts of the world, taking their language and culture with them. Some of an introduced language is absorbed into the local one or, in the case of the British Empire, the introduced language (in this case English) can become dominant in the colonised countries – especially as the language of power and government. Countries such as India still use English as the language of administration.

English has also borrowed extensively lexically to accommodate new foods and cultural experiences. We borrowed words like 'curry' and 'tea' for new foods and drink, making our own versions of these words. Travel has meant that we observe other languages and we order 'tapas' when in Spain, a 'cappuccino' or 'espresso' in Italy and a 'pain au chocolat' in France.

Globalisation in the latter part of the 20th century further developed English into a world language, not least because of the impact of technology and American English. Shopping, for example, has become a global business, with designer names and clothing brands from all countries recognisable around the world; think about English global brands like Marks and Spencer and how they are synonymous with ideas about Englishness.

Wars or invasions

The Norman Conquest and the Germanic tribes who invaded over a thousand years ago had a strong impact on how English developed – grammatically, phonologically and lexically. We now have a lexically rich language containing many synonyms because of the people who invaded; using Old English we can 'ask', from the French influences post-1066, we can 'question'. And, although the UK hasn't been invaded for a long time, the language of warfare has affected the words we use. We wouldn't

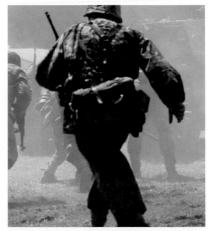

Fig. 3 *The language of warfare has affected the words we use*

have words like 'collateral damage', 'surgical strikes' and talk of an enemy being 'neutralised' without the modern lexicon of war.

The language of science and technology

In the 18th and 19th centuries there were many scientific advances and so neologisms were needed to name the latest of these. Because of the academic prestige of Latin and Greek, many of the new words were formed using these languages, for example 'biology', 'chloroform', 'centigrade' and 'claustrophobia'.

Sometimes we recycle words and use words with higher status – such as Latin or Greek words – for scientific and medical inventions: BSE (Bovine Spongiform Encephalopathy) sounds so much more serious than its colloquial counterpart used by the media ('mad cow disease').

Trade, working practices and new inventions

Throughout history people's occupations and technological developments have changed English. New words are needed to name inventions and to describe what you can do with them. 'Dishwasher' seems a logical choice for the object it names, as does the Macintosh coat for the man who invented it. But what about 'internet'? This seems more metaphorical, showing that names arise in different ways. Even our surnames have links to occupations and past working practices (think of Butcher, Baker, Cooper and Fletcher).

Social, ideological and cultural changes

Changes in attitudes often result in language alterations. When looking at older texts you can see that people held different views about certain social groups. As views have changed about the acceptability of some language use, so English lexis has accommodated them. We discriminate less against certain groups within society in our language use and are **politically correct** when talking about ethnicity, gender or sexuality.

On a less serious note, interests in fashion and culture have been consistent and, as tastes change, so does language. We don't wear 'winklepickers' or 'pantaloons' any more, but might wear 'dolly shoes' and 'thongs'. Next year, we'll need new words! But it's not just about lexis: cultural change also affects the way we sound, the registers we use and our grammatical choices.

The media

The growth of the media and the ways they reach us – print, television, internet, mobile phones – has influenced language. Arguably, a more casual, colloquial and speech-like register has evolved as media styles have become less formal.

New lexis is often introduced via the media to describe contemporary society, and perhaps persuading us to a point of view. Think of the acronym 'WAG' (used for the wives and girlfriends of footballers) and headlines such as the colloquial 'Gotcha' (used to display patriotic feelings during the Falklands War of the 1980s). This journalese-style language of hyperbole and abbreviation expresses the language of the popular press, but earlier newspapers were also less than reverential to people in society.

However, the modern media are often highly interactive. We can select the channels we watch, when we want to, and blogs allow individuals to report

Key terms

Political correctness: words or phrases used to replace those that are deemed offensive.

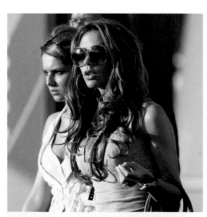

Fig. 4 *Some new words are created by the media to describe contemporary society, like WAG, for example*

events and opinions from wherever they live. Social networking sites have made personal communication possible between large numbers of people who have never met. 'Facebook' and 'MySpace' are new words created to name these sites and what they do. 'Face' and 'book' as two separate morphemes have been joined together to suggest the idea of an internet book of faces. This is interesting as it changes ideas of what books are (printed texts), linking this with the modern obsession for images rather than words. 'MySpace' puts emphasis on the individual, conveying with the possessive pronoun ('my') the sense of ownership over something that is 'virtual' and abstract when linked to the internet ('space').

Exploring lexical change

So how do we create new words for the English lexicon?

1 We borrow them from other languages, either to fill a gap in our own language or to allow us another word for the same object/idea.

2 We adapt existing words (using morphology) – either a lazy or efficient way to make a new word.

3 We create completely new ones when we don't have anything that will do – probably the least common way.

Neologism describes the creation of a new word or expression, but the term 'coinage' is also often used to describe a completely new word.

Certainly, the early invasions of Anglo-Saxons and Vikings from the 5th century onwards brought new words from Germany and Scandinavia, and the Norman invasion of 1066 brought French words. These words mixed together, along with Latin words from religious sources and educated readers, and English developed into today's language. Our rich lexical history is illustrated by these words.

Table 1 *English synonyms*

Old English / Germanic origin	French/Latin
come	arrive
ask	enquire/request
buy	purchase
motherly/fatherly	maternal/paternal
forbid	refuse/prohibit
pull out	extract

Adapted from http://en.wikipedia.org/wiki/List_of_Germanic_and_Latinate_equivalents

We have many synonyms at our disposal, precisely because of these varied influences, and we can use these in different modes (speech and writing) and contexts (with various audiences) and to create different registers (for example, in legal discourse). In some situations, particular words are more appropriate – perhaps to demonstrate knowledge and understanding. For example, a Latinate word could impress in a university interview, but a more colloquial word would be a better choice when speaking to friends. Using distinctive registers allows you to converge with, or diverge from, your audience as you wish, perhaps to gain either **overt** or **covert prestige**.

Key terms

Overt prestige: refers to the status speakers get from using the most official and standard form of a language. Received Pronunciation and Standard English are accepted as the most prestigious English accent and dialect.

Covert prestige: refers to the status speakers who choose not to adopt a standard dialect get from a particular group within society.

⇗ 💡 Where do new words come from?

New words can be created in various ways (Table 2).

Table 2 *Ways in which new words can be created*

Term	Definition	Example
Borrowing / loan word	The introduction of a word from one language to another; these can be anglicised or remain similar to the original in spelling and pronunciation	Anglicised: chocolate (from French, chocolat) Non-anglicised: pundit (from Hindi, meaning a learned person or a source of opinion) now a popular media term for a political commentator or sports expert
Eponym	The name of a person after whom something is named	Sandwich, Braille
Proprietary names	The name given to a product by one organisation becomes the commonly used name for the same product	Tampax, Hoover, Walkman

⇗ Classroom activity 1

In the following passage, borrowings, or loan words, have been underlined.

- What countries do you think they have come from? Group words into semantic fields.
- Why do you think English needed to borrow these particular words?

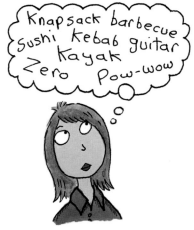

Fig. 5 *The English language contains many words borrowed from other languages*

Should I wear a poncho, an anorak or my favourite parka when I went out on the ski slope? I packed some clothing and chocolate in my knapsack. My enjoyment of tobogganing was curtailed after I kamikazed into the igloo which was obstructing my path. The anonymous owner was absent but his tattooed neighbour suggested a pow-wow. Fearing he was a cannibal or an assassin, I fled. I trekked back to my hotel and as zero hour approached, I decided some food would cheer me up greatly. What should I choose? If it had been breakfast I would have chosen marmalade and coffee, but it was evening and my mouth watered for sushi, tortilla, moussaka or a shish kebab. Strangely I also fancied a cup of tea and some sherbert. I changed into my dungarees and went to where the barbecue was being held. Next holiday I will go on safari or kayak down a river, or go on a cruise. I thought about lying on a hammock in the sun, although I don't like mosquitoes. After eating I changed into my pyjamas and strummed on my guitar.

Source for the words used: **David Crystal**, The Cambridge Encyclopedia of the English Language, *2003*

How do you research word origins? *The Oxford English Dictionary* (OED) is one of the foremost and most authoritative sources of English words, and is updated regularly. You may be able to access it free from your local library, or your school or college may have a subscription: www.oed.com. Alternatively, etymological dictionaries provide information about words' origins, allowing you to research spelling, pronunciation, origin and changes in meaning.

Here's an extract for the adjective 'nice' from the OED online. Over the centuries this word has changed from meaning 'foolish, silly' to 'pleasing' and this extract demonstrates a now archaic use of the word. Not only can you see written evidence of the word's usage from Middle to Late Modern English, but also see the changes to English syntax, orthography and spelling.

nice, adj. and adv.

3. a. Precise or particular in matters of reputation or conduct; scrupulous, punctilious. Now rare.

c1387-95 CHAUCER Canterbury Tales Prol. 398 Ful many a draughte of wyn hadde he drawe Fro Burdeuxward whil that the chapman sleep; Of nyce conscience took he no keep. c1450 (1410) J. WALTON tr. Boethius De Consol. Philos. (Linc. Cathedral 103) 98 Nyce men..Ye seken..To enbelesch youre excellent nature! a1542 T. WYATT in R. Tottel Songes & Sonettes (1557) f. 48v, He the fole of conscience was so nice: That he no gaine would haue for all his paine. ?1573 H. CHEKE tr. F. Negri Freewyl II. iii. 81 He vnaduisedly strooke the young man, and because he is altogeather scrupulous and nice, he imagineth that he can not be free from irregularitie. 1693 T. SOUTHERNE Maids Last Prayer IV. i. 35 You shall promise me, for you are so nice in points of Honour. 1703 Clarendon's Hist. Rebellion II. VII. 187 So difficult a thing it is to play an after-Game of Reputation, in that nice and jealous profession. 1709 SWIFT Project Advancem. Relig. 11 Women of tainted Reputations find the same Countenance..with those of the nicest Virtue. 1785 W. COWPER Task III. 85 Men too were nice in honor in those days, And judg'd offenders well. 1826 B. DISRAELI Vivian Grey II. v, I am not very nice myself about these matters. 1843 E. MIALL in Nonconformist 3 227 The Duke of Wellington said..'Men who have nice notions about religion have no business to be soldiers.' 1887 S. BARING-GOULD Red Spider I. xvii. 288, I should get it back again.., and not be too nice about the means. 1938 P. G. WODEHOUSE Code of Woosters xii. 261 Bertram Wooster in his dealings with the opposite sex invariably shows himself a man of the nicest chivalry. 1948 P. G. WODEHOUSE Spring Fever xiii. 127 Obtain possession of it by strong-arm tactics. Up against this dark and subtle butler, we cannot afford to be too nice in our methods.

www.oed.com

■ Extension activity 1

Using etymological dictionaries you could:

- Look up words from certain semantic fields: for example, food, clothing or music. Find out where these words came from, when they were first used and whether their usage has changed.

- Select one word (for example, nice) to see how it has changed in meaning. Do this once you have studied semantic change (see page 81).

New words can be created by abbreviating in various ways (Table 3).

Table 3 *Abbreviating words*

Term	Definition	Example
Acronym	A lexicalised word made up from the initial letters of a phrase (sounded as a word)	RADAR
Initialism	A word made from initial letters, each being pronounced	CD
Clipping	A new word produced by shortening an existing one	Edit (from editor)

Acronyms and initialisms often come from medical, military or technological fields where speed in communication can be important, or when creating an inclusive jargon forms a social identity for those in the in-group and excludes others. Look at these examples to demonstrate how abbreviations are formed in these fields:

■ DNA (**D**eoxyribo**n**ucleic **A**cid)
■ BSE (**B**ovine **S**pongiform **E**ncephalopathy)
■ RADAR (**Ra**dio **D**etection **A**nd **R**anging)
■ SWAT (**S**pecial **W**eapons **A**nd **T**actics)
■ LASER (**L**ight **A**mplification by **S**timulated **E**mission of **R**adiation)
■ CD (**C**ompact **D**isk)
■ DOS (**D**isk **O**perating **S**ystem)
■ WWW (**W**orld **W**ide **W**eb)
■ SCUBA (**S**elf-**C**ontained **U**nderwater **B**reathing **A**pparatus).

However, not all acronyms are for serious purposes. A recent example, WAG, was a media coinage, putting footballers' wives and girlfriends into a group. David Crystal sees the popularity of abbreviating words as our liking of 'linguistic economy' and the WAG acronym worked well in tabloid coverage for this reason. Space constraints and technological limitations are other motivations; text-messaging acronyms and initialisms usefully convey messages without wasting characters and reduce words so that complete messages can be seen on screen. Prior to SMS (Short Message Service, or text messaging), personal ads used abbreviations for financial, as well as linguistic, economy – WLTM (would like to meet), GSOH (good sense of humour) and NS (non-smoking) are all recognisable initialisms from 'lonely hearts' columns.

Making new words from old ones and adding to existing words are types of derivational morphological change (Table 4).

Table 4 *Re-using words*

Term	Definition	Example
Affixation – usually in the form of:	The addition of bound morphemes to an existing word	Affixes are sometimes linked to contemporary tastes
Prefixes	The addition of a bound morpheme to the beginning of a root word	Examples of prefixes: mega/uber
Suffixes	The addition of a bound morpheme to the end of a root word	Recent suffixes: (radical)ising
Conversion	A word changes its word class without adding a suffix	Text (noun and verb)

Compound	The combining of separate words to create a new word, sometimes using a hyphen to link them	Size zero Man flu Carbon footprint
Back formation	The removal of an imagined affix from an existing word	Editor became edit
Blend	Two words fusing to make a new one	Smog (smoke + fog)

Affixing and compounding are the most common ways of changing words. Lexical change is often driven by the current context. At the moment, environmental change is a key debate and so needs a host of new words; as well as 'carbon footprint' we have 'carbon offsetting' and 'carbon neutral', showing how collocations form around buzzwords like 'carbon'. Celebrity culture has also produced lexical change: the compound 'size zero' identifies the ultimate body shape and the blend 'celebutantes' describes aspiring young celebrity 'wannabes' encouraged by reality TV shows.

Blackadder, the 1980s television comedy, set one of its episodes in the 1700s, satirising Dr Samuel Johnson's *Dictionary of the English Language* by using lexical change to generate humour. In this scene Blackadder mocks Dr Johnson's achievement and the possibility of recording every word in the English lexicon. How do the writers use affixing to create the made-up words?

■ Link

You will encounter Dr Johnson's impact on English language standardisation in the topic Why does language change? (see page 108).

> **Johnson:** Here it is, sire. (*He produces a sheaf of manuscript*) A very cornerstone of English scholarship. This book contains every word in our beloved language.
>
> **Blackadder:** Every single one, sir?
>
> **Johnson:** Every single one, sir.
>
> **Blackadder:** In that case, sir, I hope you will not object if I also offer the Doctor my most enthusiastic contrafibularatories.
>
> **Johnson:** What, sir?
>
> **Blackadder:** Contrafibularatories, sir. It is a common word down our way.
>
> *Johnson takes a pencil from behind his ear. He is furious.*
>
> **Johnson:** Damn!
>
> *He starts writing in the dictionary.*
>
> **Blackadder:** Oh, I'm sorry, sir. I'm anaspeptic, phrasmotic, even compunctious to have caused you such periconbobulations.

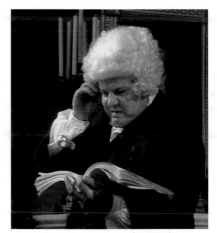

Fig. 6 *'Oh, I'm sorry, sir. I'm anaspeptic, phrasmotic, even compunctious to have caused you such periconbobulations.'*

R. Curtis, B. Elton, J. Lloyd and R. Atkinson, Blackadder: The Whole Damn Dynasty, *1998*

Blackadder parodies the coining of new words to antagonise Dr Johnson. Mainly adjectives ('anaspeptic', 'phrasmotic', 'compunctious'), they use recognisable affixes – as do the nouns ('contrafibularatories', 'pericombobulation'). Also being mocked might be the 18th-century desire to use Latin and Greek affixes ('contra-', '-otic') to show intellectual status and an elevated register.

Although humorous, this extract demonstrates some of the ways words enter English. But, of course, as words enter English, so other words

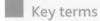

Key terms

Obsolete: no longer having any use.

stop being used and become archaic or **obsolete**. Later examples from Dr Johnson's famous dictionary show how fashionable and topical words from one period don't always stand the test of time. Table 5 lists some previously popular colloquial/slang expressions for a foolish person from the 19th and 20th centuries. How many are familiar to you? Would you use them today?

Table 5 *Change in colloquialisms*

Era of first usage	Word	Origin
1850s/1860s	thick	Schoolchildren's slang
1870s/1880s	twerp	Possibly originated from a surname
	chump	Derived from its earlier meaning – a lump of wood
1900s/1920s	Dumb Dora	Combining a girl's name with an alliterative collocation
	nitwit	An ironically rhymed link between a 'nit' (the egg of a louse) and 'wit'
1930s/1940s	bird-brain	Alliterative compound linking a bird and intelligence
	twit	Derived from the verb meaning 'to taunt'
	clot	Earlier meaning 'lump'
1950s/1960s	barmpot	Northern English dialect (a pot storing yeast)
	pea-brain	Back-formation from pea-brained (metaphorical connections)
	Herbert/ Wally/ Charlie	Using male names to symbolise connotations of stupidity

Extension activity 2

Return to this list when you have learnt the semantic change terminology (see page 81). Identify how the words in Table 5 changed from their original meaning, and suggest why they gained their new connotations.

Blends, as another way of making new words, retain some of the meanings of the original words and so link two meanings to create a neologism. However, individual morphemes are not used to create the new word, but salient parts of words are merged to create the new noun.

Classroom activity 2

Copy and complete the table below. Which words are being blended? What semantic connections exist between the component words and the newly created ones?

Blend	Blended words	Blend	Blended words
motel		skort	
brunch		Oxbridge	
Wikipedia		labradoodle	
docusoap		boxercise	
guesstimate		netiquette	
Chunnel		confuzzle	

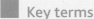

💡 Exploring semantic change

In addition to creating new words, language users are prone to recycling words and changing their meaning. Semantic change, or **drift**, can occur:

- gradually, over time, as old meanings become forgotten
- in response to a new context for a particular word, for example technology
- as current slang where a particular social group takes ownership of an existing word and changes it to suit.

Key terms

Drift: a process of linguistic change over a period of time.

Table 6 *The process of semantic change*

Term	Definition	Example	Change in meaning
amelioration	a word takes on a different, more positive, meaning than it had previously, thereby gaining status	pretty	sly: attractive
		priest	old man: church leader
pejoration	a word takes on a different, more negative meaning than it had previously, so losing status	notorious	widely known: infamous
		idiot	private citizen: someone being stupid
		cunning	learned: deceitful
weakening	a word loses the strength of its original meaning	soon and presently	immediately: in a short while
narrowing (or specialisation)	a word becomes more specific in its meaning	meat	any food: flesh of an animal
		wife	any woman: married woman
broadening (or generalisation)	a word keeps its original meaning but acquires others	place	a broad street: an area

Semantic shifts occur when words expand and contract and then settle for meanings very different to the original. To illustrate this, the word 'pants' originated from the French *pantalon* and referred to men's trousers. In British English, its meaning has shifted to mean underwear (presumably as a shortening of 'underpants', or 'undertrousers'). American English still uses 'pants' to mean 'trousers', showing that this semantic change did not occur in the USA.

More recently semantic change has occurred because of political correctness (PC), which seeks to redress some of the linguistic bias that featured in your AS study of power and gender. PC alternatives for the following two phrases remove gender bias or judgements based on physical ability or appearance: man-made (artificial); maiden name (birth name).

Other types of semantic change can also relate to less concrete changes in interpretations of words and look for new meanings and associations to be made from existing words, often combined in more abstract ways.

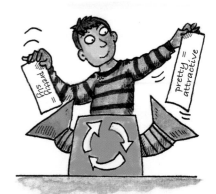

Fig. 7 *Words are often recycled and their meanings changed*

Key terms

Euphemism: inoffensive word or phrase used to suggest something less pleasant.

Idiom: a speech form or an expression of a given language that is peculiar to itself grammatically or cannot be understood from the individual meanings of its elements.

Table 7 *Metaphorical changes*

Type	Definition	Example	Description
Metaphor	A word acquires new meanings because it is used metaphorically	bug	An insect or crawling creature, or to annoy, or a fault in a system
Euphemism	A way of describing something unpleasant in a more pleasant manner	down-sizing passed away surgical strikes	Making workers redundant Died Bombing people in a war
Idiom	A speech form, or an expression, that can't be understood literally from the meanings of the individual parts	pull your socks up bull in a china shop	Try harder Clumsy

Classroom activity 3

Copy and complete the table below, identifying the semantic change/s represented by the words given. Use etymological dictionaries to help you.

Word	Semantic change	Word	Semantic change
doctor		web	
gay		mouse	
virus		a domestic	
guts		friendly fire	
punk		hoodie	
vulgar		starve	

Key lexical changes across Late Modern English

Table 8 *Influences on word creation*

Century	Some neologisms	Some influences
18th	sandwich vaccination torpedo mob	Science and medicine Classical languages (Latin and Greek) Attitudes to class and social roles
19th	biology chloroform claustrophobia	Industrialisation and new inventions Latin and Greek Science and medicine British Empire Travel
20th/21st	genocide laser McWorld doodle-bugs chavs pukka	Technology (especially IT) Globalisation World wars American English Consumerism and leisure time Social attitudes – gender, ethnicity, sexuality Youth sociolects and non-standard forms Ability to record speech

🔍 Exploring words and contexts together

Linking contextual influences to language change explains many coinages or changes in semantics. Looking at these recent words brings together some of the new terminology you have acquired in this topic with the reasons for their introduction or semantic shifts.

Table 9 *Words and their contexts*

Word	Meaning	Contextual influence
phishing	You might recognise this word from its internet usage as meaning obtaining personal and banking details fraudulently through emails and fake websites. It's a metaphorical extension relating the activity of fishing to the hope of catching, or baiting, an unsuspecting victim. Orthographically, the 'ph' instead of 'f' uses a contemporary slang-style spelling, differentiating it from the original word.	Neologism resulting from technology.
metrosexual	Here two morphemes are joined by affixing 'metro', probably an abbreviation of 'metropolitan' meaning 'city', as a prefix to 'sexual'. This media term describes a new type of urban man interested in shopping and appearance, embodied in well-known personalities such as David Beckham. For retail and fashion industries this stereotyping offered marketing potential, also providing a catchy word for journalists.	You can see the influence of the media, fashion and society here.
blog	Another term resulting from technological developments, blending 'web' and 'log' and then clipping the word. Similar to a diary, it is posted publicly on the internet.	In addition to technology influencing language change, this word highlights how people's desire for social networking in a virtual, rather than real, world has changed language.
bootylicious	A term of praise meaning sexually attractive (and usually directed at women), that derives from rap music and blends 'delicious' and 'booty', US slang for buttocks. Interesting, too, how the noun 'booty' has extended metaphorically and broadened from its origin; it was associated with goods or property seized by pirates or in wars and 'booty' was a valuable prize, usually for men.	American musical and cultural impact on English is demonstrated with this word.

Exploring lexical and semantic change through Late Modern English

As applying linguistic methods systematically is an important skill being tested, looking for changes to words and meanings is crucial. Identifying such features can be invaluable for assessments focusing on diachronic change, so here are three recipes for further investigation:

■ Hannah Glasse, *The Art of Cookery made Plain and Easy* (1747)
■ Charles Elme Francatelli, *A Plain Cookery Book for the Working Classes* (1852)
■ Ainsley Harriott, *Meals in Minutes* (1998)

To make a **Currey** *the* **India Way.**

TAKE two Fowls or Rabbit, cut them into fmall Pieces, and three or four fmall Onions, peeled and cut very fmall, thirty Pepper Corns, and a large Spoonful or Rice, brown fome Coriander Seeds over the Fire in a clean Shovel, and beat them to Powder, take a Tea Spoonful of Salt, and mix all well together with the Meat, put all together into a Sauce-pan or Stew-pan, with a Pint of Water, let it ftew foftly till the Meat is enough, then put in a Piece of Frefh Butter, about as big as a large Walnut, fhake it well together, and when it is fmooth and of a fine Thickness difh it up, and fend it to Table. If the Sauce be too thick, add a little more Water before it is done, and more Salt if it wants it. You are to obferve the Sauce muft be pretty thick.

Hannah Glasse, The Art of Cookery made Plain and Easy, *1747*

No. 3 Economical Pot Liquor Soup.

A thrifty housewife will not require that I should tell her to save the liquor in which the beef has been boiled; I will therefore take it for granted that the next day she carefully moves the grease, which will have become set firm on the top of the broth, into her fat pot, and keeps it to make a pie-crust, or to fry potatoes, or any remains of vegetables, onions, or fish. The liquor must be tasted, and if it it found to be too salt, some water must be added to lessen its saltness, and render it palatable. The pot containing the liquor must then be placed on the fire to boil, and when the scum rises to the surface it should be removed with a spoon. While the broth is boiling, put as many piled-up table-spoonfuls of oat-meal as you have pints of liquor into a basin; mix this with cold water into a smooth liquid batter, and then stir it into the boiling soup; season with some pepper and a good pinch of allspice, and continue stirring the soup with a stick or spoon on the fire for about twenty minutes; you will then be able to serve out a plentiful and nourishing meal to a large family at a cost of not more than the price of the oatmeal.

Charles Elme Francatelli, A Plain Cookery Book for the Working Classes, *1852*

wan kai thai-style red curry

Thai-style curries are very 'in' at the moment. We all seem to love the combination of exotic spices with that creamy coconut taste. And to think you can have all this in about 15 minutes – it's well worth trying. The curry paste I use is available in most large supermarkets.

Serves 4 PREPARATION: 5 MINS | COOKING TIME: 15 MINS

1 tablespoon sunflower oil
1 onion, thinly sliced
2 tomatoes, roughly diced
400 g (14 oz) can coconut milk
1 tablespoon Thai red curry paste
500 g (1 lb 2 oz) cubed, skinned white fish such as cod, haddock or coley
juice of 1/2 lemon
1 tablespoon soy sauce
a handful of fresh basil or coriander leaves
salt and pepper
cooked rice and steamed sugar-snap peas or mangetout, to serve

Heat the sunflower oil in a large, non-stick pan and cook the onion over a high heat for 4–5 minutes until beginning to brown. Add the tomatoes and cook for 1 minute then stir in the coconut milk and curry paste. Bring to a gentle simmer and add the fish; cook gently for 4–5 minutes until the fish is just tender.

Stir in the lemon juice, soy sauce and fresh herbs and season to taste. Spoon the rice into serving bowls and gently ladle over the fish curry; serve with sugar-snap peas or mangetout.

NUTRITION NOTES PER SERVING:
calories 172 | protein 23.3g | carbohydrate 9.3 g | fat 4.9 g | saturated fat 0.62 g | fibre 1.7 g | added sugar none | salt 1.47 g

Ainsley Harriott, Meals in Minutes, *BBC Worldwide, 1998*

Classroom activity 4

Read the preceding texts carefully, jotting down all the words from the recipes that you think show examples of lexical change (neologisms, compounds, borrowings, for example) or illustrate semantic change (broadening, narrowing, etc.).

Although you can recognise many words that are specific to cookery, evidently some semantic change has occurred. Some narrowing has taken place – 'fowls' now refers only to chickens or game birds, but previously meant all birds, and has become archaic; 'liquor' has now narrowed to mean alcohol by most, although as chefs still use it in this way the term could be considered more specialist. The noun 'shovel' has narrowed to be primarily used to refer to a garden, rather than a kitchen, implement. The **archaism** ('broth') might still be used dialectally but would be likely to be simply termed 'soup' by most nowadays. Most interestingly, the noun 'scum' has broadened. For chefs it can still be used in the cooking sense to describe the unpleasant matter that rises to the surface of liquid, but its slang use has transferred this to refer to people despised by others in society. Look, too, at the use of 'in', a colloquial term used to describe something popular, presumably an abbreviation of the phrase 'in fashion'.

Lexically some compounds ('Tea spoonful', 'sauce-pan', 'Stew-pan') have become single words; this process is still evident in the 1852 compounds ('table-spoonfuls') but by 1998 the new hyphenated compound is 'non-stick', showing the influence of technological development. Also in the 20th century the way that we shop has affected the lexis with the noun 'supermarket' created to describe the place we go to buy our ingredients. (Incidentally, the linguist Steven Pinker describes the affix 'super' as being 'promiscuous', as it can be attached to any word class.) Scientific neologisms ('nutrition' etc.) are more evident in the latest recipe, as are the number of borrowings, especially from East Asian countries. And what about the word 'currey' itself? Hannah Glasse's recipe is the first recorded for it in England, so it must have been a fresh, anglicised borrowing.

Adjectives in 1852 are used differently. Today we might find something too salty, rather than 'too salt' and 'saltiness' would be used rather than 'saltness'. The 'y' is a common manner of creating an adjective but so too is the suffix 'ness' – perhaps the 'i' was added for phonological effect! The title, too, uses the proper noun 'India' as an adjective.

Now use these recipes to relate lexical and semantic change to their contextual influences.

- What examples can you find of science and technology affecting the recipes?
- Is there evidence for social and cultural attitudes having changed towards cooking?
- What impact have travel and globalisation had?

Science and technology

In 1747 measurements are imprecise, where cooking is until 'the meat is enough'. In 1852 the indicated time period ('twenty minutes') suggests either a greater awareness of time or an ability to measure it, and by 1998 timings and nutritional information are precise. Both the older texts show the limited technology available: in 1747 the seeds are browned 'over the Fire in a clean Shovel', whereas in 1852 the soup is stirred 'with a stick or a spoon on the fire'. By the 20th century, cooking implements have advanced to being 'non-stick'. Layout, too, has been affected by

 Examiner's tip

Learning the new lexical and semantic terminology for language change will help you precisely and effectively explain the key features of texts, helping you meet the main assessment objectives (AO1 and AO2).

■ Key terms

Archaism: an old word or phrase no longer in general spoken or written use.

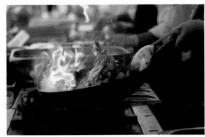

Fig. 8 *Cookery is an example of one area where a great deal of lexical change has occurred over the years*

advances with computerised printing, where fonts can be varied for the various sections of the modern recipe, becoming part of the discourse structure as well as a graphological device.

Social and cultural attitudes

1747's 'Send it to table' imagines that a servant creates the dish, demonstrating a class-based and hierarchical society, whereas in 1852 the economical soup is being produced by women for their own families. Both chefs use the same adjective ('plain'), understanding the type of cooking that will appeal to their audience – one perhaps because the 'currey' is more exotic than the audience is used to and the other for economic reasons. Today we seem to want more exotic dishes ('wan kai thai-style curry'), which are considered fashionable ('in'), to serve for smaller numbers ('serves 4'). The detailed instruction for the modern audience also suggests either inexperienced or leisure-time cooks, who cook for pleasure rather than necessity. Even the purposes of the recipes have been affected by culture, with Harriott representing the modern TV/celebrity chef who is marketing his book – see the persuasive introduction, an added feature to the typical discourse structure of an instructional recipe. However, both Glasse and Francatelli were 'celebrities' and well-known in their own time.

Travel and globalisation

Clearly the ingredients have become more varied as people have travelled more and it has become easier to import them. But, even in 1747, this was happening with coriander used to flavour the dish – an influence of the emerging British Empire and colonisation of India. Other ingredients, such as the rabbits, show that people were still sourcing food locally.

Extension activity 3

The BBC and OED joined forces recently to search for the origins and semantic changes of particular words. This was recorded in the accompanying programme, *Balderdash & Piffle*. Lists of words and findings are on: www.oed.com/bbcwords or www.bbc.co.uk/history/programmes/wordhunt. Look at the words they are seeking. How do you think these were created lexically and how have they have changed semantically?

Changes in written style

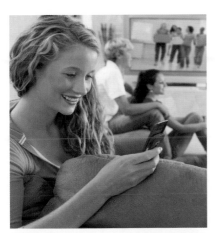

Fig. 9 *Technological advancements, such as mobile phones and text messages, help to shape language change*

Exploring orthographical, spelling and punctuation change

Although there was a big drive in the 18th century to prescribe all aspects of written language use, spelling had already gone through some standardisation from Old English onwards. Caxton's introduction of the printing press to England in the 15th century had a huge influence on standardisation: spelling could be codified because the technology allowed it. With more people having access to the written word, rules became sensible to enable clearer communication.

English spellings have taken centuries to establish. Today it is recognised that some people find accurate spelling difficult. Some spellings have to be memorised because of irregularities (such as homophones) and rules learnt for common patterns such as doubling consonants (sit/sitting). Our spelling heritage reflects old pronunciations, and some rules and oddities have, like grammar and lexis, resulted from the influences of other languages on the evolution of English.

In the 21st century, technology has caused spelling changes, showing that language, despite efforts to retain elements of it in a fixed form, constantly changes. Think how you spell words differently when you text, rather than in other forms of writing, and you can see that even when you know what is 'correct', you choose to flout conventions for linguistic economy or speed, or just because it's easier!

🔍 Classroom activity 5

Look at the three texts below. The first is an extract from John Gabriel Stedman's *Narrative of a Five Years Expedition Against the Revolted Negroes of Surinam* which also provides an interesting anti-slavery story. The second is from Dorothy Wordsworth's private journal; she was the sister of the famous poet, William Wordsworth. The third is a series of comments posted by a Facebook member in response to photos her friends have posted.

- What features of the orthography/spelling seem non-standard?

- Can you identify the 'rules' being used by the writers for their orthographical/spelling choices?

During the ſtay in this place the companies frequently walked on ſhore, and I accompanied them in their excurſions; but the pleaſure I had flattered myself with, from exchanging the confinement of a ſhip for the liberty of ranging over a delicious country, was damped by the first object which preſented itself after my landing. This was a young female ſlave, whoſe only covering was a rag tied round her loins, which, like her ſkin, was lacerated in ſeveral places by the ſtroke of the whip. The crime which had been committed by this miſerable victim of tyranny, was the non-performance of a talk to which ſhe was apparantly unequal, for which ſhe was ſentenced to receive two hundred laſhes, and to drag, during ſome months, a chain ſeveral yards in length, one end of which was locked round her ancle, and to the other was affixed a weight of at leaſt a hundred pounds. Strongly affected with this ſhocking circumſtance, I took a draft of the unhappy ſufferer, and retained a dreadful idea of the inhumanity of the planters towards theſe miſerable ſubjects to their power.

John Gabriel Stedman, Narrative of a Five Years Expedition Against the Revolted Negroes of Surinam, *1796*

"…I sate with W[illiam] in the orchard all the morning and made my shoes. In the afternoon from excessive heat I was ill in the headach and toothach and went to bed – I was refreshed with washing myself after I got up, but it was too hot to walk till near dark, and then I sate upon the wall finishing my shoes." (26/7/1800)

"I made pies and stuff the pike – baked a loaf. Headach after dinner – I lay down. A letter from Wm rouzed me, desiring us to go Keswick. After writing to Wm we walked as far as Mr Simpson's and ate black cherries. A Heavenly warm evening with scattered clouds upon the hills. There was a vernal greenness upon the grass from the rains of the morning and afternoon. Peas for dinner." (3/8/1800)

Dorothy Wordsworth, *private journal, 1800*

haha we planned 2 wear as little as poss :P lol

Thanks lol i dont think i am!!! x

I nooo i havent even seen you round school recently lol

Am good lol you?

Omg we look different now lol x

Lovin the hat haha x

gawjess : P x

I no!! it looks sooooooooo cool!!!!! (:

www.antimoon.com

Key orthographical and spelling changes across Late Modern English

Table 10 *Orthographical changes in Late Modern English*

Century	Practices	Some influences
18th	ʃ/s: ʃ was left over from Old English and continued in use into Late Modern English. It was used initially (at the beginning) and medially (in the middle), but the short 's' was always used at the end of words. Spelling forms become more regular, although often still idiosyncratic.	The long ʃ was used until 1800, when it was replaced by the short 's'. As it didn't have a phonological function, the phoneme didn't need a different grapheme and, because of printing practices when pages (and letters) had to be individually set, it was deemed unnecessary. Dictionaries.
19th	More consistent and standardised spelling evolving.	Increasing standardisation, the availability and number of dictionaries and the drive for a more literate society, with schooling beginning to be offered to all children.
20th/21st	Standardised spelling rules. More recently, non-standard forms have become more extensively used.	Educational practices and government interventions. Emergence and development of information and computer technology, specifically text messaging and instant messaging.

What are the reasons for orthographical change?

Why has spelling changed? For three main reasons: phonological, technological and for purposes of standardisation.

Phonological

As the sounds of English changed, so the written word needed to accommodate this. For example, our modern 'silent e' rule evolved from old inflectional endings where sounds were pronounced to show the word's function; it now marks long vowels. In Middle English the terminal –e was a key feature, often used at the end of words where we would now omit it ('roote', 'soote'). This –e may have been linked to Middle English pronunciation, but died out in Early Modern English as people became unsure whether to write it as it was no longer sounded. However, you might think of the irregularities of English spelling and reflect on how they differ from pronunciation!

Technological

Printing practices in the 1800s shaped the presentation of letters in the long 's' and throughout Late Modern English technological advances have driven graphological opportunities so now we can choose to use non-standard forms depending on the medium (e.g. text messaging), the audience (e.g. friends) and the function (interactional); or, as in advertising, non-standard choices can send a message about the product ('Beanz Meanz Heinz', 'milk's gotta lotta bottle', 'finger lickin' good'). Earlier than this Caxton's printing press in the 15th century encouraged spelling standardisation because it facilitated mass printing. But in the Early Modern English period (1450–1700), individual printers established their own conventions and styles – as did writers – so uniformity was not deemed important at first. Printers wanted to fit words neatly on a line, so they began to drop letters such as the terminal –e. At other times they added letters because they got paid by the number of letters. You can see another resonance with text messaging: writers want words to fit neatly on a screen, or change spellings to keep within the required number of characters.

Standardisation

During Late Modern English, spelling was further standardised and codified in dictionaries and spelling books. Before this, spelling had been determined by individual choices, rather than by commonly agreed rules.

Changing punctuation

Punctuation has both grammatical and rhetorical functions. It separates clause elements, and gives weight and emphasis to points we wish to make. Like other linguistic aspects it also has gone through notable changes and developments.

A process of expansion in the number of punctuation symbols occurred as the written mode became more important but it has simplified again, with a more informal, sparser writing style being popular in recent years. Most punctuation marks have a long history. Caxton used the period (.) and the colon (:). He also used the oblique stroke (/) – called the virgule – a punctuation symbol we now call the 'slash' and use in our technological communications; it was replaced by the comma during the 16th century.

However, not all punctuation was used as we use it now, even if the symbols look familiar. In texts from early in the Late Modern period:

- commas are more liberally used to link long, extended clauses and full stops are not always where we would expect them
- colons and semicolons are common features to separate clauses, thus creating more sentence complexity
- apostrophes extended to signifying the possessive and to representing missing letters
- speech marks began to be used to differentiate between speech and writing
- contractions occur in various ways. (Poets typically used contractions such as 'ow'st'; however, some of these might be for the poetic metre, as the contractions alter syllable length.)

Nowadays we use punctuation differently when using discrete forms of communication. When texting, which has more of a speech-style, you may find that you use punctuation only to mark prosodic features, but use them in non-standard, multiple forms (!!!) and at the end of sentences (.) but not in contractions (dont) and with limited capitalising of first words in sentences or for names (meet at james house 18er). However, in your academic essays you apply standard forms to create the right effects.

Research point

Lynne Truss's 2003 book *Eats, Shoots and Leaves* provided a humorous but cautionary reflection on the state of English punctuation. Here is one of her anecdotes to persuade readers of the importance of using punctuation correctly.

> A panda walks into a café. He orders a sandwich, eats it, then draws a gun and fires two shots in the air.
>
> 'Why?' asks the confused waiter, as the panda makes towards the exit. The panda produces a badly punctuated wildlife manual and tosses it over his shoulder.
>
> 'I'm a panda,' he says at the door. 'Look it up.'
>
> The waiter turns to the relevant entry and, sure enough, finds an explanation.
>
> 'Panda. Large black-and-white bear-like mammal, native to China. Eats, shoots and leaves.'

Lynne Truss, Eats, Shoots and Leaves, *2003*

She also credits some of the current misunderstanding of punctuation rules to the fact that before the 19th century it was customary to put an apostrophe before the plural inflection on foreign, borrowed words ending with a vowel, such as 'banana'.

Thinking points

1. What does this joke suggest about the important function of punctuation?

2. Why can other forms of punctuation, for example the apostrophe, cause the same confusion?

Changing capitalisation

By Late Modern English capital letters had begun to be capitalised according to the rules we follow today – mainly because 18th-century grammarians felt that a system was needed. Previously, in Early Modern English, capital letters were used, as now, at the beginning of every sentence and every proper name. They were also used rhetorically for personified and abstract nouns; indeed, writers capitalised any noun that they considered important. However, you may still see some of these practices in texts from the early 18th century. To show how capitals were used, here is a 1676 text about a herbal remedy, St John's Wort, from *The English Phyſitian Enlarged* by Nicholas Culpeper.

> Government and Vertues. It is under the Coeleſtial Sign Leo and under the Dominion of the Sun. It hath power to open Obſtructions, to diſſolve Swellings, to cloſe up the lips of Wounds,and to ſtrengthen the parts that are weak and feeble. The Decoction of the Herb and Flowers,but of the Seed eſpecially in Wine, being drunk, or the Seed made in a Powder,and drunk with the Juyce of Knot-graſs, helpeth all manner of Spitting and Vomiting of Blood,be it by any Vein broken inwardly by Bruiſes, Falls or however. The ſame helpeth thoſe that are Bitten or Stung by any venomous Creature: and is good for thoſe that are troubled with the Stone in the Kidnies : or that cannot make Water; and being applyed, provoketh Womens Courſes. Two drams of the Seed of St. John's-wort made into Powder,and drunk in a little Broth,doth gently expel Choler or congealed Blood in the Stomach : The seed is much commended being drunk for forty dayes together,to help the Sciatica, the Falling-ſickneſs and the Palſie.

Nicholas Culpeper, The English Phyſitian Enlarged, *1676*

Extension activity 4

In the 21st century advertising often deliberately breaks orthographical, punctuation and spelling rules for effect. Collect examples of recent adverts from magazines. You could also see whether this has been a recent phenomenon by looking at older 20th-century adverts on websites such as www.cyber-heritage.co.uk.

Classroom activity 6

Investigate punctuation, orthographical and spelling changes by comparing the texts below. The three extracts are from John Gabriel Stedman's *Narrative of a Five Years Expedition Against the Revolted Negroes of Surinam*; Mary Kingsley's book, *Travels in Africa*; and a 2008 blog from www.travelblog.org.

How is punctuation used differently in each text? How do these add to the writers' intended effects on the audience and their message, as well as to grammatical complexity? What has changed orthographically? Can you suggest why these changes have occurred?

Here I ſlepped on ſhore, with my officers, to wait on Captain Orzinga, the commander, and delivered three of my ſick men into his hoſpital; where I beheld ſuch a ſpectacle of miſery and wretchedneſs as baffles all imagination; this place having been formerly called *Devil's Harwar*, on account of its intolerable unhealthineſs—a name by which alone I ſhall again disſtinguiſh it, as much more ſuitable than that of Slans Welveren, which ſignifies the welfare of the nation.

Here I ſaw a few of the wounded wretches, who had eſcaped from the engagement in which Lieutenant Lepper, with ſo many men, had been killed; and none of them told me the particulars of his own miraculous eſcape: " I was ſhot, Sir," ſaid he, 'with a muſquet-bullet in " my breaſt; and to refit or eſcape being impoſſible, as " the only means left me to ſave my life I threw myself " down among the mortally wounded, and the dead, " without moving hand or foot. Here in the evening " the rebel chief, ſurveying his conqueſt, ordered one of " his captains to begin inſtantly to cut off the heads of " the ſlain, in order to carry them home to the village, " as trophies of their victory: this captain, having al- " ready chopped off that of Lieutenant Lepper, and one " or two more, ſaid to his friend, *Sonde go ſleeby, caba* " *mekewe liby den tara dogo tay tamara*; The fun iſ juſt "going to ſleep, we muſt leave thoſe other dogs till to- "morrow.

Vol.　　I.　　　　　　T

John Gabriel Stedman, Narrative of a Five Years Expedition Against the Revolted Negroes of Surinam, *1796*

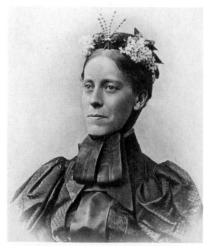

Fig. 10 *Mary Kingsley (1862–1900) travelled alone in Africa from 1893 and wrote about her experiences*

I left Calabar in May and joined the Benguela off Lagos Bar. My voyage down coast in her was a very pleasant one and full of instruction, for Mr. Fothergill, who was her purser, had in former years resided in Congo Francais as a merchant, and to Congo Francais I was bound with an empty hold as regards local knowledge of the district. He was one of that class of men, of which you most frequently find representatives among the merchants, who do not possess the power so many men along here do possess (a power that always amazes me), of living for a considerable time in a district without taking any interest in it, keeping their whole attention concentrated on the point of how long it will be before their time comes to get out of it. Mr. Fothergill evidently had much knowledge and experience of the Fernan Vaz district and its natives. He had, I should say, overdone his experiences with the natives, as far as personal comfort and pleasure at the time went, having been nearly killed and considerably chivied by them. Now I do not wish a man, however much I may deplore his total lack of local knowledge, to go so far as this. Mr. Fothergill gave his accounts of these incidents calmly, and in an undecorated way that gave them a power and convincingness verging on being unpleasant, although useful, to a person who was going into the district where they had occurred, for one felt there was no mortal reason why one should not personally get involved in similar affairs.

Mary Kingsley, Travels in West Africa, *1897*

Been raining on/off all day, that kind of light rain that soaks. Cant see anything of Mt Fuji, last time I momentarily saw it was on a bullet train coming here at 200+ KPH, selected action mode on the camera, pushed the continuous rapid photo button & off it went. Managed 1 reasonable photo. We purchased a Hakone 2 day pass for transport, much cheaper than individual tickets. First port of call was the Glass Forest Museum. Its French, what a grand building. It has a wonderful inner green garden [something I cant picture in Oz these days] It takes U back to Venice & has innovative glass designs. The grounds have glass trees with lights, what a sight. Later I heard a smash in the souvenir shop, turned around & a Japanese lady knocked over an item. Time to go I thought.

Next was the Hakone Botanical Gardens. it was established in 1976 – it was formally a rice paddy & is now a specially designed ecosystem consisting of man made hills with rockeries, streams, ponds & moors.

We then went to Samurai Art Museum, it was quite small and of marginal interest. Checked out the cable car, followed the mist up the mountain & rejoiced at the sight of rhododendrons. Around 5 pm we decided to return to our accommodation, thats when we felt confident about the transport system & decided to be brave & take the ubiquitous short cut. WRONG, such a beast doesn't exist [unless you are Darren or Chris & know how to use a compass] We arrived home near dark, transversed the great Southern Ocean & made it home.

Now time 4 that nasty bottle of red I bought, [its red vinegar – Inge likes it!]

www.travelblog.org

Exploring grammatical change

When you read texts from early on in the Late Modern English period you probably feel that there is something very different about them – not only the vocabulary, but the formality of style seems to use some unusual syntax. But most noteworthy grammatical changes had already happened before this period as the language grew from its early influences from other European invaders. Standardisation, a key event in the 18th century, was a major factor in 'fixing' English grammar, even if it is clear that not all of these practices have made it to the present day.

This extract from Hester Thrale Piozzi's 1789 work *Observations and Reflections Made in the Course of a Journey Through France, Italy and Germany*, compiled from her travel journals, reveals some fundamental changes in grammar and syntax. As you read it, jot down the phrases that seem 'strange' to you.

The cold weather continues ſtill, and we have heavy ſnows; but ſo admirable is the police of this well-regulated town, that when over-night it has fallen to the height of four feet, no very uncommon occurence, no one can ſee in the morning that even a flake has been there, ſo completely do the poor and the priſoners rid us of it all, by throwing immenſe loads of it into a navigable canal that runs quite round the city, and carries every nuiſance with it clearly away—ſo that no inconveniencies can ariſe.

Italians ſeem to me to have no feeling of cold; they open the caſements—for windows we have none (now in winter), and cry, *che bel freſchetto!* while I am ſtarving outright. If there is a flaſh of a few faggots in the chimney that juſt ſcorches one a little, no lady goes near it, but ſits at the other end of a high-roofed room, the wind whiſtling round her ears, and her feet upon a perforated bras box, filled with wood embers, which *cavailer fervente* pulls out from time to time, and repleniſhes with hotter aſhes raked out from between the andirons. How fitting with theſe fumes under their petticoats improves their beauty of complexion I know not; certain it is, they pity *us* exceedingly for our manner of managing ourſelves, and enquire of their countrymen who have lived here a-while, how their health endured the burning *foſſils* in the chambers at London. I have heard two or three Italians ſay, *vorrei anch' io veder quell' Inghilterra, ma queſto carbone foſſile?* To church, however, and to the theatre, ladies have a great green velvet bag carried for them, adorned with gold taſſels, and lined with fur, to keep their feet from freezing, as carpets are not in uſe here. Poor women run about the ſtreets with a little earthen pipkin hanging on their arm, filled with fire, even if they are ſent on an errand;

Hester Thrale Piozzi, Observations and Reflections Made in the Course of a Journey Through France, Italy and Germany, 1789

Key features you may have noticed about the grammar are:

- **Negation**: constructing a negative in the 18th century is unlike the modern use of **dummy auxiliary** verb 'do'. Examples here are 'no very uncommon occurrence', 'I know not', 'for windows we have none', 'Italians seem to me to have no feeling of cold'.
- **Syntax**: in this text the syntax differs from modern usage, for example with 'certain it is' the complement comes before the main subject and verb and in 'continues still' the adverb comes after the verb.
- **Pronouns**: Piozzi's choice of 'one a little' employs a pronoun that we now view as archaic and representing a Received Pronunciation (RP)-type accent.
- **Prepositions**: choices seem odd, such as 'at London' instead of in London.
- **Contractions**: here the lack of contractions throughout the text seems noteworthy, for example 'while I am starving' would be more likely to be presented today using a contraction. This could connote a more formal style or a change in practice in later Modern English to adopt more conversational tones in writing.

Looking at this extract, you can see that the punctuation enhances the complexity of the text for a modern audience. The majority of the sentences are compound or complex and the extract shows the fashionable style of the time in its multi-clause sentences with colons and semicolons joining runs of connected sentences.

Key terms

Dummy auxiliary: the verb 'do' which is used to form questions and negatives or to add emphasis in a statement.

The Late Modern English period also contains some important changes in grammatical usage. Literary texts from the 18th and 19th centuries demonstrate stylistic differences from 20th-century literature. Grammatically, sentences were likely to be longer, with embedded clauses and phrases, but these have become simpler. Using more subordinate clauses, influenced by Latin, became a fashionable way to make discourse more elaborate and to display one's learning. This style continued well into Late Modern English but has perhaps reversed now with many writers adopting a simpler style.

■ Classroom activity 7

David Crystal in *The Cambridge Encyclopedia of the English Language* uses examples from Jane Austen's *Emma* to illustrate some characteristic grammatical qualities of the 18th and early 19th centuries. Match the right grammatical feature in Table 11 with Crystal's examples.

Table 11 *Jane Austen and 19th-century grammar*

Example from Austen	Grammatical feature
He told me in our journey … She was small of her age	Irregular verbs
She say you to the day? She doubted not …	Tense usage
It is a nothing of a part … To be taken into the account …	Contracted forms
Fanny shrunk back and much was ate …	Prepositions
I am so glad we are got acquainted. So you are come at last!	Articles
The properest manner … The richest of the two …	Auxiliary verbs
Will not it be a good plan? It would quite shock you … would not it?	Adverbs
I stood for a moment, felling dreadfully. It is really very well for a novel.	Comparative/superlative adjectives

Adapted from David Crystal, The Cambridge Encyclopedia of the English Language, CUP, 2003

Some features of modern grammatical change are being affected by speech practices as the boundaries blur again between the spoken and written mode:

■ adverbs are being replaced by adjectives – for example, 'you've done great!'

■ prepositions – bored of / down to / talk with

■ irregular verbs are still altering – for example, 'I've wrote it down for you.'

■ pronouns – 'whom' is disappearing as the object pronoun, being replaced with 'who'.

⚤ Key grammatical changes across Late Modern English

Table 12 *Late Modern English: grammatical changes*

Century	Practices	Some influences
18th	Formal style with complex sentences, multiple subordination and embedded clauses	Standardisation Hierarchical and formal society with emphasis on conventions and rules Writing valued as separate from speech
19th	Grammatical formality still evident, although sentences less complex than in 18th century	Continuing standardisation Changes in class attitudes Beginnings of universal education Dialectal voices represented in literature (for example, Dickens)
20th/21st	Simpler syntax and coordination, including minor and simple sentences, more popular in media/advertising Non-standard spelling and punctuation used in text/email forms	Worldwide and American English Technology Social levelling and equality Oral language/forms affecting writing styles Growing informality Growth of entertainment and leisure industries

Currently, persuasive media such as advertising use pronouns as synthetic personalisation, creating a pseudo-relationship with their audience. Think also about how political speakers use pronouns to play on their audience's feelings and make direct appeals – 'we' as including the audience in their opinion or to take responsibility and 'you' to appeal to the audience directly. However, despite the fact that we only have one second person pronoun, subtle distinctions can be made between the authorial tone and voice.

■ Research point

Norman Fairclough, a contemporary linguist, coined the term 'synthetic personalisation' to describe how advertisers use direct address to create a sense of a personal and individual relationship with an intended audience. This persuasive device often results in a more conversational text and so seems more appealing to the intended audience as it pretends a close, friendly relationship with them.

Thinking points

1 Why do you think Fairclough calls it 'synthetic'?

2 What other persuasive texts use this kind of personalisation to appeal to their audiences?

■ Language change and gender

■ Classroom activity 8

Compare these three extracts from magazines from consecutive decades of the 20th century. The first is an article from a 1950s magazine. The second is a 1960s magazine article. The third is a 1970s problem page from *Jackie*. Not only do these provide an opportunity to look at specific linguistic features, they also offer scope to focus again on one of your key social contexts: gender.

■ Which pronoun forms are used and how do they add to the authorial tone?

It's a joy to think about summer dresses, isn't it? Lovely to greet those first sunny days with a brand new frock.

I think we can all manage at lease one new dress this summer, even with close budgeting . . . so here is a selection of the latest styles from which to choose. I have chosen these dresses for their variety of design, for their reasonable price, for their obvious wearability, and because they are washable. There's someting for every occasion, so I feel sure you'll find one which is just right for you.

They will give you a clear picture of the new season's styles, and help you to get ready now for sunny days ahead.

Let's see what they have in common, so that we can recognize fashion trends for the new season. Lines generally are slender, but there is comfortable fullness in the skirts; sleeves are very short and abbreviated; waists are well-defined, with stiffened or inset belts; skirts are a little shorter than last year.

There's a good choice of fabrics — ranging from fine taffeta and rayon jersey, to hard wearing gingham and cotton spun.

If you are looking for something for best, there's 'Norma', in non-creasing silky rayon jersey. The midriff fits smoothly, and the bodice is gathered into a high, drawstring neckline, forming brief cap sleeves. This is a pretty style for the girl with a good figure, and excellent, too, for her friend with a smallish bust, as the gentle gathers successfully conceal any deficiency in measurements. The bold flower print comes in a wide variety of colours, on a white ground.

Smart enough for a wedding, or for a summer dancing date, is 'Susannah', in finely striped taffeta. Row upon row of honeycomb hand-smocking at the waist-line gives an expensive-looking touch to the swirling skirt. A draped collar turns back from the squared neckline, and matching buttons trim the bodice. Colours are green or tan and white.

For the perfect holiday dress, I choose 'Malibu' in an attractive leafy print. The low neckline is edged with an elasticized ruffle, to be worn on or off the shoulders. There are big patch pockets on the gathered skirt.

For the teens and twenties, there is 'Louisiana'—the ever-popular gingham, in this year's large duster check. The full skirt has shirred pockets placed squarely on the hips, the high neckline is trimmed with a saucy frill, and puff sleeves complete the picture.

As I said before, all these dresses can be washed and ironed in an evening—an important point to remember, and they are coming into the shops now. Write to me if you would like further details.

'Summer Preview', 1950s magazine article

I could go on and on—like I always do—about pretty things in a girl's bedroom. How about dolls? I know you can't use them, but little traditionally-dressed dolls are so pretty to scatter in odd spots. And how about pretty chocolate boxes for stockings and hankies?

And candlesticks are not just for lighting romantic, cosy tête-á-tête meals. They also look gorgeous on either side of a mantlepiece.

Oh, and just before we finish off our little chat—well, my chat—let's get really personal. We all use hair rollers—don't try to deny it—it does no good! And, let's face it, these rollers are about the most unfeminine things you can use. Someone once said that they were like a rocket base on top of a woman's head—and that about sums it up!

'Beauty is Where Beauty is', 1960s magazine article, *1965*

DEAR CATHY & CLAIRE – I'm 14 and badly want to go to college when I leave school. Art is my best subject and my art teacher encourages me a lot, so I'd like to have a career to do with that.

The trouble is, my parents are dead against it. They say I have to leave school next year and get a job to help out at home. I just can't get through to them that this is something really important to me and that I could do well if I have the correct training.

We're not that badly off, although there are three younger than me and the thought of a dreary office job or working in a factory repels me. Please tell me what to do for the best as we keep having rows about it and it's making me very unhappy.

When somebody has an obvious talent for something and is getting forced into something they don't want to do, it's very frustrating. The fact that you're encouraged at school means you can make something of yourself in that line of work, and we think it's a crying shame to see talent being wasted.

We sympathise, but we think you should also look at it from your parents' point of view. Their reasons are obviously financial – and the fact that you don't think so is probably due to your mother's good management!

We suggest that you ask your art teacher to have a talk with your parents and let them know that your chance of success in this field is very real. If they decide to let you stay on, they will be giving up a lot for you, and we hope you appreciate it, and do your bit to help, too. A Saturday job, for instance, would provide you with your own pocket money and keep you in tights and all the little extras that you take for granted, but which raise the bill for your parents that little bit higher.

Find out from your careers officer at school about grants for further education – we're pretty sure you'd qualify. And don't be afraid to give up a few things. It's all in the cause of Art! Good luck!

The Cathy and Claire page, Best of Jackie magazine, *Prion Books, 2005*

As you analyse these texts you might also want to reflect on how gender is represented. The magazine excerpts are of particular interest because they cover three decades of the 20th century; however, finding texts from the two earlier centuries of the Late Modern English period aimed at advising men or women will reveal important changes in attitudes.

Table 13 *Key features of gender representation in the three magazines*

Era	Linguistic features
1950s	■ Lexical choices ('lovely') seem typical for women, along with the tag question (isn't it?). ■ Much focus is placed on practicality ('wearability', 'washable') with pragmatic implications for women's domestic roles ('can be washed and ironed in an evening'). ■ It is assumed that women understand specific terms for clothing design ('abbreviated', 'inset belts') and for material ('taffeta'). ■ Judgemental comments are made about physical shape ('a deficiency in measurements'). ■ The graphology and descriptions of the dresses connote appropriate ways to behave and focus on the right stance. ■ References to styles ('low neckline', 'short skirts' and 'saucy frill') hint at changes in styles to come. ■ There are named dresses for different ages – suggesting ideas about suitability or a lack of individuality. Contexts: post-war Britain, recovering from war but beginning of decades of consumerism. Women in domestic roles, but technological advances (such as the washing machine) helping release women from the kitchen.
1960s	■ Lexical repetition of the adjectives 'pretty' and 'gorgeous' supports ideas about women's use of 'empty adjectives'. Baby talk-type lexis ('hankies') reinforces the impression of women in a less powerful position. ■ References to talking ('our little chat' and 'I could go on and on like I always do') reinforce notions of women using an 'inferior', or deficit, language style. ■ Words ('romantic, tête-à-tête', 'candlelight') emphasise girls' interest in love rather than serious topics, adding to the pragmatics of femininity and feminine behaviours running throughout the text; the pre-modification used for dolls ('traditionally-dressed') connotes the desire for conformity and overt prestige. The comparison of rollers ('a rocket base') suggests an undesirable look, with 'rocket' having more masculine connotations. Contexts: more liberation and opportunities for women emerging. The decade of the mini-skirt!
1970s	■ The problem-page topic is career opportunities, although the options for the girl are initially limited because of her parents' attitudes ('a dreary office job' or 'factory'), creating an implied sense of difference from boys' aspirations. ■ Sense of different socialisation with the verbs ('appreciate', 'help'), which imply how the girl should behave if she is allowed to continue at school. ■ Domestic finances are still linked to the female role ('mother's good management') and even the suggestion of a Saturday job seems to be to contribute only to frivolous female items ('to buy tights'). Contexts: educational attainment for girls improving and more career opportunities.

■ **Extension activity 6**

Collect articles and problem pages from modern girls' magazines and compare them with these texts. Adverts offer another good data source for similar comparisons; there are now numerous websites with a range of adverts from past centuries. Focus on power or gender as another way of interpreting the data, applying AS theories, as well as concepts connected to language change.

🔍 Exploring layout and text design changes

Of course, the visual appearance of texts has always been important to readers, and the ability to lay out a text has changed with technology. Early manuscripts were handwritten but the visual appearance of a text was also important, with colour and pictorial images used to bring the text to life. Printed fonts developed, and mass production replaced the laborious handwritten process for major works. Graphic design has evolved through Late Modern English, really expanding with computer technology and the ability to reproduce photographic images. Graphic symbols now have a semantic function, with this field of study defined as typography.

■ **Classroom activity 9**

Look at the same words in different fonts. What are the connotations of each font and how does it affect the message contained in the text?

Graphology is important

Graphology is important

Graphology is important

Graphology is important

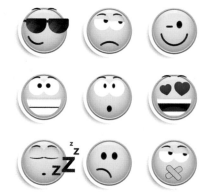

Fig. 11 *Using emoticons is one way of connoting our feelings in the texts that we create*

Graphological features of 18th-century texts included the use of italics for stress, but today, we have great graphological freedom with the ability to adapt word-processed texts easily for a specific audience and purpose. Advertisers use this to influence us, but we also play with the meanings of texts we create. This is evident in text messages, blogs and entries on social networking sites, where we manipulate graphological features for a particular effect. Smileys :-) and other **emoticons** connote our feelings. Underlining suggests how strongly we feel about something and colours can be decoded for our moods. Internet texts have also changed the way texts are read, no longer in the linear form of printed books but in a non-linear manner as we focus on areas of text that visually appeal to us or scan texts for the content we seek.

Here illustrations from newspapers dated 1761 and 1806 demonstrate the changes to graphological presentation, especially in the density of text and lack of separation between articles.

■ **Key terms**

Emoticons: the online means of showing facial expressions and gestures.

The LEEDES Intelligencer.

Printed by GRIFFITH WRIGHT, at New-Street-End.

Nᵒ 369   TUESDAY, May 19, 1761.   [VOL. VII.]

THURSDAY NIGHT's POST.
From the EVENING-POSTS, May 12.
Arriv'd the MAILS from HOLLAND and FLANDERS.

Constantinople, March 9.

THE Grand Signior applies himself indefatigably to business, and has taken a resolution to see every thing with his own eyes; which, however, is not like to be very beneficial to other people; since the first visit he made to the Arsenal, produced the strangling of three principal officers of the navy, for the trifling offence of having minded their own business better than that of their master's; who, to make himself amends, has also seized their estates.

Naples, April 4. The following is a translation of the Turkish manifesto against the Maltese.

" By the mighty powerful Grand Sultan Osman, &c. &c. &c. The great Amurath, illustrious Sultan of the Turks, our predecessor, and well beloved brother of immortal memory, had conceived the design of wresting the little rock of the Knights of Malta from the Christians, and destroying their ships which cover and infest our seas : but death snatched him off, and prevented his project from taking effect. To us he left it in charge by his will to see his design put in execution. Perhaps we should have deferred the enterprize, had we not been obliged to it by our just wrath against these Knights and their ABETTORS; the behaviour of whom, in regard to our ships, is but too shocking. Therefore, taking a quick and lawful resolution, we ordain by this present ordinance, that our subjects appear at Constantinople in the moon of March, with their galleys, and their other armed vessels ; and that all ships in our arsenals be ready at the same time, that we may embark our army, in order to imprint terror in the Universe ; that the whole Christian world may feel our just indignation ; and that by our invincible power may be made the last massacre of the Christians, &c. &c. &c."

Vienna, April 25. We expect soon some very interesting

him over to London:—Thus we have the destination of the yatcht, which some people here fancied, was gone to bring over from France, such a man as Monsieur Bussy.

Paris, April 27. The public is impatient to learn the crime of the Advocate who drew up the memorial for Ambrose Guy against the Jesuits. The Court of the Chatelet condemned him to be publickly whipped, and branded, and sent to the galleys for three years. This sentence being read to him the 22d, he cut an artery that evening in prison, and was found expiring next day. His body was drawn on a hurdle to the place of execution, and hung up by the feet, for his self murder.

Paris, May 1. The St. Anne, the Tigre, the Deal-Castle and and other armed ships, are arrived at our American Colonies. We hope the Vierge de Sante, and the St. Francis de Paule, which failed lately from Toulon, will be more fortunate than the Oriflamme. They are going to Cape Francois with a prodigious quantity of merchandize.

——, *May 2.* The Council of State, have condemned the Jesuits to pay to the heirs of Ambrose Guy, who died a little unaccountably under their management about thirty years ago, the sum of eight millions of livres. Before the Council they insisted, that never any such man existed ; and it is fresh in every body's memory, that the gazettes, under their influence a few years ago, insisted there never was any such suit.

Sixteen men of war are ordered to be equipped in all haste at Brest, and several Captains have received orders to repair thither forthwith.

Two rumours are this instant spread ; that all the garrison of Belleisle, consisting of 2000 men, has been put to the sword by 12000 English, who were irritated by the brave resistance they had made ; the other, that a respectable northern power has consented, on condition of being paid a certain subsidy, to put 20,000 men and 10 or 12 ships of war into our pay ; but this second piece of intelligence is much more probable than the first.

A M E R I C A.
N E W-Y O R K, *March 23.*

sea, in sending it home ; the consequence of which is, that the French merchants being better acquainted with the country than the British, the former engross all the fur trade, and even import goods of the manufactures of France, by the way of Guernsey and Jersey, by which means they will always be enabled to engross the fur trade, and laugh at all the efforts of the British merchants to share it with them ; so that if a stop is not put to the French exportation of furs, and to their importation of French goods by the way of Guernsey and Jersey, adieu to the British trade in Canada ; it will be in vain to import any thing more than the trifle that may be wanting for the use of the troops.

SHIP-NEWS.
Admiralty-Office, May 9.
Extract of a Letter from Vice-Admiral Saunders to Mr. Cleveland, dated in Gibraltar Bay, April 6, 1761.

" I have the satisfaction to desire you will acquaint their Lordships, that his Majesty's ship Isis fell in with the Oriflame on the 1st instant, off Cape Tres Foreas, and, after a running fight of some hours, took her ; and they are now both arrived in this Bay. She had been 29 days from Toulon, and one from Oran. The particulars of her lading are not yet known, as her papers of that fort are not found.

" I am extremely sorry to acquaint their Lordships, that altho' the Isis had only four men killed, Captain Wheeler is unfortunately one of that number, who, with two others, (a Midshipman and Quarter-Master) were killed by one shot very soon after the beginning of the action. The Isis had nine wounded, two of them badly. The numbers killed and wounded in the Oriflame are not yet ascertained, but are supposed to be between forty and fifty.

" They began to engage at six in the evening, and continued a running fight to half past ten ; the Oriflame endeavouring to get to the northward of the Isis, in order to get over to the Spanish shore, to prevent which, Lieutenant Cunningham, (commanding officer of the Isis) found it necessary to run on board her, which he did, with no other damage to either ship than the loss one of his own anchors, very soon after which she struck. She had 40 guns mounted, 26 of twelve pounders, and 14 of eighteen, and upwards of

The Leedes Intelligencer, 19 May 1761

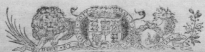

The Times, 10 January 1806

Compare visually the older newspapers with this edition of the *Yorkshire Evening Press* from 2 May 1945.

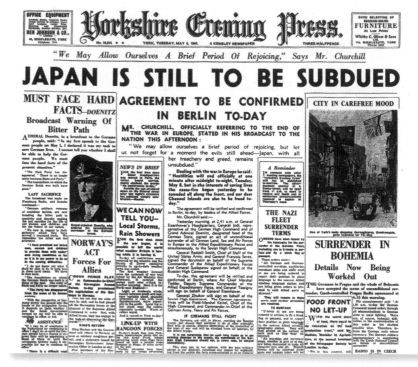

Yorkshire Evening Press, *2 May 1945*

In 20th-century newspapers, headlines have become important, although you could consider the entertaining styles of headlines that modern tabloid papers adopt. This one is very factual ('Agreement to be confirmed in Berlin today'). The use of fonts is perhaps surprising as many techniques are used – bold (**'Dealing with the war in Europe …'**), capitals (MR. CHURCHILL, OFFICALLY …'), and varying sizes of print and boxes. These add to the structure as they separate articles, as well as highlighting the main sections. Graphology has assisted readers as important information and the manner to read the text effectively has now become clear.

This text is also good to illustrate another key social context – power. Both **influential** and **instrumental power** combine within the newspaper. For example, using the modal verb and the pronouns in the headline ('We can now tell you') indicates the instrumental power in the legal restrictions imposed on providing information on even the weather in wartime, and the relief felt by all about the ending of the war is in the lighthearted pragmatics of the non-standard and exclamatory concluding sentence (And it rained in York today!'). Unlike today, little journalistic comment is given in the main article and Churchill's own words in direct speech carry the influential message of the agreement made in Germany but the warning of future danger in Japan. But, if you compared this to journalism now and coverage of recent conflicts, you might see a contrasting tone with less reverential media attitudes to senior politicians.

Key terms

Influential power: power used to influence or persuade others.

Instrumental power: power used to maintain and enforce authority.

Extension activity 7

Graphological change is another interesting area of study. You could investigate synchronic change by looking at a variety of today's websites, or investigate changing graphology in adverts and newspapers. Much is accessible online but local archives are a good source of data.

Changes in speech style

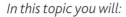

Key terms

Omission: the leaving out of a phoneme in a group of phonemes clustered together.

Assimilation: the influence exercised by one sound upon the articulation of another, so that the sounds become more alike.

Informalisation: the way in which language is becoming increasingly informal in all areas of society.

Received pronunciation (RP): the prestige form of English pronunciation, sometimes considered as the 'accent' of Standard English.

Exploring phonological change and changing speech styles

During Late Modern English the spoken mode has risen in status and value and is another form that shows how language has changed. However, as the development of recording technology has only been relatively recent, the sounds of English before the mid-19th century have to be worked out from written clues. That the sound of English has changed considerably is not in dispute, but why it has is more hotly debated.

First, what about the phonological aspects of your own spoken language? Do you say 'hanging' or 'angin'? 'Football' or 'foo'ball'? 'Handkerchief' or 'hankerchief'? These examples highlight the main ways in which spoken language changes:

- **Omission**: Where sounds disappear from words. Often this involves the clipping of the final consonant. In the example of the slang word 'hanging' (suggesting something is not very nice!) the omission can be at the beginning as well as the end. Also, we tend not to pronounce the medial 'g', preferring to say 'hanin'.

- **Assimilation**: The pronunciation of one phoneme is affected by an adjacent phoneme: 'don't you' is usually pronounced 'dohnchu' in natural speech.

Jean Aitchison, in *Language Change: Progress or Decay*, cites this as a natural tendency occurring within all languages. So why have speech styles changed? The main reasons for phonological change are the following:

- **Ease of articulation**: As you saw above, we often make spoken words and phrases easier to say. We also abbreviate words. You don't often refer to your 'mobile telephone', instead probably preferring to call it your 'mobile' or your 'phone'. Some people would view changing phonology as a sign of laziness rather than an inevitable process. The big phonological changes of previous centuries, such as the Great Vowel Shift of 1400–1600 where the sounds of the vowels changed (for example, 'sight' would have been pronounced with the 'ee' sound in modern 'meet'), occurred across all English society as the language evolved from its mixed heritage and made the spoken language more like today's oral form.

- **Social prestige and changes in society**: People move around more and, along with mass communication, the result is less regional variation. The impact of radio and television has grown over recent decades and the **informalisation** of these media has affected the spoken language. Also, some people's desire to create cultural identity has caused more sociolectal variations and a move against 'correct' speech.

Even in the 20th century, speech styles changed. In the early days of radio, BBC presenters used **Received Pronunciation (RP)**, the prestige accent associated with the upper classes. Clearly there has been a significant change: now the regional diversity of presenters is celebrated and you can list a host of television personalities from all parts of Britain. Even the Queen has apparently adapted her speech. A report in the scientific journal *Nature* in 2000 cited a study that noted how her accent had changed between the 1950s and the 1980s. Analysis of her vowel sounds showed that whereas her pronunciation of 'had' used to almost rhyme with 'bed', it is now closer to 'bad'. The study concluded that the blurring of accents was occurring throughout the media, with a downwards convergence towards the language styles of younger people, rather than for any geographical reason.

Research point

Convergence is part of Howard Giles' accommodation theory, which centres on pragmatics and how speakers adjust their speech behaviours to accommodate others, showing their need for approval.

However, divergence is the opposite. When people diverge from others, it may be to make their accent stronger or to adopt exaggerated speech behaviours in order to distance themselves from other speakers – or to reinforce their different identity.

Convergence and **divergence** can be upwards (towards RP) or downwards (to a regional or sociolectal variation).

Key terms

Divergence: when a person's speech patterns become more individualised and less like those of the other person in a conversation.

Thinking points

1. Why do you think the Queen might be downwardly converging?
2. If it is happening, what could the general trend towards downwards convergence in society suggest?
3. In what situations might you want to converge or diverge from others?

The term 'Estuary English' was coined in the 1980s by David Rosewarne in his *Times Educational Supplement* articles, and described the effect of London accents spreading through counties adjoining them along the Thames. Estuary English – a mixing or 'ordinary' London and south-eastern accents with RP – is seen by some as RP's possible successor as the Standard English pronunciation. It conforms to Standard English grammatically and lexically, but has distinct phonology. Another feature that distinguishes it from being just another regional variation is that, like RP, speakers from all regions use it. Some of its key features are:

- glottal stops ('foo'ball', 'Ga'wick')
- 'l' vocalisation, where the 'w' sound replaces 'l' ('foo'baw')
- yod coalescence, another common feature of Estuary English, where the 'y' sound (as in 'yod') is changed because of the preceding consonant ('fortune' used to be pronounced 'fortyoon' and is now pronounced 'forchoon').

What may be happening is the desire to accommodate other people's speech styles and dialect levelling, where the distinctions between different accents and dialects are becoming less apparent.

Research point

Norman Fairclough, the linguist responsible for synthetic personalisation (see page 96), believes that this is part of what he terms conversationalisation. He believes that there have been 'shifting boundaries between written and spoken discourse practices, and a rising prestige and status for spoken language'. Many linguists see this informalisation and personalisation of language in today's language use and credit spoken language with driving changes in the written mode.

Thinking points

1 What types of written communication might provide evidence for these 'shifting boundaries'?

2 Do you think that these linguists are right in their view that language is more informal now? How would you support this?

However, regional accents are often judged against people's attitudes and feelings about them. Dennis Freeborn, in *Varieties of English*, summarises them into three views:

- **The incorrectness view**: All accents are incorrect compared to Standard English and the accent of RP. Freeborn refutes this, citing evidence that accent's popularity originates in fashion and convention; RP became the standard because it had social prestige, rather than being more correct than any other variety.

- **The ugliness view**: Some accents don't sound nice. This seems to be linked to stereotypes and negative social connotations, especially as the least-liked accents seem to be found in poorer, urban areas.

- **The impreciseness view**: Some accents are described as 'lazy' and 'sloppy', such as Estuary English, where sounds are omitted or changed. Freeborn offers the glottal stop as an argument that some sound changes are logical and governed by linguistic views.

Dialectal representations of speech (**eye dialect**) have developed in prose throughout Late Modern English. Writers have experimented with realistic 'voices' for characters, including famous writers like Charles Dickens who, in the 19th century, created distinctive, idiolectal voices for his characters. These showed not only their social status and class, but also gave them individuality. The extract below, from *Great Expectations* (1860), depicts a young boy's meeting with an escaped convict.

> After darkly looking at his leg and me several times, he came closer to my tombstone, took me by both arms, and tilted me back as far as he could hold me; so that his eyes looked most powerfully down into mine, and mine looked most helplessly up into his.
>
> 'Now lookee here,' he said, 'the question being whether you're to be let to live. You know what a file is?'
>
> 'Yes, sir.'
>
> 'And you know what wittles is?'
>
> 'Yes, sir.'
>
> After each question he tilted me over a little more, so as to give me a greater sense of helplessness and danger.
>
> 'You get me a file.' He tilted me again. 'And you get me wittles.' He tilted me again. 'You bring 'em both to me.' He tilted me again. 'Or I'll have your heart and liver out.' He tilted me again.
>
> I was dreadfully frightened, and so giddy that I clung to him with both hands, and said, 'If you would kindly please to let me keep upright, sir, perhaps I shouldn't be sick, and perhaps I could attend more.'

www.bibliomania.com

Key terms

Eye dialect: a way of spelling words that suggests a regional or social way of talking.

Classroom activity 10

How does Dickens use eye dialect, elision and assimilation here to represent the convict's accent? How does he make the boy sound different from the convict?

These two versions of the same story, one from 1956 and the other from 2002, illustrate changing speech styles, as well as representing changing contexts.

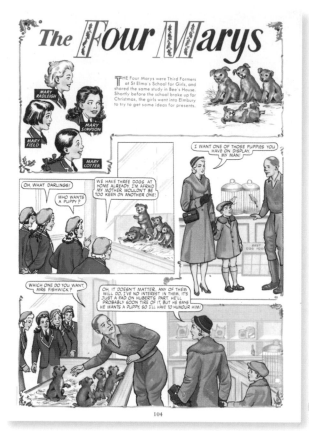

'The Four Marys' from Bunty, **D.C. Thompson**, 1956

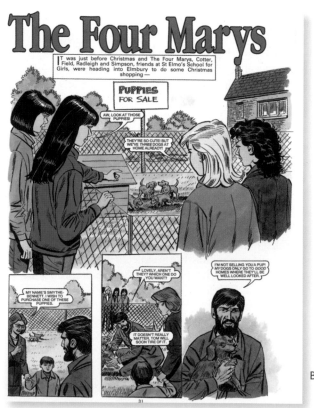

'The Four Marys' from Bunty, **D.C. Thompson**, 2002

Table 14 *Comparing the two versions of 'The Four Marys'*

1956	2002	Comment
Oh, what darlings! We have three dogs at home already. I'm afraid my mother wouldn't be too keen …	Aw, look at those puppies! They're so cute! But we've three dogs at home …	Interjections (oh, aw) represent a changing phonology. Lexical choices represent the age of the young girls ('darlings', 'cute'); 'cute' implies an American influence. Both words seem 'typical' of female language, according to some gender theorists (e.g. Lakoff). Negative politeness ('I'm afraid') is a feature of 1956 compared with the more direct and non-standard style of the recent text ('But …').
I want one of those puppies you have on display, my man.	My name's Smythe-Bennett. I wish to purchase one of these puppies.	The 1956 mother's choice of vocative ('my man') connotes class attitudes, along with her imperative tone ('I want'). This contrasts with the more equal, and polite, tone of her introduction and verb choice in 2002 ('my name's', 'I wish').
Which one do you want, Mrs Fishwick?	Lovely, aren't they? Which one do you want?	So too has the man's address to the mother changed. Instead of using her title ('Mrs Fishwick') in a respectful manner he simply says 'Which one do you want?', again suggesting a more equal relationship in the service encounter between customers and service providers.
Oh, it doesn't matter … It's just a fad on Hubert's part. He'll probably soon tire of it.	It doesn't really matter. Tom will soon tire of it.	Note the alteration to the boy's name. An unfashionable name now, 'Hubert' was probably chosen to represent a stereotypically spoilt boy and this would have been understood by the 1950s audience. In 2002 the choice is 'Tom', a popular name with no particular connotations.

 Extension activity 8

You can access real sound recordings via the internet, enabling you to conduct your own study into the changing sounds of English. For example, the Downing Street website has MP3s of prime ministers and you could compare the spoken styles of politicians from different points in the 20th century.

There's also archive material of people discussing their experiences. Pathé news broadcasts are good for hearing the RP style of newsreaders. Advertisements and cartoons are good resources for further investigations into changes in the representation of spoken English. Melvyn Bragg's Radio 4 programme, *The Routes of English*, provides opportunities to hear his research into the changing nature of English speech.

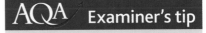 **Examiner's tip**

As Unit 3 is a synoptic module, revise the theories you covered in AS for Unit 1, Section B – power, gender and technology. You will be rewarded in the exam for applying these relevantly to A2 data. Other key concepts to revise are register, mode, dialect, sociolect and idiolect.

 Extension activity 9

Websites such as www.cyber-heritage.co.uk have an excellent collection of 20th-century adverts. Investigate how gender, power and technology are represented in them. What contexts and social attitudes seem important in the adverts from different decades?

Why does language change?

Key terms

Prescriptivism: an attitude to language use that makes judgements about what is right and wrong and holds language up to an ideal standard that should be maintained.

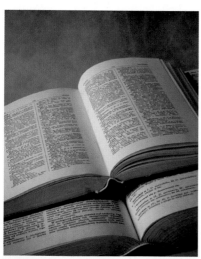

Fig. 12 *Dictionaries are one reason why spelling is more rule-bound than it used to be*

The focus, so far, has been on changes to specific linguistic features of English, and some of the reasons for these. However, the changing attitudes of language users themselves are also interesting. It is important to consider how, and why, we arrived at the Standard English used now, and to think about people's views about the varieties of English we can use. Throughout your study you will encounter diverse attitudes to the ways in which language changes, and you should become accustomed to interpreting these, not only for the ideas expressed but also for their impact on English over time and the historic contexts in which they were expressed.

Exploring language standardisation

You cannot look at texts from all language periods without seeing that a process of standardisation has occurred. As you become familiar with Late Modern English texts (your main study focus) you can see the transitions in style and usage from 1700 to the present day. Language has been standardised in all the key linguistic areas:

- **Lexis and semantics**: Dictionaries have attempted to 'fix' the meanings of words, or reflect semantic changes.
- **Grammar**: Printing and **prescriptivism** have fixed some syntactical rules, captured in grammar books.
- **Spelling**: Dictionaries, spell-checkers and the teaching of spelling rules make spelling more 'correct' and rule-bound than it used to be.
- **Graphology**: Printing has allowed for more uniformity, and even cursive handwriting styles are taught to children in school.

You might suggest that recent technological developments have affected language standardisation, with people making more idiolectal choices over things like text spelling. But does this simply create another standardisation opportunity?

Perhaps it is worth starting by posing some questions, allowing you to reflect on the reasons for standardisation.

- Why standardise a language?
- Who is responsible for standardising language?
- How is language standardised?

The first one is the easiest to answer. Your response might be that standardisation is essential so that speakers and writers of a language can communicate with one another effectively, and their messages can be understood. Standardisation also places value on a particular dialect of a language, giving it prestige and a national identity. The second and third questions are linked: standardisation has a long history; it happened gradually as the result of some key factors:

- printing allowed conventions of spelling and punctuation to evolve and, as many argue, gave southern dialects supremacy in creating Standard English
- people's desire to stabilise, fix and codify the language became stronger and resulted in grammar books and dictionaries that recorded rules for written English.

So you can see that standardisation was driven by people for social and political reasons and supported through technological advances that made it possible to codify language and create rules. However, standardisation is very much caught up with attitudes and values, such as those of prescriptivism that you considered in the last section, and notions of what is 'correct' and 'poor' English usage. Good practices are reinforced through teaching and educational standards, agreed by government bodies. Much political and media rhetoric is heard concerning raising literacy standards and maintaining English grammatical rules. Even your assessment objectives embody ideas about the way you should be writing. The wording of AO1 demonstrates the emphasis placed on your written English:

> 'Select and apply a range of linguistic methods, to communicate relevant knowledge using appropriate terminology and coherent, accurate written expression'.

For some people, standardisation itself is not a problem, but the notion of 'fixing' the language to rules from the past – specifically the 18th century in grammatical terms – is more difficult to justify. And the biggest challenge to English comes from the nature of language as a dynamic force that constantly evolves and changes because speakers use it differently.

Emerging standardisation

The drive for standardisation had been a gradual process over centuries, enabled by printing technology and the establishing of a particular dialect (Standard English) for printed texts and assisted by the crucial changes to English grammar, lexis, punctuation and phonology occurring in Early Modern English and during the **Renaissance**.

But it was in the 18th century, at the start of Late Modern English, that standardisation was more firmly established. The grammarians of the 18th century left a more lasting effect on English, and their work has resulted in many of the 'rules' you apply when you use written Standard English; famous examples are not using double negatives and not ending a sentence with a preposition.

In 1755 Dr Samuel Johnson recorded and described the words in use at the time in the first major dictionary. The rise of traditional grammar in the 18th century was the result of all the pressures to make language conform and to set down rules, driven by grammarians. Bishop Robert Lowth's *Short Introduction to English Grammar* (1762) and Lindley Murray's *English Grammar* (1794) contributed to trying to order and 'fix' the English language into a prestigious and standard form. Part of this prestige involved the revering of Latin and incorporating some of its rules into English. The spoken language and the language used by ordinary people was judged inferior by 18th-century standards, linking ideals about English usage to class attitudes.

Jonathan Swift, another respected writer of this period, disliked the new colloquial language and phrases which included such fashionable features of pronunciation as the clipped and contracted words used particularly by poets (Drudg'd, Disturb'd, Rebuk't, Fledg'd). Here extracts from his 1711 letter to an influential MP entitled 'A Proposal for Correcting, Improving and Ascertaining the English Tongue' set the tone for 18th-century attitudes to making English a pure and standard form. Following this is an extract from the Preface to Johnson's 1755 dictionary.

■ Key terms

Renaissance: from the French for rebirth, it refers to a cultural movement in European history from middle of the 14th to the 17th century which looked back to the classical age for its inspiration.

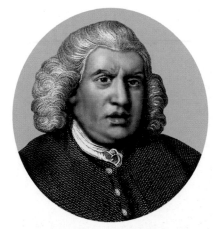

Fig. 13 *Although not the first to compile a dictionary, Dr Johnson's was the most ambitious and started a trend for dictionaries*

■ Classroom activity 11

As you read these extracts, check words that seem archaic to you in the *OED*, or another etymological dictionary. What are Swift's main criticisms in this extract? How does this differ from Johnson's feelings about his ability to 'fix' language, especially words?

My LORD; I do here in the Name of all the Learned and Polite Persons of the Nation, complain to your LORDSHIP, as *First Minister*, that our Language is extremely imperfect; that its daily Improvements are by no means in proportion to its daily Corruptions; and the Pretenders to polish and refine it, have chiefly multiplied Abuses and Absurdities; and, that in many Instances, it offends against every Part of Grammar. But lest Your Lordship should think my Censure to be too severe, I shall take leave to be more particular.

Several young Men at the Universities, terribly possed with the fear of Pedantry, run into a worse Extream, and think all Politeness to consist in reading the daily Trash sent down to them from hence: This they call *knowing the World*, and reading *Men and Manners*. Thus furnished they come up to Town, reckon all their Errors for Accomplishments, borrow the newest Sett of Phrases, and if they take a Pen into their Hands, all the odd Words they have picked up in a Coffee-House, or a Gaming Ordinary, are produced as Flowers of Style; and the Orthography refined to the utmost. To this we owe those monstrous Productions, which under the Names of *Trips, Spies, Amusements*, and other conceited Appellations, have over-run us for some Years past. To this we owe that strange Race of Wits, who tell us, they Write to the *Humour of the Age*: And I wish I could say, these quaint Fopperies were wholly absent from graver Subjects. In short, I would undertake to shew Your LORDSHIP several Pieces, where the Beauties of this kind are so prominent, that with all your Skill in Languages, you could never be able either to read or understand them.

Jonathan Swift, 'A Proposal for Correcting, Improving and Ascertaining the English Tongue', 1711

That it [the Dictionary] will immediately become popular I have not promised to myself; a few wild blunders, and risible absurdities, from which no work of such multiplicity was ever free, may for a time furnish folly with laughter, and harden ignorance in contempt; but useful diligence will at last prevail, and there can never be wanting some who distinguish desert; who will consider that no dictionary of a living tongue ever can be perfect, since while it is hastening to publication, some words are budding, and some falling away; that a whole life cannot be spent upon syntax and etymology, and that even a whole life would not be sufficient; that he, whose design includes whatever language can express, must often speak of what he does not understand; that a writer will sometimes be hurried by eagerness to the end, and sometimes faint with weariness under a task, which Scaliger compares to the labors of the anvil and the mine; that what is obvious is not always known, and what is known is not always present; that sudden fits of inadvertency will surprize vigilance, slight avocations will seduce attention, and casual eclipses of the mind will darken learning; and that the writer shall often in vain trace his memory at the moment of need, for that which yesterday he knew with intuitive readiness, and which will come uncalled into his thoughts to-morrow.

Dr Samuel Johnson, from the preface to A Dictionary of the English Language, *1755*

Johnson's *A Dictionary of the English Language* offered definitions of about 40,000 words. Although earlier dictionaries had existed, this was the most ambitious, starting the trend for dictionaries that culminated in the *Oxford English Dictionary* in the 19th century. These examples from Johnson's dictionary show how words come into fashionable usage, then sometimes fade away: 'blatherskite' (nonsense); 'fleer' (a mocking word or look); 'gulosity' (greediness); 'kickshaw' (something ridiculous) and 'tonguepad' (a great talker). These could all now be classed as obsolete, rather than archaic.

The 19th century simply built on the standardisation process, and mass education and literacy programmes reinforced the 'ideal' standards in written English. Indeed the focus for centuries of standardisation has been on written English, creating a distance and difference between this mode and spoken English.

The seemingly constant conflict between some people's desire for stability and purity in language use and the reality of the world we live in is exemplified in this cartoon strip.

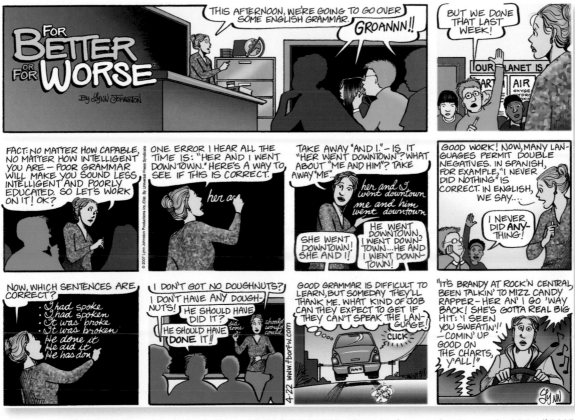

Lynn Johnston, 'For better or for worse' cartoon strip, 22 April 2007

Some major dictionaries and grammar books that have played an important part in standardisation include:

■ **1755**: Dr Johnson, *A Dictionary of the English Language*
■ **1762**: Robert Lowth, *Short Introduction to English Grammar*
■ **1794**: Lindley Murray, *English Grammar*
■ **1884**: First **'fascicle'** of the *OED* (*Oxford English Dictionary*)
■ **1926**: Henry W. Fowler, *Modern English Usage*

■ Key terms

Fascicle: one of the divisions of a book published in parts.

AQA Examiner's tip

Understanding diverse attitudes towards language change and the impact of standardisation are important areas of focus in the specification. Knowing the key historic developments and evaluating the attitudes presented by writers from different periods will help you respond to data perceptively.

What attitudes affect standard and non-standard language use?

Having had the opportunity to study the history of standardisation and some 18th-century attitudes towards English usage, it is important to consider how attitudes to standardisation and the changing nature of English have developed. A good starting point is to look at your own use of English. What do you think affects your use of English?

What you considered important is possibly much concerned with your identity – where you come from and the social groups you belong to – and part of this is linked to standard and non-standard forms or your views of prestige. Language choices we use in our speech and writing reveal much about us as individuals and as members of wider cultural or social groups.

Classroom activity 12

Before finding out linguists' views, reflect on your own. Read the following sentences, then rewrite them in Standard English. Some of the changes are grammatical, others are lexical. Think about your responses to both forms. When would it be more, or less, acceptable to use one form rather than the other?

- I didn't do nothing wrong.
- Who are you going out with?
- Can you borrow me this pen?
- You was right, wasn't you?
- That was sick.
- r u goin 2 james house l8er.
- Den im goin 2 da cinemas.

Exploring prescriptive or descriptive attitudes

This activity assessed what you knew about rules. Now think about how you felt about the differences. Do you think the version is right, or that it doesn't matter as the non-Standard English versions are perfectly understandable? Do you think it's important to write correctly or do you think it is fine to adapt your language according to the context or medium of communication – for example, if you are speaking or texting as opposed to writing a formally assessed essay for your English Language A Level? Ask yourself which of the statements in Figure 15 best describes how you feel about language.

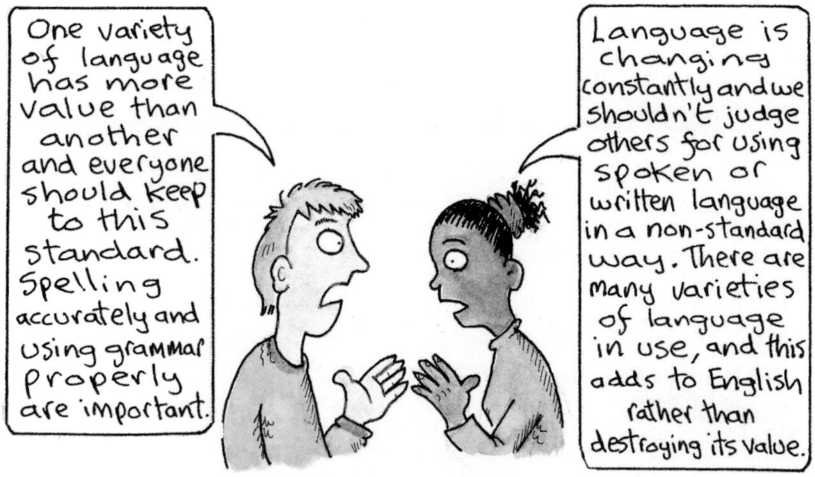

Fig. 14 *Prescriptive versus descriptive attitudes*

If you agreed with the statements in the boy's point, then you are taking a prescriptive view, believing that high standards should be maintained. This point of view places value on the purity of language and that there is both 'good' and 'bad' language. Prescriptivism is about looking at the past and seeing current English usage as showing declining standards. Judgements are made about regional dialect and sociolectal forms, such as slang, as being inferior to the main dialect of written English, Standard English.

Agreeing with the girl's point shows that you take a descriptive view of language, believing that change is inevitable and necessary, and should be embraced instead of resisted. Variation in English, whether regional or social, is valued and judgements are not made on the basis of best or worst. Different forms of language are legitimised as providing variation, rather than being inferior. **Descriptivism** gives spoken English the same status as written forms.

Descriptivism is a more recent approach, resulting possibly from English as a global language and from linguists' research into how language is actually used. There are many English speakers all over the world and the different varieties add to the lexicon and the repertoire of grammatical structures.

■ **Key terms**

Descriptivism: an attitude to language use that seeks to describe it without making value judgements.

■ **Research point**

Jean Aitchison, in her 1996 Reith Lectures (The Language Web), posed the question 'Is our language in decay?' She used a series of metaphors to suggest people's worries and fears about language change:

■ **Damp-spoon syndrome**: Language changes because people are lazy, like leaving a damp spoon in the sugar bowl, which is vulgar and in bad taste. This view presupposes that one type of language is inferior to another.

■ **Crumbling castle view**: Language is like a beautiful castle that must be preserved. However, language has never been at a pinnacle and a rigid system is not always better than a changing one.

■ **Infectious disease assumption**: Bad/poor language is caught like a disease from those around us and we should fight it; but people pick up language changes because they want to, perhaps in order to fit in with certain social groups.

Thinking points

1 What aspects of language do some people find inferior?

2 In what ways do people try to preserve language?

3 Do you think we can 'catch' language use from others?

■ Exploring language debates

It might surprise you that the view that English is in decline and not being used properly isn't new. Here are some historical opinions that could be compared with the views being expressed by some of today's writers:

■ In the 18th century, the age of prescriptivism, many writers proposed that an Academy of English be set up to establish the rules of English usage, although this never happened. The main fears were: the speed of change, the lack of official control over change, and writers' disregard for grammar and spelling.

■ In the 20th and 21st centuries there seems to have been a greater informalisation, as fewer distinctions are made between the spoken and written mode, and non-standard forms of English (such as dialects or text language) are valued. Debates have centred on society's attitudes towards language used about specific groups, hence the notion of using politically correct English. Other altered attitudes are to the use of taboo language, as you only have to contrast television programmes of the 1950s with the language allowed on television now. The 20th century marked the popularity of the descriptivist attitude to language change among linguists, although other influential members of society (the government and the media) often offer prescriptivist ones.

Placing these feelings in an earlier context, in Early Modern English, some people in the 16th century were upset that writers and scholars borrowed words from Latin, Greek and other European languages to name inventions and ideas. Others saw this as a criticism of English vocabulary, calling the new words 'inkhorn' terms (presumably because they were associated with scholars). Even earlier, in the 14th century, many worried that English was changing because of the French influence (brought over as the language of the ruling classes when the Normans invaded in 1066), fearing that English would disappear as a distinctive language.

Extension activity 10

Thinking about these debates and people's fears over language change, evaluate these points:

■ How do the debates of previous centuries compare with arguments put forward today about language change?

■ In Johnson's preface to his dictionary he said that no lexicographer 'shall imagine that his dictionary can embalm his language, and secure it from corruption and decay'. To what extent do you think he was right? What evidence would you give to support your viewpoint?

■ Although we follow many rules today, what evidence is there that grammar hasn't been completely fixed?

💡 Key changes in attitudes across Late Modern English

We can compare the opening pages of the three textbooks below (written between 1750 and 1996) to show how much attitudes to grammar have changed: Ann Fisher, *A Practical New Grammar with exercises of bad English* (1750); John Ash, *Grammatical Institutes, or an Easy Introduction to Dr. Lowth's English Grammar* (1760); David Crystal, *Rediscover Grammar* (1996). As you read, think about the following:

■ What are the writers' attitudes towards English?

■ How does each text reveal its descriptive or prescriptive attitude in its language?

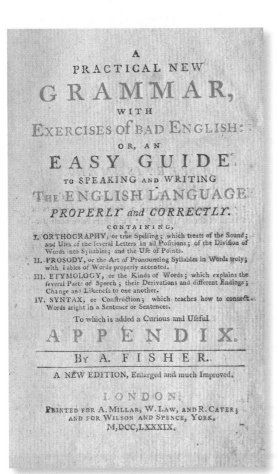

Ann Fisher, A Practical New Grammar with exercises of bad English, *1750*

THE Importance of an *English Education* is now pretty well underſtood; and it is generally acknowledged, that not only for Ladies, but for young Gentlemen deſigned merely for Trade, an intimate Acquaintance with the Properties and Beauties of the *Engliſh* Tongue would be a very deſirable and neceſſary Attainment; far preferable to a Smattering of the learned Languages.

John Ash, Grammatical Institutes or, An Easy Introduction to Dr. Lowth's English Grammar, *1760*

> ### What is grammar?
>
> Grammar is the business of taking a language to pieces, to see how it works. Its study has fascinated people for over 2,000 years – since the time of the Ancient Greeks. But in recent years, grammar has come to be unpopular. People have become uncertain about its value, and many schools have ceased to teach it, or they teach it very selectively.
>
> Currently, the topic is controversial. Some argue strongly that the teaching of 'old-style' grammar (along with multiplication tables) would be a solution to the supposed problems of deteriorating standards in modern education. Others, remembering with dread their first close encounter with grammatical study, argue equally strongly that to reintroduce grammar in its old form would be a disaster.
>
> The aim of this book is to explain what English grammar is about, so that people can make up their minds on the matter. My own view is that the study of grammar is something that *everyone* can find fascinating, fruitful, and even entertaining. It taps the same instincts for thinking about language that are used when people play Scrabble, complete a crossword, or fill in gaps in sentences, as they do in TV game shows likes *Blankety Blank*. But grammar, compared with these activities, turns out to be rather more useful, socially and educationally.

David Crystal, Rediscover Grammar, *Longman, 1996*

Ann Fisher's use of the pre-modifier 'bad' for English in the title of her book immediately sets the tone for the text and announces it as a prescriptive standpoint. She emphasises that it is a guide to speaking and writing 'properly' and 'correctly', both adverbs describing the appropriate manner of communication with 'properly' repeated to describe the right stresses ('accent') to be placed on spoken words. To us the phrasing seems odd, showing that some aspects of style, grammar and lexis have changed since 1780 ('connect words aright'), but 'right' links with the adjective 'true' applied to spelling and the notion of correct language that runs through the opening of her textbook.

Interestingly, Ash's text reveals much about 18th-century gender and class attitudes to language study; note that both 'Ladies' and 'young Gentlemen designed merely for trade' are singled out as benefiting from this book about practical English. The pragmatic assumption is the value placed on 'the learned languages' (Latin and Greek) for higher-class men. The phrase 'intimate acquaintance' makes the learning of English sound highly personal and easier to acquire for the types of people studying this than 'a smattering' of Latin. This text, from this extract, does not put forward explicitly the prescriptive view, but it is suggested in the nouns ('properties', 'beauties').

Crystal is defensive of grammar study, using negative words ('unpopular' and 'uncertain', 'old-style grammar') to describe people's attitudes to studying it, suggesting that for many English seems to have lost its 'value'. This is a post-prescriptive point of view stressing that people's fear and dislike of grammar ('dread', 'disaster') may be rooted in their educational experiences of being taught it. This formal teaching was exactly what the 18th and 19th centuries wanted to achieve in order to 'prescribe' the teaching of 'proper' grammar. In the 19th century these teaching methods were enshrined in school practices. Crystal discusses people's enjoyment of words and word-games and uses adverbs ('socially', 'educationally') that could be compared with some of the benefits that Fisher and Ash saw. Arguably, Crystal does not take a descriptive attitude himself here but talks about other people's responses to grammar.

However, by acknowledging their feelings rather than imposing his solution seems to be a descriptivist stance.

�️ Changing attitudes and changing contexts

As you study language change and texts from different eras and sources, you can see how attitudes have changed with regard to your key social contexts of power, gender and technology. For example, issues of political correctness might be evident in contemporary texts discussing gender, for example using 'birth name' instead of 'maiden name' so as not to judge a woman by their sexual status. With power along with other key changes you might see different formality levels used by writers and speakers to suggest a changed relationship with their audience. Good examples would be to compare political speeches from 1700 to the present, to see differences between politicians' rhetoric; or to look at the language of advertising for the tone used to address their target audiences.

Taking the technological context and recent ICT developments as a particular focus, you will be aware that texting and instant messaging have polarised views lately, reviving the prescriptivist and descriptivist debates. In an article in the *Daily Mail*, 'I h8 txt msgs: How text messaging is wrecking our language' (September 2007), John Humphrys (a respected broadcaster on *Today*, a Radio 4 current-affairs programme) aired his views about text-speak, and his disappointment with the OED for taking hyphens out of words because they think people don't have time to use them.

Classroom activity 13

Read this extract from Humphrys' article and focus on these two aspects:

1 What evidence is there that he is taking a prescriptivist approach? Support your points by identifying specific features of his language choices that suggest this, for example the semantic field of violence.

2 Analyse the language in the article for features of lexical/semantic and orthographical change, for example the noun 'vandal' is interesting to look at for its etymology and its semantic change.

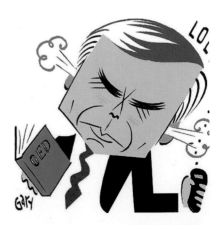

AQA Examiner's tip

Don't assume that all Unit 3 texts are genre-based. Some may be articles like this one, which exemplify different points of view, asking you to evaluate attitudes towards language change and link to ideas discussed throughout your study of language change.

It is the relentless onward march of the texters, the SMS (Short Message Service) vandals who are doing to our language what Genghis Khan did to his neighbours eight hundred years ago.

They are destroying it: pillaging our punctuation; savaging our sentences; raping our vocabulary. And they must be stopped.

This, I grant you, is a tall order. The texters have many more arrows in their quiver than we who defend the old way.

Ridicule is one of them. 'What! You don't text? What century are you living in then, granddad? Need me to sharpen your quill pen for you?'

You know the sort of thing; those of us who have survived for years without a mobile phone have to put up with it all the time. My old friend Amanda Platell, who graces these pages on Saturdays, has an answerphone message that says the caller may leave a message but she'd prefer a text. One feels so inadequate.

(Or should that have been ansafone? Of course it should. There are fewer letters in that hideous word and think how much time I could have saved typing it.)

The texters also have economy on their side. It costs almost nothing to send a text message compared with a voice message. That's perfectly true. I must also concede that some voice messages can be profoundly irritating.

My own outgoing message asks callers to be very brief – ideally just name and number – but that doesn't stop some callers burbling on for ten minutes and always, always ending by saying: 'Ooh – sorry I went on so long!'

But can that be any more irritating than those absurd little smiley faces with which texters litter their messages? It is 25 years since the emoticon (that's the posh word) was born.

It started with the smiley face and the gloomy face and now there are 16 pages of them in the texters' A–Z.

It has now reached the stage where my computer will not allow me to type the colon, dash and bracket without automatically turning it into a picture of a smiling face. Aargh!

John Humphrys, *'I h8 txt msgs: How text messaging is wrecking our language'*,
Daily Mail, *24 September 2007*

Research point

David Crystal, in *Rediscover Grammar*, sees what he calls a tridialectal future for us, an extension of bidialectism, where people use their national standard and a regional dialect. He says that we move comfortably between three dialects in various situations:

- at home we will use the dialect of the region from which we come
- travelling around Britain, for work or pleasure, we will use Standard English
- travelling around the world we will use World Standard English.

Thinking points

1. On what variety of English do you think World Standard English will be based?

2. Can you evidence this tridialectism from your own experiences?

Extension activity 11

As a final Thinking point, reflect on your own experiences of studying English Language. Do you think that this course offers a descriptive or prescriptive view? Base your evaluation on a consideration of:

- the topics covered in the different modules
- the discussions you have had in class around some of the topics
- the assessment objectives and what aspects of language study they reward.

Examination preparation and practice

In this topic you will:

- understand what you will be asked to do in the examination

- learn how you will be assessed in the examination

- use student responses and examiner feedback to improve your performance in the exam.

AQA Examiner's tip

As the texts are all data-based, don't be tempted into essay-like responses detailing the historical background of language change. Remember to work with the data in front of you.

Assessment

As part of the $2\frac{1}{2}$ hour examination you will spend half of the time allowed on Section A: Language acquisition and half the time allowed on Section B: Language change. You need to answer one question from each section, so this will give you 1 hour and 15 minutes for each.

You will have the choice of two questions for Section B: Language change. There are a variety of data types that you can expect to see. These include:

- written and spoken data

- comparisons of similar genre texts from different dates within Late Modern English – testing your knowledge of diachronic change

- extracts from dictionaries

- articles about language change.

All questions are data-based, meaning that you will have facsimiles of written material produced from 1700 onwards.

Assessment objectives

AO1: Select and apply a range of linguistic methods, to communicate relevant knowledge using appropriate terminology and coherent, accurate written expression (7.5%)

AO1 is worth up to 24 marks. You are credited at the highest level if you are systematic in your approach to the data in front of you. Read the question carefully, note the main parts of it and annotate the exam paper before you start writing. Focus particularly on identifying relevant linguistic features, using the linguistic methods that are familiar from your English language study (grammar, phonology etc.). Make sure you write clearly and accurately in the exam, as this shows the examiner that you are able to use English yourself effectively.

AO2: Demonstrate critical understanding of a range of concepts and issues relating to the construction and analysis of meanings in spoken and written language, using knowledge of linguistic approaches (5%)

This is worth 16 marks. It is testing what you know about the theories and concepts you have studied in English language, from both AS and A2. Getting high marks for this assessment objective is about being selective in your choice of theories and theorists to discuss. Unlike language acquisition, there are fewer specific theorists to learn for language change, and your discussion will be more on the ideas and attitudes to language change in Late Modern English. You do not need to learn historical dates in detail, but having some understanding of what had happened to English by the dates of the texts you have to analyse will inform your comments.

AO3: Analyse and evaluate the influence of contextual factors on the production and reception of spoken and written language, showing knowledge of the key constituents of language (2.5%)

This is worth 8 marks. Read both the question and the data carefully, noting down the significant features of context you can see. Such information could include the historical period, the social and political attitudes of the times, and the ways people lived and accessed the types of text you have in front of you to interpret. All the factors that you have looked at that affect language change (technology, travel, fashion, etc.) could be relevant to link to your interpretation of features within the data. So consider how the context affects the language used and don't make a discussion of context separate from your analysis of the data.

↰ Practising for the exam

In this section you have the opportunity to practise the types of question that you might meet in the Unit 3 examination. Practising small tasks, as you have done throughout the topics, has been important to ensure your understanding of all the different linguistic areas and methods you can use in your analysis. However, practising extended writing tasks is the most useful thing you can do, as it tests your ability to look in detail at data, and assesses your ability to apply what you know about language change.

Write your answer to the question below, keeping the assessment objectives and mark scheme in mind. Check your answer against the sample response that follows and read the examiner's comments, matching these to the Mark Scheme extracts provided. Add these to your own ideas to see what a comprehensive answer could have included. Evaluate your own answer to decide what you could have done differently to maximise your marks.

Preparing wisely

Knowing the topic thoroughly will be the biggest help to you, giving you confidence when you face the previously unseen data. You know what revision methods work best for you, but remember the assessment objectives and their weightings when you are revising, and in the examination when you are constructing your answer.

Examination question

Q3)   **Texts E** and **F** are letters written home by soldiers on active service. **Text E** is from a word-processed version of a handwritten letter sent during the Crimean War in 1854. **Text F** is an email written during the Iraq War in 2003.

Refering to both texts in detail, and to relevant ideas from language study, explore how language has changed over time.

You may wish to comment on some of the following: choices of vocabulary and grammar and their effects; the organisation and development of ideas; the wider contexts of historical language change.

AQA January 2005

Text E

Camp before Sebastopol

Nov 20 1854

Dear father,

i only received your kind letter and newspaper for wich i am extremely thankful i was glad to find that you was all in the enjoyment of good health as thank god it leaves me att present When I wrote To you last i stated that i had orders to proceed to the siege of sebastopol we landed on the crimea on the 14th of sept and marched for our scene of operations that night without any tents and the only covering we had was a single blanket in addition to our great coats and to make matters worse there was a fal of heavy rain the very first night of our bivuoaking wich Though a bit of a Damper in the most of us however we proceed joyful on our way elated with the hopes of meeting the Russians – We had turned out severall nights the pickets having been alarmed with the Cossacks that lurks in the neighbourhood of our camp

We have had a very severe Storm on Tuesday last it blewe down nearly every tent in the encampment leaving them in pieces if such weather was continuing it would kill the most of us i hear that we lost 20 vessels and one of them called the Prince containing all the warm clothing for the army also 200 000 in [unclear] it is a serious los to the whole of us as we are nearly naked John Macklin of the Royal artillery was taken to hospital from this and i hear since he is dead i have only received 2. of the papers and 3 letters that you have sent and i wish you would be kind enough to send me a newspaper occasionally and a copy of this to sisters and brother as i have no time to write To them we are now before sebastopol and god knows when we will take it and there is a talk of our remaining Here for the winter if so it will kill half of us please to give my kind love To all relations and accept the same of me from your affectionate Son J Honey

Directions
    Private J Honey
    10 Com R S & Miners
    British army Crimea
    Before Sebastopol

P.S. please to give this piece of [unclear] to Miss Clark She is a much loved cousin

The Military Museum of Devon and Dorset

Text F

> HOLA PEOPLE!
>
> BEEN MEGA REDDERS 2DAY FIRST HOT SUNNY DAY FOR 2 WEEKS, HAS JUST BEEN OVERCAST + WINDY AND THE ODD MEGA HONKING SANDSTORM WHERE U CAN SEE (?), UR TENT TRIES TO BLO DOWN AND EVERYTHING INSIDE + OUTSIDE OF TENT FILLS UP WITH SAND.
>
> APART FROM SAND IN EVERY ORIFICE AM DOING FINE AND STILL PLAYING THE WAITING GAME, BUT ON STANDBY ALL THE TIME AND COULD BE GOING OFF WHENEVER, WHEREVER SO WE HAVE TO 'STAY BENDY' AS WE KEEP GETTING TOLD. GOT SKY TV ON CAMP SO KEEP TRACK OF WHATS GOING WITH THINGS [personal information omitted]
>
> SAY HELLO TO MY MILLIONS OF FANS WHO KEEP PHONING UP! AND TRY NOT TO WORRY TO MUCH, HAVE A DRINK FOR ME INSTEAD (DID HAVE BEER BUT NOW DRY DUE TO OBVIOUS REASONS)
>
> LOADS OF LOVE [personal information omitted]

Georgina Foss

Student answer

With this response the candidate has chosen to approach the data through contextual factors (AO3), but linking the main point about the effect of technology to a quotation from the texts shows close reading of the actual data.

The obvious change that has occurred between the two texts is the use of technology in the email. This makes communication much quicker and easier for the soldier in 2003, as it is less time-consuming and does not require typical letter conventions, such as the sender's address and date found in the later texts is automatically inserted in an email. Also it is evidently more efficient as J Honey says in his letter 'I have only received 2 of the papers and 3 letters that you have sent', implying the postal service was less reliable than a guaranteed email. However the soldier in Text F also comments on the parcel being left in the rain and so clearly this is still relevant to soldiers today despite the 150 year difference.

The approach to the question remains comparative, a helpful approach in these types of data sets, allowing the response to be systematic in style and based on applying linguistic methods (AO1).

The register of the handwritten letter is much more formal as he addresses it to 'father' showing a respectful relationship and also it is interesting that Text F addresses the email to 'people', whereas in 1854 this would not be typical of a letter, to address it to several people. Text F also uses 'hola', which is unusual as it is a Spanish borrowing, but shows that the soldier is trying to be lighthearted and upbeat with his email.

Some of the contextual factors (AO3) are perhaps a little speculative, but they seem valid and sensible interpretations in light of the data.

AO3 is strength of this response but, as it is the least weighted Assessment Objective, more of these contextual factors could be linked to explicit features of the data in order to show AO1 knowledge.

The content of Text E is very informative, describing all the current status of the army, and the weather and problems they had encountered. This is possibly due to the fact that this sort of news was unavailable at the time, whereas now the army can be monitored on the news online etc. It could also be that the soldier in E is writing to his father and so would be expected to share this information whereas in Text F the solider writes to a collective audience and thinks they do not necessarily need to know this information, preferring to reassure them that he is fine by making jokes (sand in every orifice) to keeping an informal and upbeat tone to show that he is happy and not scared to be at war. However in Text E the solider expresses his worries at his ill-health and does not try to reassure his father, which shows that this was not expected of a relationship between father and son in 1854.

Both use non-standard language but for different reasons. There are mistakes from the soldier in E with his verb formations, such as 'you all was' and with the relative pronoun 'Cossacks that lurk'. There is also non-standard punctuation with a lack of commas and full-stops, despite being well after standardisation. I think this is because this letter preceded mass literacy and education and it is highly possible that this soldier was not taught in a school for long. However in Text F the soldier uses non-standard spellings such as 'ur' and '2day' and graphological features such as the + sign, heavily influenced by technology. These are a form of spelling using homophones and numeric substitutions used to save time and characters within the message. The soldiers here would have limited time to write their emails because others probably need access to the computer too. Even the choice of capitals for the whole text indicates that it might have been competed in a hurry.

Text E still has evidence of Early Modern English, with older syntax such as 'on Tuesday last' and the spelling of 'blewe' with the terminal –e, 'att' with a now obsolete double consonant and 'wich' without the 'h'. As standardisation was a long, continuing process it's possible these words and rules were still becoming standardised.

Both texts contain army jargon and field specific lexis. Text E uses 'siege', 'bivouacking' and 'encampment', although Text F uses less: 'standby', 'bendy', perhaps because it is possible for the audience of F to see what's happening on television and the writer needs to be less explicit. Text F is much more colloquial and informal. The way Text F is written represents speech in its spontaneous and colloquial style, shown in the exclamatory sentences and the humorous comments 'say hello to my millions of fans', possibly to reassure his reader using his typical idiolectal style. His imperatives at the end 'say', 'try', and 'have' all seem to have pragmatic meanings for his readers to keep positive for him. Indeed, this text seems more interactional, a result of the immediacy of email contact as compared to a letter sent from Russia to Britain in wartime in the 19th century. The 1854 soldier describes his situation in a more matter-of-fact tone and does not try to euphemise his thoughts, such as 'if so it will kill half of us', although uses politeness features such as modal verbs 'I wish you would' also indicating respect for his father.

Examiner's comment

This answer's strength lies in its contextual awareness, interpreting the context thoughtfully in the light of the data (AO3). There is a range of linguistic methods (AO1) – including lexis, grammar, orthography – and the written expression is fluent. Some awareness of language concepts (AO2), especially in relation to language change (using relevant terminology such as register, idiolect, mode), suggests a clear understanding of the areas the candidate has studied. This is a strong, engaged response given the time constraints of an exam.

There is, of course, more that could be said about the texts and this is an opportunity for you to select other features of the two letters that could be discussed.

This paragraph takes the response back to a more detailed application of a range of linguistic methods (AO1), with non-Standard English, grammatical, punctuation and spelling choices grouped together effectively. AO3 is again evident with connections made with specific features, showing the ability to select 'judicious examples' (AO2). An understanding of language concepts and issues underpins this whole section.

Sensible and well-observed points here showing AO2 strengths. An understanding of language change as an ongoing process shows good understanding of the changes to English over time. Generalised historical observations are avoided in favour of close focus on specific details of syntax and spelling.

Again the clustering of exemplified linguistic features shows the ability to evaluate the data and combine the demands of the Assessment Objective to maximise the data; this also suggests that the candidate has used their time helpfully to plan their response.

■ Further reading

Aitchison, J. (1991) *Language Change: Progress or Decay?*, CUP

Beard, Adrian (2004) *Language Change*, Routledge

Bragg, M. (2004) *The Adventure of English*, Sceptre

Crystal, D. (1995) *The Cambridge Encyclopaedia of the English Language*, CUP

Elmes, S. (2000) *The Routes of English*, BBC Books

Freeborn, D. (1991) *Varieties of English*, Macmillan

Games, A. (2006) *Balderdash & Piffle*, BBC Books

- AO1 Select and apply a range of linguistic methods, to communicate relevant knowledge using appropriate terminology and coherent, accurate written expression (5 per cent of the A Level mark).

- AO2 Demonstrate critical understanding of a range of concepts and issues relating to the construction and analysis of meanings in spoken and written language, using knowledge of linguistic approaches (5 per cent of the A Level mark).

- AO3 Analyse and evaluate the influence of contextual factors on the production and reception of spoken and written language, showing knowledge of the key constituents of language (2.5 per cent of the A Level mark).

- AO4 Demonstrate expertise and creativity in the use of English in a range of different contexts informed by linguistic study (7.5 per cent of the A Level mark).

Key terms

Synoptic: bringing together a full range of skills and viewpoints.

Investigating language is a fundamental process to the study of the English language and this coursework unit is your opportunity to immerse yourself in a particular language topic, carry out your own linguistic research, and reflect upon your findings. Although you have engaged with the research of other linguists in your AS and A2 study, and will have carried out some data-gathering and data-analysis activities in your work so far, this unit will probably be the first time you undertake a language project that is quite as independent, structured and academic in its approach. In this sense you might find the skills involved are more like a social science subject, like sociology or psychology.

This unit is designed to be **synoptic**, which means that it draws upon all of the skills and material that you have encountered so far in the course. The coursework is assessed in the form of two pieces that you will produce, which are linked by the topic you have investigated: a language investigation and a media text.

Section A: Language investigation

The language investigation is where your coursework unit begins in earnest, and forms its major part. With the guidance of your supervisor (likely to be your class teacher), you will be able to choose any topic that will lead to a fruitful focus on language. You might find there is a particular topic you would like to pursue that you have covered in the course so far – for example, gender, power and technology, and the language of particular genres from AS, or child language acquisition and language change from A2. However, your choice does not have to come from these previously studied areas, and you may want to explore an area of particular interest to you – for example language variation in accent and dialect, or language and conversational interaction.

Once you have chosen your topic, this section will help you to navigate your way through the process of investigation. This includes learning how to: read around your chosen subject; collect, present and analyse data; and discuss your findings, placing them within the wider debate of the subject.

Section B: Media text

The media text is the smaller section of the Investigating language coursework, both in size and in terms of how many marks it is worth. It shares some ground with the AS coursework you have done, in that you will write for a specific audience, purpose and context – for example, a newspaper editorial or magazine article – all for a non-specialist audience this time, unlike the more technical investigation write-up. Having explored a particular topic in your investigation, this piece gives you the opportunity to engage with a related linguistic debate.

A Language investigation

Introduction

In this section you will:

- learn what makes a successful investigation focus

- consider the stages involved in an investigation

- acquire some of the terminology relevant to investigating language.

Key terms

Data: examples of any kind of language in use collected, sourced, or presented for analysis.

Reliable: used to refer to data that is an accurate reflection of real language use.

Empirical: work that comes from observation and experience, rather than pure theory.

Objective: an unbiased, factual view of a subject.

Subjective: a view of a subject that includes personal opinion.

Hypothesis: a statement of theory to be tested by research and data analysis.

Methodology: the design of an investigation and the stages it goes through.

Qualitative: data analysis that focuses on individual instances of language use and analyses them closely and in context.

Quantitive: data analysis that summarises findings in larger sets of data and presents statistical findings.

The investigation you are embarking on is about trying to find out new things about language by using a clear and open process that others can understand and learn from. In a sense, this involves finding out some sort of 'truth' about how language works – so be prepared to work with what your **data** throws up, even if it isn't quite what you were expecting (assuming it is **reliable**).

Your investigation can be on any topic whatsoever, so long as it is focused on language – in fact, it is important that you choose something that motivates you and that you have a personal interest in. However, it is vital to remember that your investigation should take an **empirical** approach, grounded in data, and lead to **objective** conclusions, rather than **subjective** opinions – so you must avoid allowing any preconceived ideas to prejudice what you can find out about a topic you know well.

In all, your final investigation should be up to 2,500 words in length (which doesn't include your data or appendices). Because the investigation is a more scientific piece of work, it should go through a series of particular stages, and be presented in a way that deals with each of them deliberately. These stages are:

- **Introduction**: This allows you to discuss the topic you have chosen, including your reasons for choosing it, and any links to existing research. You will also present your **hypothesis** here, and set out your overall aims, in terms of what aspects of language you will analyse.

- **Methodology**: A description of the process you went through from beginning to end in your investigation, including a reflection on any issues that you encountered.

- **Analysis**: This is the most important part of your investigation, involving a systematic analysis of your data using linguistic terminology, which can be a blend of **qualitative** and **quantitive** approaches. You should also include details about the contextual factors involved in your data.

- **Conclusion and evaluation**: Here you will interpret the analysis of your data and present your conclusions in relation to the hypothesis you set out. You will also have the opportunity to make points about the overall successes and challenges involved in your investigation in the evaluation, and give ideas for further study.

- **Bibliography and references**: Details of any sources you used to help you: books, websites or articles.

- **Appendices and data**: This is where you will include the data that you collected, as well as copies of any other material needed to fully understand your investigation (e.g. a particular piece of existing research that you based it on).

Make sure that you include all of the named parts of the investigation detailed here, and that they are clearly labelled in your final draft: these are sections specifically set out by the examination board.

Focusing your investigation

Key terms

Primary data: spoken or written data collected by a researcher.

Corpus: a large, text-based collection of data, usually stored electronically so that it can be quickly analysed and searched.

Ethically sound: this refers to the methods of gathering data and conducting an investigation that make sure it won't mislead or offend anyone.

Link

There is more information about data collection in the 'Methodology: collecting your data' topic on pages 141–143.

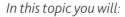 Possible subjects

The range of possible areas of language use you can investigate is virtually limitless; the only restrictions on the subject of your investigation are that it must have a clear language focus, and be based on the collection and analysis of 'real' **primary data**. This usually means gathering or accessing specific, real examples of language in use. These may be print-based sources and/or the recording and transcribing of speech, or even accessing a collection of 'raw' data already in existence, known as a language **corpus**.

Before you start to settle upon potential investigation topics, take on board the following three additional guiding principles that will help steer you towards a successful idea:

- **The investigation must be of manageable scope:** With only 2,500 words available for your academic analysis and report, you will have to limit yourself to a specific area of enquiry, and a limited quantity of data. It is impossible, for example, to explore the entire history of the English language, to compare the styles of two whole magazines, or carry out a comprehensive survey of the writing produced by 20 primary school children.

- **It must be practical:** This means the material you wish to collect needs to be reasonably accessible. The project must also be realistic in terms of the time and resources you have available to you – tackling lots of heavily detailed transcription, for example, might prove too much.

- **It must be ethically sound:** It is not usually acceptable to base your investigation on the study of material that would be considered offensive, or to use unethical methods of data collection.

This still leaves a potentially vast range of possibilities, and you might well ask 'where do I start?' This topic will encourage you to begin to create a shortlist of your own potential choice of topics.

Building on existing units

One approach is to revisit some of the topics you have already studied, and to use the work you carried out for the AS units and in Unit 3 as a starting point for Unit 4. As you do so, it is useful to frame a number of questions arising from a particular topic, any one of which could become the basis of an investigation.

Unit 1: Categorising texts

Unit 1 equipped you with a strong foundation in the form of the range and depth of linguistic concepts and terminology it introduced and applied to texts – your investigation should make purposeful use of a linguistic register throughout, so use your notes and glossary work from last year to help you establish this.

In addition, Unit 1 was based around the analysis of a range of different texts and genres, and work with existing research was begun in the form of the topics of gender, power and technology.

Text varieties

The Text varieties section of Unit 1 foregrounded the importance of audience, purpose and context (these can be considered a part of the **social variables** that will affect the data you work with) in shaping particular texts, and the range of textual varieties available across spoken, written and mixed modes.

You will be analysing closely some form of spoken or written data in your investigation, and the way that the Unit 1 examination asked you to isolate particular linguistic features translates well into the need to identify particular **linguistic variables** in your investigation.

In general, the most successful investigations of this type are based on a question or an issue which can be explored by comparing two or more pieces of data, with a focus on one or two controlled variables at a time. This means comparing like with like: if, for example, you were interested in how the language style of radio presenters on different stations (say Radio 1 and Radio 2) reflected their different target audiences, you would need to record examples of similar programmes from each station (perhaps the morning breakfast show or a phone-in), rather than trying to compare a music programme with the chairing of a political discussion or a celebrity interview.

For example, a question like 'How does the presentation of the news reflect the needs and interests of different audiences?' would need to try and keep all other variables the same by limiting the data to a single medium (print-based, web-based, radio or television) and by comparing the way the same stories are presented on the same day. Television news offers many possibilities: you could compare the language of the children's news programme *Newsround* with the *BBC 1 Six o'clock News* bulletin of the same day, concentrating on the headlines and perhaps two or three of the major news stories they both cover. Or you could compare the language of the main bulletins on the major terrestrial channels – BBC1, ITV1 and Channel 4 – with a focus on one or two news (or sports) items.

Print-based news has traditionally offered many possibilities for study: these include the rather predictable comparison of language styles between tabloid and broadsheet papers (eliminate other variables by sticking with papers of similar political stance, such as the *Daily Mirror* and *The Guardian*, or the *Daily Mail* and *The Times*). Alternatively, you could consider how political bias is reflected in the coverage of the same story by papers of contrasting loyalties, comparing, say, the *Daily Telegraph* and *The Guardian*. Or you could consider how news output with a local audience (whether print-based, radio or television) differs from the national media. You could, for example, compare the coverage of your local team's football match in your local paper with the report in a national publication.

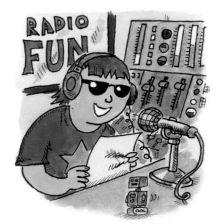

Fig. 1 *Comparing differing language styles, such as those of DJs, would be a possible language investigation*

AQA Examiner's tip

The examination board is keen to see unique investigations that reflect a student's own interests in language – not least because something a student has shown a personal interest in often turns out to be a more involved, original and sophisticated piece. It is essential to make sure you keep your focus closely on language and aim to meet all the success criteria. Work closely with your supervisor to turn your own ideas into a real, working language investigation.

Key terms

Social variables: the ways in which the context of data differs by social factors like age, gender, ethnicity and social class.

Linguistic variables: specific linguistic features identified as markers for possible variation in an investigation.

Classroom activity 1

Listed below are four further broad questions which might be the starting point for an investigation. They all need narrowing down to a manageably precise focus. Using the 'one variable' principle discussed above, suggest for each of them examples of suitable data that might be collected as the basis of the study.

1. How far does the language of advertising vary according to the gender of the target audience?

2. How does a 'live' commentary on radio differ from one on television?

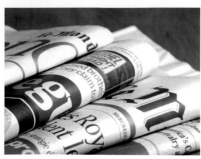

Fig. 2 *Newpapers offer many possibilities for study*

Key terms

Secondary data: data that has already been collected by another researcher, which is made use of in a new investigation.

3 How do the publishers of popular magazines use language to appeal to readers of different ages?

4 How do teachers vary the language they use according to the class they teach?

Language and social contexts

These core topics from Unit 1 first brought you into contact with another important element of your investigation, in the form of **secondary data**, when examining the research and theories of other linguists. Unit 4 offers you the chance to incorporate secondary data sources by putting a particular linguist's ideas or findings to the test, or bringing in work from others to add depth to your own.

Table 1 suggests a range of issues from your AS work on gender, power and technology, and related questions that you could take further in an investigation:

Table 1 *Possible investigation ideas related to Unit 1*

Gender and language use	Are women better listeners and do men interrupt more?
	How true is it that males use less phatic talk than females?
	Are males more likely to be competitive, and females cooperative?
	Are there significant gender differences in the styles of texting preferred by males and females?
	How early in their development do gender differences in language start to appear in boys and girls?
Representation of gender in language	How does language represent and construct ideas of masculinity and femininity in magazines?
	How do males and females differ when they describe themselves and members of the opposite sex?
Power and conversational discourse	How is status and dominance shown in domestic, social or professional discourse?
	How do people in authority control and manage conversations in formal situations such as meetings?
Power and written texts	How does the language of legal texts convey power and authority?
Power, persuasion and rhetoric	How do politicians use persuasive language to exert influence and achieve impact?
Language and new technology	To what extent has a set of conventions emerged in areas such as texting, blogs, webpages or MySpace?
	Are texting and email more like speech or writing?
	How similar to or different from 'real' interaction is the 'conversation' in chat rooms and online forums?
Radio, television and phones	How do phone conversations differ from face-to-face talk?

Classroom activity 2

Choose one of the specific questions from Table 1 and suggest the kinds of data you would collect in order to investigate it well. Note any observations you have about the collection process and the nature of the data needed.

Unit 2: Creating texts

The skills and study in Unit 2 will be of considerable use in Section B's media text, but they also provide rich pickings for potential investigations into the language of particular genres of texts. Consider the suggestions in Table 2, arising out of the main purpose areas you studied in Unit 2.

Table 2 *Possible investigation ideas related to Unit 2*

Texts to persuade	How is language used to persuade in radio advertisements?
Texts to inform	What methods are used by the writers of software instruction manuals to present complex information to non-specialist audiences?
Texts to instruct	How is advice and instruction delivered by a teacher in the feedback they write on assessed work?
Texts to entertain	How close to 'natural' conversation is the scripted dialogue of *EastEnders*?

 Extension activity 1

Look back at some of the texts you studied as part of your original writing work for Unit 2, Section A. Make a note of at least one potential area for further investigation that might emerge from any of the texts you surveyed or your wider interests and reading. For example, if you studied a number of speeches in preparation for your 'Writing to persuade' piece, you could develop this into a study of political oratory and rhetoric.

Unit 3: Developing language

Unit 3 opens up two very rich areas for language investigation in the form of language acquisition and language change. Table 3 lists just a few of the possibilities in these areas.

Table 3 *Possible investigation ideas related to Unit 3*

Child speech development	In what ways does a child's language develop between the ages of 18 months and 24 months (or 24 and 30 etc.)?
	What part does a carer/parent play in the development of early language?
	What similarities and differences are there in the early language acquisition of twins/siblings?
	How does the language acquisition of a child with learning difficulty/hearing impairment differ from that of other children?
Child literacy studies	How do early reading books/schemes support and develop early reading?
	What does a child's reading aloud, and the mistakes they make, reveal about the process of learning to read?
	What variations are there in the rate at which children acquire early writing skills?
Language change	How has the language and style of news reporting changed during the last 100 years?
	What linguistic changes have taken place in children's literature over the 19th and 20th centuries?
	How does teenage slang and colloquial language differ in children's television drama from the 1970s to the 2000s?

AQA Examiner's tip

If you opt to carry out an investigation into one of the Unit 3 areas of language acquisition and language change, you do not need to observe the same restrictions specified for the examination of texts written after 1700, or children's spoken language up to the age of 7.

■ Key terms

Longitudinal study: a data-gathering exercise for investigation that takes place over a significant period of time, for example recording the same child's language use over several weeks or months.

Care giver: the term used to refer to the main adult who looks after a child.

Child directed speech: a distinctive form of language use employed by adults when interacting with young children.

Cockney: a distinctive accent spoken in London.

Scouse: a distinctive accent spoken in Merseyside.

Accent: the distinctive pronunciation patterns used by a particular group of people.

Dialect: the lexical, semantic and grammatical patterns of language use distinctive to a particular group of people.

Non-standard: language use of any kind that differs from standard grammatical, lexical, semantic, phonological or graphological uses.

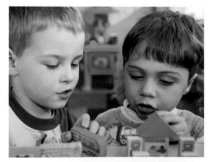

Fig. 3 *Child language development provides wide scope for an investigation*

As an example, child speech development investigations could take the form of a **longitudinal study** of one or two children, given the time period that may well be available to you. This would involve observing their progress by making several recordings (perhaps at monthly intervals) over a period of around six months, with the children engaged in similar activities. Studying children at any period between the age of approximately 15 and 40 months is likely to reveal tangible and interesting developments. A related focus could be to extend data collection to include the interaction of child and **care giver**, to examine the role of **child directed speech** and the nature of carer support, once again ensuring that you arrange to record and study similar types of interaction.

■ Classroom activity 3

Examine the other topics in Table 3, and for each suggest some specific examples of data you would collect in order to answer them scientifically, in a similar way as decribed for the treatment of child speech development.

Wider investigation topics

Outside of the topics that you have studied so far, there are many other profitable areas of the English language that you might choose to investigate further, including those of accent and dialect variation, World English issues and some other specialist areas, discussed below.

◉ Accent and dialect

When the word 'accent' is mentioned you may well conjure with ideas of some of the more recognisable regional accents like **Cockney** or **Scouse**, which you can often hear in day-to-day life, or through the media. However, **accent** and **dialect** is potentially a much wider area of investigation than this: not only could you look into variation in the language of people from different parts of the country; you could also include all sorts of sociolect forms: the ways people use language depending on their occupation, race, social class and other social factors.

The terms 'accent' and 'dialect' are often used to differentiate between phonological, pronunciation differences (accent) and wider lexical, semantic and grammatical differences in the language people use (dialect), which will give you an idea of the scope for both range and depth of analysis. Investigations of this kind are usually based around identifying **non-standard** usage of English in a particular accent, dialect or sociolect. They are also usually based on spoken data, although it is possible to find examples of such varieties in written forms too.

■ Data response exercise 1

The following data is a transcript of two young Scouse speakers. Read it closely and:

■ identify any non-standard language features you can see

■ describe each one you find as linguistically as you can.

Transcription conventions are given on page v.

A:	'ow do you know I was gonna friggin' tell 'im
B:	I just knows (.)
A:	youse better promise |me | YOU won't tell
B:	|wha'|
B:	I ain't never gonna |tell | (1.0) am I
A:	|you better|

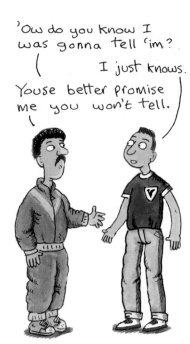

In addition, investigating accent and dialect can bring you into contact with some lively current research and debate into areas like **Estuary English** (see page 104), and some excellent resources, like the accent recordings archive on the Collect Britain website, and BBC Voices project. It could also be a source of considerable personal interest as you may well have family or friends who have strong accents or dialects of some kind, and who would make ideal subjects for collecting your data.

Fig. 4 *Different accents, dialects and sociolects often contain non-standard language features*

 Extension activity 2

Undertake some wider reading into accents and dialects to see if it is an area that interests you for investigation. Use the BBC and Collect Britain websites as a starting point:

■ www.collectbritain.co.uk

■ www.bbc.co.uk/voices

 Language around you activity 1

Make a mind map of the varieties of language use you come into contact with each week, be it from friends, family, colleagues, television, radio, the internet or another source. Use it to identify any potential areas of investigation around you.

🔍 World English

The issue of World English is related to the idea of accent and dialect varieties. Under this umbrella term are the range of different forms of English spoken across the world, from the more obvious examples of the differences between American, British and Australian English, through to **creole** forms that use English in combination with other languages to create new English language hybrids.

Possible investigations in this area might be to compare the language of American, British or Australian English soap operas, newspapers, magazines or websites, focusing on the different pronunciation patterns, lexical items, word meanings and grammatical structures used.

■ **Key terms**

Estuary English: a variety of English with its roots in the Thames estuary area, but seen to be spreading to many other parts of the UK

Creole: a language variety created by contact between one or more language forms and becoming established over several generations of users.

■ Key terms

London Jamaican: a distinctive variety of language blending Cockney, Jamaican creole and Standard English forms.

Code-switching: a language skill that enables the user to change between different languages and language varieties while speaking.

Creole-based forms tend to be a more specialised area, but there is a good deal of rich spoken and written data available, and even literary sources. The linguist Mark Sebba has investigated the language of Caribbean immigrant communities in England, and the phenomena of **London Jamaican** and **code-switching**.

■ Classroom activity 4

The extract from John Agard's poem 'Listen Mr Oxford don' makes use of Jamaican creole forms as well as Standard English. Read through it and make notes on some potential investigations that you could see rising out of it, if combined with other data.

> I ent have no gun
> I ent have no knife
> but mugging de Queen's English
> is the story of my life
>
> I don't need no axe
> to split up yu syntax
> I don't need no hammer
> To mash up yu grammar

John Agard, 'Listen Mr Oxford don', Mangoes and Bullets, *Serpent's Tail, 1997*

Specialist areas

There are also many specialist interests that you could look to for inspiration for your investigation. These could be something that you have a particular enthusiasm for and knowledge of yourself, for example in graphic novels, computer programming languages, or the lyrics of particular genres of music, or particular kinds of writing.

■ Extension activity 3

Research the following examples of specialist English language which could be a focus for your investigation:

- Leet (language used by 'hackers' and other online computer groups)
- Polari (language used by homosexual men in the 20th century).

■ Look around you

An alternative way of choosing a subject to investigate is to think of the many language experiences you encounter in your own daily life and which interest you – there is certain to be some original raw material here. From there, it's a question of pursuing some aspect of language use which has attracted your attention or curiosity.

Let's take the case of Mark, who is currently studying English language. Consider his profile in Table 4, and the examples of potential data and investigations around him.

Take your time to settle on the ideas you would like to follow for your investigation. Use the examples and methods suggested here to explore widely and don't be afraid to keep several different potential projects open, until you settle on the best choice.

Table 4 *Profile of Mark Hudson, an English Language student aged 17.*

Details about Mark's life	Potential investigation ideas
Current occupation: Student at a sixth form college.	Interactions between friends at college, singling out a variable of age or gender in particular. Or perhaps an investigation into the official literature of the college and how it communicates with students, or promotes itself in comparison to other, similar institutions. Or a comparison of the internal emails written by students and teachers.
Location: Has lived in Manchester since he was 11. Previously lived in Birmingham.	Perhaps he has relatives in the Midlands – potential for study of regional dialect/accent in their use, or in his local area, or a comparison of the two.
Subjects studied: English language, History, Sociology and Maths.	Mark's academic subjects also offer possibilities: apart from the speech styles of his teachers (already suggested) he might look at the ways teachers write their reports, or provide feedback on work, or present information via handouts … or look at the language of the textbooks he is required to read.
Family: Lives with mum (secretary), dad (market-stall holder) and two younger brothers (aged 10 and 13). He has three surviving grandparents and one surviving great-grandmother.	Mark could compare the language use and attitudes of the various generations in his family. This could include an investigation into their accents and dialect use, or their attitudes towards slang.

Classroom activity 5

Copy and complete the table below, which contains details of three further aspects of Mark's life. For each of them, suggest potential data sources and investigation ideas that you can see arising.

Details about Mark's life	Potential investigation ideas
Part-time job: Helps out on his dad's market stall on Saturdays.	
Interests and hobbies: Football – plays for local team in Sunday league and supports Manchester City. Cars – has recently passed test. Music – plays guitar in a band with friends.	
Media habits: Enjoys a variety of music; reads car magazines; contributes to online Manchester City supporters' forum. Favourite programmes: enjoys reality TV shows such as *I'm a Celebrity* … and *Big Brother*.	

Extension activity 4

It is possible that your school or college has a selection of investigations from previous years available; although the examination specification from 2010 has changed from the previous syllabus you can still learn a lot by studying the topics, methodology and data used by previous students. Ask your teacher if you can look at some for more examples of suitable topics, hypotheses and questions.

🔍 Framing a focus for your investigation

In most examinations you have little control over the questions you have to answer, but for Unit 4, the choice is yours. Once you have some ideas about the kinds of language areas you might like to investigate, you need to define precisely what it is that you are going to find out, and the sort of data you will need.

The best investigations go beyond mere description of the data, and engage in some *issue* or *debate* arising from it. For example, you may decide to test out some of the ideas associated with language and gender you encountered in Unit 1, or explore the controversy about the use of phonics in the teaching of reading.

With this in mind, there are two ways in which you can provide yourself with a sufficiently precise focus for your investigation – by framing it as a hypothesis, or as a question.

Your focus as a hypothesis

Setting up your investigation around a hypothesis creates an investigation that seeks to test one or more assumptions or expectations against the data that you produce. Look at the following example:

■ Female speakers will use more politeness strategies than males in informal mixed gender conversation.

This will guide the structure of your investigation and will be foregrounded in your introduction section as you set out the aims and hypothesis there. An investigation that takes this tack is particularly appropriate for challenging existing research, or for testing a stereotype.

When it comes to structuring your analysis section and concluding your findings, the hypothesis will be an important factor. You might like to consider setting more than one hypothesis, in order to allow you to be more systematic. For example, the hypothesis above could be broken down into the following group of hypotheses that 'unpick' a couple of distinctive features that might be seen to contribute to 'politeness strategies':

■ **H1:** Female speakers will use more positive lexis towards other speakers than males in informal mixed gender conversation.

■ **H2:** Female speakers will use more fluent turn-taking strategies than males in informal mixed gender conversation.

■ **H3:** Female speakers will give more back channel support than males in informal mixed gender conversation.

From this perspective, each hypothesis can be tested individually in the analysis, and the conclusion can bring the findings together to reflect upon the extent to which the 'politeness strategies' hypothesis is true.

Your focus as a question

Sometimes an investigation is less explicitly based on testing a particular theory of language, and more to do with exploring actual language usage. In this case, it would be more appropriate to structure your investigation around a particular question. For example, if you are setting up a comparison:

■ What differences are there in the language used by David Cameron and Gordon Brown to describe the issue of climate change?

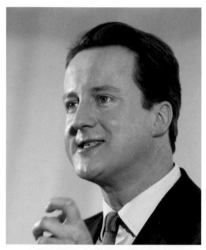

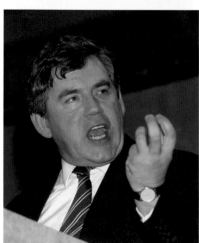

Figs. 5 and 6 *Your investigation could be based on a comparison, for example, the differences in language use between politicians.*

As was the case with the hypothesis, you might also want to consider setting more than one question to cover the related areas of enquiry you would like to pursue in your research. For example, this might allow you to break down the linguistic coverage, or to open up a related debate attached to your investigation.

■ **Q1:** What differences are there in the language used by David Cameron and Gordon Brown to describe the issue of climate change?

■ **Q2:** Does the language that David Cameron and Gordon Brown use reflect differing attitudes towards the issue of climate change?

In this case, a particular process to the investigation becomes evident, and helps to structure the analysis and conclusions of the research as a whole.

Classroom activity 6

Below are some questions and hypotheses suggested by students as possible starting points for their investigations. Comment on their suitability and suggest the kinds of data they might go on to collect.

1 **Topic**: A comparison of newspaper reports of shipping disasters from the *Titanic* (1916) to *The Herald of Free Enterprise* (1987).
Hypothesis: That the reports will reveal lexical, grammatical and graphological evidence of an increasingly informal, populist and visually-oriented style of reporting.

2 **Topic**: A study of how members of my family interact in different situations.
Question: What differences are there in the way members of my family address and talk to each other in different domestic contexts?

3 **Topic**: A comparison of the oratory techniques of Tony Blair and Winston Churchill.
Question: What linguistic features do the speeches of Tony Blair and Winston Churchill have in common?

💡 🔍 Your investigation proposal

When you begin to settle on a number of specific areas that you could investigate, it is a good idea to write up your thoughts, to look at how viable each proposal is, and to submit it to your supervisor for advice. Keep your mind open at this stage and aim to put forward at least three ideas, to give each one the room to grow and allow you to decide which will be the best to pursue into a full investigation.

Your proposal doesn't need to take any particular form (your supervisor may well ask you to use a form or system he or she is used to), but it does need to provide as clear an account as possible of the following aspects:

1 Your link to, or interest in the investigation area.

2 The sort of data you plan to collect – if you can provide a sample, even better.

3 Where and how you plan to gather your data.

4 The main areas of language and features you aim to work with.

5 The question or hypothesis at the heart of your idea.

6 Details of any related linguistic research or theories.

Look at the following proposal by an A2 student, Maxine. Table 5 shows to what extent she has provided insight into each of these six strands, and it is followed by a sample of the sort of advice a supervisor would give at this stage.

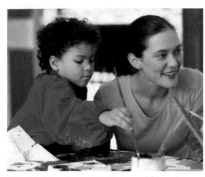

Fig. 7 *Your investigation could involve an area you are interested in pursuing a career in, e.g. teaching.*

■ **Proposal 1**: I am interested in training to be a primary school teacher as I love getting involved with helping really young kids learn. My mum works in a primary school and I sometimes go in and help her. For my investigation, I would like to find out more about how the creative writing of children in the early years of primary school compares with the later years. I would collect examples of their writing – this could be writing that has already taken place and is in the students' folders, or my mum would be able to help me set up opportunities to produce some new work. The writing would be stories, hopefully of the same subject and would be handwritten. The main frameworks that I would be using would be lexis and grammar, but I would also like to look at some semantic and phonological devices as this is something that the pupils work on developing. Other than expecting the later writing to be better, I'm not sure what my overall aim would be, so I'd really like some advice on that!

Table 5 *A breakdown of Maxine's investigation proposal*

Investigation criteria	Information given
1. Your link to, or interest in the investigation area.	She is interested in training to be a primary school teacher and loves getting involved with helping really young kids learn.
2. The sort of data you plan to collect – if you can provide a sample, even better.	She gives examples of handwritten stories, and aims to be able to keep the subject constant to allow better focus on linguistic variables.
3. Where and how you plan to gather your data.	Her mum works in a primary school and can go in to help and get new or existing data, so she should find opportunities to collect data easy to arrange.
4. The main linguistic methods and features you aim to work with.	She is aware that lexis and grammar will be essential, but also has ideas about semantic and phonological devices.
5. The question or hypothesis at the heart of your idea.	She is expecting the later writing to be better and wants to find out how the children develop their writing ability across these age groups.
6. Details of any related linguistic research or theories.	She had not mentioned any at this stage.

Here is an example of the sort of advice a supervisor would give at this stage:

■ This looks like it could work well, Maxine:
  – Your strong personal interest and link should help make the project involved and enjoyable.
  – It would probably be better to gather new data yourself as you could also interview pupils to gain some insight to their writing alongside.

– Written data would be good to work with, and you could take some time to collect a 'good' set before moving forward.

– It would be a good idea to link the investigation to some sort of research background, or even details from the National Curriculum or Literacy Strategy to give it some perspective.

– Begin thinking about more specific language features that you would like to focus on from the frameworks that you mention.

Classroom activity 7

Below are two more proposals submitted by a student, Maxine, for her supervisor to advise on.

1 Read each one and test that it covers each of the six points above by making notes (you might like to draw up a basic table to help compare them).

2 Decide on the advice you would give Maxine about each proposal.

■ **Proposal 2:** My favourite topic from AS was the language and gender research we looked at, in particular the Robin Lakoff handout about women using more words for colours. I think this is true, and I would be interested in testing it out with students at college. My idea would be to show males and females a series of colourful pictures and ask them to describe what they see. I would be working with semantics in detail and also lexis.

■ **Proposal 3:** As you know, my family and I are originally from Birmingham before we came to London. I was 8 and my sister was 6 when we moved here and I've noticed that, although I still have traces of a Brummie accent, me and my sister now speak much more like my friends who have lived in London all their lives. My mum and dad both still have really strong Birmingham accents, like my grandparents back in Birmingham, although my grandma says they have changed a bit. I would like to compare my accent with my parents and grandparents to see how it has changed, and if mum and dad's have also changed. I think this relates well to the idea of Estuary English, although I would need to research this more. I would expect to have to analyse phonology in great depth, but I think I would need to look at other areas as well.

🔍 🗨 Secondary sources

A useful source may introduce you to some of the most interesting or controversial aspect of a given topic, just as Fairclough's ideas about power and Tannen's ideas about language and gender did in Unit 1. You can use it as a point of departure and a basis for comparison with your own study, referring to it in both your investigation report and your media text – perhaps in your introduction, or just in passing as you proceed with your analysis. It will certainly be useful in your conclusion to show that you are aware of the work that other researchers have carried out, and to discuss your findings in relation to these.

Here are some of the main ways that examining existing research can help you with your own investigation:

■ **Useful approaches and terminology:** The kinds of areas of language and terminology used in published research can provide a suitable style model for your own academic analysis.

Extension activity 5

The following ideas and research frameworks about language were all introduced in Unit 1. For each, design an investigation that would test, apply or develop them:

1 Fairclough's three-part method for analysing advertisements in terms of power.

2 Levinson and Brown's application of face theory and other aspects of politeness.

3 Ideas about 'women's language' proposed by Lakoff, Holmes and Coates.

Link

There is more information about bibliographies and sources in the Coursework preparation and practice topic at the end of this section on pages 163–164.

Classroom activity 8

Give the same sort of treatment to the secondary source described below, that of Otto Jespersen's research on language and gender from 1922. As above, evaluate the possible value and credibility of the source and discuss the potential of the source as a starting point for a new language investigation.

■ **Secondary source:** The respected linguist Otto Jespersen claimed in a work on language and gender published in 1922 that women 'shrank from coarse and gross expressions' and preferred 'veiled and indirect expressions'. Limited empirical evidence was presented in support.

■ **Methodologies for experimental research:** Some experimental or survey-based research may provide you with a useful model for carrying out your own investigation; look in particular at how the data collection was arranged to ensure it was ethical and valid.

■ **Results or hypothesis to test:** The conclusions and results of earlier research could inform your own hypothesis or focus question. You could decide to test these earlier findings.

The dangers of plagiarism

The nature and dangers of plagiarism have already been noted as you prepared your Unit 2 coursework. In your investigation and media text, as with your original writing last year, you must distinguish between legitimate research of secondary sources, which you explicitly acknowledge, and intellectual theft, which includes any unacknowledged 'cutting and pasting' and other presentation of such material as if it were your own. When researching, it is all too easy to note down/cut and paste whole phrases and sentences from a source, and to incorporate these, advertently or otherwise, into your own writing. This is malpractice, and the penalties are potentially severe.

Bibliography: keeping notes and references

For both the investigation report and your media text, you will need to include a comprehensive bibliography of sources consulted. So whenever you consult a source of information, whether print-based or online, you need to keep careful notes. This means:

■ noting down the author, title, publisher and date of any publication you consult

■ noting down the full web address of any online source and the date you visited it

■ in your notes, if you are quoting/copying directly from the source, *always* showing this with speech/quotation marks

■ reproducing this information in your bibliography when you write your final texts.

Whatever sources you are using, don't forget to use them *critically*: check out the credentials of the author, the webpage or publication, and note the date when the material was compiled, to assess whether it is still valid for your research. As an example, consider the discussion below on the validity of Jenny Cheshire's Reading research in 1982.

■ **Secondary source:** The sociolinguist Jenny Cheshire published a study in 1982 based on recordings and interviews with teenagers in Reading. She claimed they revealed that boys and girls differed in the way they used local, non-standard speech forms, and that there was evidence of social class differences in the language use of groups of children with different backgrounds and values.

■ **Commentary:** Cheshire's study was based on primary data and there is good evidence for her findings, that could be systematically compared with your own research into the area. The study is more than 25 years old and not only may differences in gender behaviour have been eroded further, but trends in non-standard regional speech could also have changed. The idea of interviewing and recording boys and girls from a similar social background to investigate possible gender differences remains a useful model for a potential investigation, though you may wish to extend the focus beyond the question of the use of non-standard forms.

Methodology: collecting your data

AQA Examiner's tip

It can take time to collect good data, so start off early. You will probably be introduced to the investigation at the end of your AS year, and the summer vacation is an excellent time to gather data, particularly if you are working with spoken data, or sifting through large amounts of written text. Starting early will also give you the opportunity to collect further or new data, if your initial material doesn't offer much potential.

Your data is the key to a productive investigation, and you should not underestimate the time and effort required to gather 'good' data. This means that as well as being ethical and valid, it is sufficiently rich to support detailed linguisitic analysis.

Some ethical issues

All research is inevitably constrained by ethical considerations, and when planning your investigation you need to bear these in mind. As a general rule, it will probably not be acceptable to undertake investigations involving:

- the use of offensive or indecent material
- any activity that is potentially harmful or illegal
- covert surveillance and recording.

Always follow these guidelines:

- When recording 'live' speech, always obtain permission from your participants before recording them, and confirm this with them again afterwards. Assure them that the recording is being made for academic purposes only and that confidentiality is guaranteed.
- When transcribing speech, delete from the transcript all names, places and other references that would enable the participants to be identified, replacing these with numbers or initials.
- With written materials, make sure you have the permission of the owner to use and quote from the texts. As with the transcripts, if necessary remove any personal references that might compromise the anonymity of the source.
- When investigating children's language, permission from either the school or the parents should be obtained.
- If in doubt, consult your supervisor.

The following two examples of student investigation proposals include a commentary on the ethical issues involved in each and the sort of advice a supervisor would give each student.

Table 6 *Ethical issues in investigation proposals*

Student investigation proposal	Commentary on ethics
Fathema is proposing to investigate the language of voice messages by collecting and transcribing all the messages left on her home phone over a period of several weeks.	As the messages have all been knowingly recorded (and most people avoid leaving unduly personal messages when they know they might be accessed by any family member), there is probably not much of a problem here. However, Fathema would need to assure the householder that all messages would be rendered anonymous by substituting any names or other references that would allow them to be identified.
Gillian visits a primary school regularly for work experience and proposes to film a group of children engaged in a collaborative learning task.	Gillian would need to secure the written permission of the school to use any material produced by the children, and where filming is involved, the school is likely either to refuse point blank or insist on parental permission being obtained. Although video is generally preferable as a source, in this case Gillian is likely to encounter fewer possible objections by sticking to audio recording.

Classroom activity 9

Here are some further ideas for investigations proposed by students. For each of them, identify any ethical issues involved and suggest what, if anything, the students might do to make their investigation ethically sound.

1 Alice is interested in the effects of alcohol on speech patterns. She proposes to invite a group of volunteers to take part in a series of interactive games during which she will serve them alcoholic drinks, and make recordings at half-hourly intervals.

2 Gabrielle wants to investigate her own father's language repertoire by recording examples of his interactions at work (with colleagues and customers) and at home (with his wife and their children).

3 Michael has discovered a number of diaries and personal letters passed down through his family from his great-grandparents. He is interested in examining them for evidence of change in the language and style of personal communications since the early 20th century.

■ The observer's paradox

Given the prohibition of covert recording, there is an immediate problem with any spoken data: as soon as our volunteers are aware they are being recorded, the 'natural' quality of spontaneous speech can be replaced by an embarrassed self-consciousness which immediately invalidates the data recorded. In certain circumstances, this can also affect written data. Hence the so-called **observer's paradox** – we can only study our material by observing it, but the very act of observing it changes the very thing we are trying to study.

There are a number of ways in which you can try to take this into account in spoken recordings in particular:

1 Do not participate in the situation, and leave the room with the recording device running.

2 Limit yourself to data recorded from reality TV shows, radio or other sources.

3 Obtain permission from the volunteers to make recordings at unspecified times and check with them afterwards that they are happy for the data to stand.

4 Disregard the first section of any recording and only use material produced when the participants have started to 'forget' they are being recorded.

Unfortunately, each of these strategies can have its own pitfalls. For example:

5 In the first strategy, unless the investigation depends on interviews with subjects, it is usually good practice for the investigator not to be a participant in the data; it would be all too easy for them to influence what was happening. However, it may not always be possible to leave your volunteers unattended, as in the case of young children.

6 In the second instance, data from reality TV shows may strike you as ideal, as the participants are all willing 'victims' and after days at a time we might assume they begin to 'forget' the presence of the cameras. However, the situations created by shows such as *Big Brother* are so abnormal that this is an unsafe assumption, and unless you record from the unedited coverage, you may also be at the mercy of skilful editing. It might be possible to find some better material, from radio phone-in shows or similar.

■ Key terms

Observer's paradox: the difficulty of gaining examples of real language data, when the presence of an observer or a contrived situation might change the way people would normally use language.

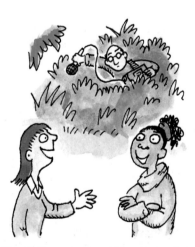

Fig. 8 *One way of avoiding observer's paradox … but is it ethical?*

Classroom activity 10

Consider the options listed above for offsetting the effects of the observer's paradox. For each of them, list any advantages/disadvantages you can see in the methodology proposed.

■ Obtaining a representative sample

All investigations must, by definition, be based on 'samples' of data, as it is never possible to study every available example of language use. It is therefore important to ensure that the samples you collect are indeed reasonably typical of the vast amounts of material which cannot be studied. If so, you can legitimately start to **extrapolate** from your data. For example, one student decided to study the variations in writing standards of children in a Year 4 class. A sensible plan would be a selective sampling of the best and weakest examples (according to specified criteria) of a particular piece of work, with perhaps two or three in between.

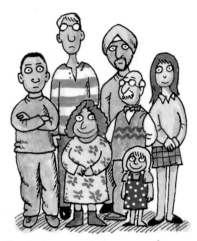

Fig. 9 *A representative group of interviewees?*

■ Some data collection methods

There are several ways to set about collecting data and you will need to think carefully about the most appropriate method to get close to the data you need. Look at the details of five main types of data collection below, with an example of past research that has used each method.

Surveys and questionnaires

Tony Thorne published the findings of research into student slang use at King's College London (KCL). This involved an ongoing **survey** from 1995 onwards where students at KCL and other London universities submitted examples of slang terms in current use, together with an explanation of each term's meaning and use. By the year 2000 around 4,500 terms had been gathered and some semantic analysis had been carried out to place the terms in a range of categories.

Obviously you would not be able to conduct a survey over many years, although you could use this methodology in miniature very effectively. Alternatively, it might be possible to make use of an existing survey to help provide data for your investigation.

Interviews

An A Level student, Tobias, wanted to gather some data on opinions towards the representation of males and females in popular magazines, to support his analysis of written data taken from a selection of male-targeted and female-targeted magazines. He used **interviews** with fellow students who represented part of the target audience of the magazines he was analysing, recorded them and took notes from the recordings to compare with his findings.

You can make use of interviews both to provide the main data for your investigation, if you are seeking to work with spoken transcripts, and to provide additional insight into your research.

Key terms

Extrapolate: to draw conclusions based on a sample of data which might apply more widely.

Survey: gathering data on attitudes or knowledge by asking many people to respond to questions and information through a questionnaire or some other method.

Interview: an interaction between two or more people for a specific purpose.

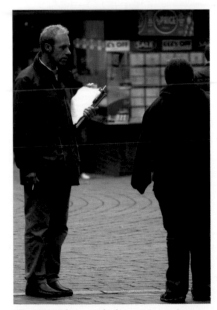

Fig. 10 *Where and when an interview takes place can affect results*

Ethnographic study: a research method involving observing the 'real life' behaviour of the people being studied.

Experiment: an artificial and controlled situation or activity designed to test a specific idea or hypothesis.

Corpus analysis: conclusions and findings drawn from running tests against a fairly large body of language material, often stored and assessed electronically.

■ Link

There is more information about the quantitative results from Cheshire's research in the 'Analysis: exploring your data' topic on page 152.

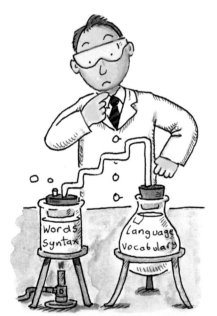

Fig. 11 *Experiments can be set up to test aspects of language use*

Ethnographic study

An **ethnographic study** is one in which a researcher finds an opportunity to observe people using language in as close to a natural, real-life setting as possible. Jenny Cheshire undertook research in Reading that compared the use of certain non-standard grammatical variables by different groups of boys and girls. She got to know a group of children and observed them interacting and playing over time, whilst recording their use of the linguistic variables her research focused on.

The distinctive features of an ethnographic study are not so much the way that you record the data (this could be recorded in transcription, or a survey table) but in creating a situation where the language used is happening as 'normally' as possible, meaning that you avoid the observer's paradox.

Experiment

An **experiment** is in some ways the direct opposite to an ethnographic study in that a deliberate situation is set up in order to test a particular aspect of language or see what happens to language use in a particular circumstance. Howard Giles carried out a linguistic **experiment** when he tested people's attitudes towards Received Pronunciation and regional dialects. He arranged for students to observe presentations on capital punishment by speakers of each of these language varieties, asking their views for and against capital punishment before and after the presentation, as a way of measuring the effect of the different accents upon them.

Although they take some thought and design, experiments can produce some excellent data, particularly if you are looking to create an investigation that tests something or seeks to find out people's attitudes – rather than one that tries to describe a particular form of language in use.

Corpus analysis

A significant amount of recorded, real language data is known as a corpus – and once it has been collected any number of tests and analyses can be carried out on it. As an example, an A Level student, Christobel, copied the text from 20 different web-based news reports on her favourite sport, the equestrian events, from the Beijing Olympics. Half of her reports were from specialist sports sites, and half from popular, general interest sites. She pasted the reports into a word processor and used it to quickly find and record the use of specialist lexis related to equestrianism, and the way that key nouns in the event had been used and modified.

A **corpus analysis** can be used with spoken or written language sources – the difficult part is putting one together, as this may well be too time-consuming for the timeframe you will be working with. However, there are corpuses available online and electronically which you could base an investigation on. Computers and the internet make it possible to get hold of many electronic texts quickly and easily, and these could lend themselves to this kind of methodology.

When it comes to applying one or more of these methodologies to your own research, you will find that several could be purposefully used – and perhaps even a combination, in certain stages, would work well. For example, if you were following an investigation into the differences between the ways girls and boys use language to interact with each other in a Year 8 secondary school classroom, in order to gain authentic data of children interacting, some sort of ethnographic study would be ideal, recording their language use for later transcription and analysis. Follow-up interviews or surveys with the children would also add value to the methodology of the investigation, although the crucial part would be the spoken data gathered by the ethnographic approach.

Classroom activity 11

Read the description of the following two different kinds of investigation and decide what sort of data-gathering methodology you think would be most appropriate for each. Make a few notes in each case, using the different methodologies set out above:

1 An investigation into the way in which the language of a Jane Austen novel has been incorporated within a film adaptation.

2 An investigation into the way that people of different ages use text messages to communicate with others.

For some investigations, the data already occurs 'naturally' and the only practical task is for you to arrange to collect it, ensuring it is both ethical and valid. For other studies, however, you may need to create a context or stimulus which will enable the data to be produced.

Look at the investigation proposal in Table 7, set alongside an appropriate methodology and commentary on why this would fit well.

Table 7 *Applying an appropriate methodology*

Investigation proposal	Method	Commentary
To test some received ideas about differences between how males and females use language to negotiate, argue and persuade.	Set up a 'ranking' exercise in which you instruct your volunteers to reach agreement as a group on a task you provide. Examples might be: Placing in order of merit a number of films / TV programmes / activities. Discussing a rank order of merit for the following holiday activities: sunbathing, watersports, visiting museums, outdoor pursuits, visiting funfairs/ theme parks, sightseeing.	This kind of ranking exercise can be an effective way of eliciting many kinds of interaction. As far as the participants are concerned, you are mainly interested in the result of the discussion, perhaps as part of some kind of opinion survey; as the experimenter, of course, you are much more interested in how your participants arrive at it.

Classroom activity 12

Listed on the following page are some more examples of student investigation proposals and suggested models for experimental data collection. They are jumbled up, and your task is to match up each investigation proposal with one of the numbered methods that you think might be suitable.

Investigation proposals	Methods
A. To investigate evidence of change in language and style in oral narratives produced by local residents of different ages.	**1.** Invite your volunteers to respond (orally or in writing) to a stimulus you provide – it could be pictures, statements, or objects.
B. To investigate the development of social talk among 5- and 6-year-olds.	**2.** Invite your volunteers to take part in a game (or other activity) that involves verbal communication.
C. To test some received ideas about possible differences in the ways males and females use colour vocabulary, vulgarism and non-standard constructions.	**3.** Invite your volunteers to relate (orally and/or in writing) a particular memory, anecdote or story. Some possibilities might be: ■ What was it like growing up in your neighbourhood during the war? ■ Tell me about an incident from your childhood when you were really scared. ■ Can you describe your earliest memories of Christmas? ■ Can you tell me a joke you have heard recently?

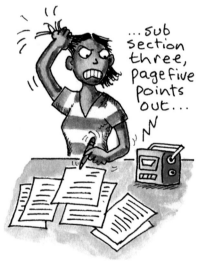

Fig. 12 *Making accurate transcripts of recorded speech can be frustrating and time-consuming!*

■ Transcribing spoken language data

Making an accurate transcript of recorded speech is an important part of many investigations, but it can be a frustrating and time-consuming process. You will probably have recorded a lot more material than you can analyse in detail, so first you will need to select the extracts to transcribe. You may only be able to do justice to two or three minutes' worth of material in all.

The most basic transcriptions simply provide a record of the words spoken by the speakers with pauses and turn-taking clearly shown. If you intend to analyse a range of phonological features (such as the significance of prosodic features, or the distinctive pronunciation of some speakers), a more sophisticated transcription is required. Similarly, if you wish to comment on specific pronunciation/accent features, you should make selective use of the International Phonetic Alphabet to transcribe just the individual words concerned, or just make use of phonetic spelling to reproduce non-standard pronunciations.

You can explain the level of detail you have chosen to use in the methodology section of your investigation report. There is a brief introduction to transcription conventions at the start of this book (on p. v), but the following example of a transcript shows you something of the range of transcription conventions that you could use:

K:	HEYA (.) you coming out tonight
G:	yeah (1.0) have you seen ↑Tommo↑
K:	↑mm↑ (.) what happened *(coughs)* to you │th. │
G:	│went to football│ │*(laughs)* │
K:	│?? │
K:	any good (2.) did you WIN=
G:	=yeah (.) four nil (1.) it was GO::::D stuff

Key:

HEYA	using capital letters to show an emphasis of louder volume
heya	**phonetic spelling** of the pronunciation of a word
(.)	a **micropause** of half a second or less
(1)	a longer pause, with the amount of seconds given as a number
↑mm↑	raised pitch
[*coughs*]	**paralinguistic** features like laughing, coughing, etc.
│went│	vertical lines show simultaneous speech
th.	a full stop showing a word clipped short
??	inaudible speech
=	running on from one speaker to another without pause
GO::::D	elongation of a sound

Extension activity 6

Record a short clip of you talking with your friends – just 30 seconds to a minute will be fine. Then use it to play and replay and practise creating a transcript of a few utterances.

Key terms

Phonetic spelling: a way of writing down speech to show the way it was pronounced by using letters and symbols to represent single sounds.

Micropause: a pause of about half a second or less.

Paralinguistics: aspects of speech in addition to the actual words and word-sounds said.

Analysis: exploring your data

In this topic you will:

■ learn how important the analysis section is to your investigation

■ follow and apply a method for exploring language data

■ develop a systematic approach to the analysis of data

■ consider several ways of structuring the presentation of your analysis

■ learn how to use quantitative and qualitative methods of analysis.

AQA Examiner's tip

Make sure that your analysis addresses a range of linguistic features and that it shows some real depth within the methods that you are using. A strong analysis section is important to all investigations, and particularly to achieving top band grades.

Key terms

Anomalies: strange, one-off or unexpected results in your data.

■ The importance of the analysis

The analysis section is the most important part of your investigation, and should be approximately half of the overall word count. It is an objective presentation of the features that you find in your data, following the structure of analysis that you set out in your aims.

It is a good idea to think about the style of writing in your analysis in a similar way to the advice you will have been given for your language analysis essays in the examination: that is, to keep a three-fold analytical structure in mind of evidence, linguistic description and explanation of meaning or effect. This way, you might like to think of producing 'analytical paragraphs' when you write up your analysis and ensure that they contain these three elements.

Once you have collected and assembled your data, you can start to get down to the really important work – the close scrutiny and analysis of the material. It's a good idea to make a couple of copies of the data so that you can keep a clean set free of notes and annotations to include in your final submission.

The exploratory process that you will go through will be guided by the aims you have set out, but whatever that is, you will be looking to get an overall feel for what your data is presenting, whilst at the same time carrying out more detailed, systematic analysis.

Getting a feel for your data involves looking for emerging patterns that seem to stretch across your data as a whole, or perhaps even **anomalies** that need to be understood or explained later, that you perhaps were not expecting.

A good way into analysing your data is to write an overview of the data (in just a few sentences) which sums up what you find interesting about it, and what issues it raises in relation to your stated investigation aim. Then go on to give a detailed initial line-by-line commentary on its significant features, either in the form of annotations/bullet points or continuous prose. The example that follows deals with this treatment of a 1930 car advertisement from the following investigation:

■ **Area for investigation:** Student interested in the changing styles of advertising language during the 20th and 21st centuries.

■ **Focus question/hypothesis:** How has the language of advertising, as reflected in print-based car adverts, changed in the 20th and 21st centuries?

■ **Key ideas/issues/contexts:** Informalisation (and trend towards more colloquial registers). Move from print-based to visual culture. Status/democratisation of car ownership. Changing car driving technologies. Discourse structure of adverts (Desire – fulfilment? Problem – solution?).

■ **Methodology:** A set of six adverts for Ford saloon cars collected from non-specialist magazines from the 1930s to the 1980s, one from each decade.

■ **Data source:** This is the earliest of the six pieces of data: from *Punch Magazine*, 30 July 1930.

Here is a facsimile of the original printed advertisement:

PUNCH, OR THE LONDON CHARIVARI.—JULY 30, 1930.

THE NEW FORDOR SALOON (3-WINDOW) £225, AT WORKS, MANCHESTER

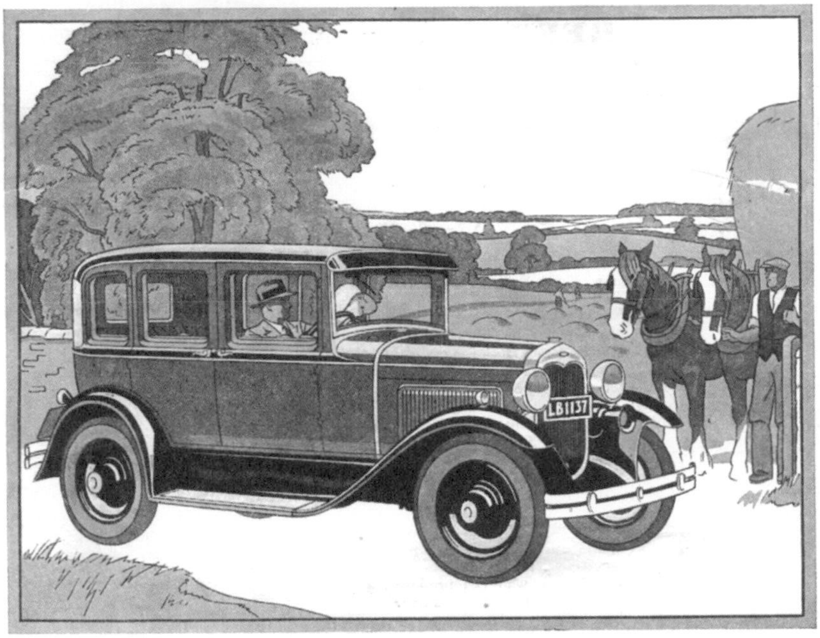

GROWING PRIDE OF OWNERSHIP

MEN WHO ARE owners of new Ford cars appreciate their advanced, modern design — also the unusual uses of fine steels — for strength and safety.

Men like the robust chassis of the new Ford car. The strong steel bodies. The practice of avoiding seasonal models. The policy of building the cars to last a long time.

Men like the new Ford's low petrol consumption, low insurance and depreciation costs.

Women, perhaps even more than men, appreciate the ease of handling and steering the new Ford. The little need of gear changing in traffic. The ease of parking when shopping.

Women like the new Ford's positive four-wheel brakes with stop light. The quick acceleration and speed with safety. The unsplinterable glass windscreen. The protecting steel bumpers and steel running boards.

Women, especially, like the pleasing choice of colours. The graceful low streamlines. The everlasting brightness of the rustless steel lamps, radiator shell and hub caps. They like the quality of the upholstery. The roominess and comfort of the car.

We recommend that you study the new Ford cars at your dealer's. Then, in one of the new closed or open body styles, enjoy a trial run to-day.

Prices (investigate low Ford insurance charges): Tourer £180; Tudor Saloon £195; Coupé £215; Cabriolet £225; Fordor Saloon (3-window) £225; De Luxe Fordor with sliding roof £245. All prices at Works, Manchester.

FORD MOTOR COMPANY LIMITED, London & Manchester

LINCOLN Ford Fordson

Here is a transcription of the printed text:

Growing pride of ownership

Men who are owners of new Ford cars appreciate their advanced, modern design – also the unusual uses of fine steels – for strength and safety.

Men like the robust chassis of the new Ford car. The strong steel bodies. The practice of avoiding seasonal models. The policy of building the cars to last a long time.

Men like the new Ford's low petrol consumption, low insurance and depreciation costs.

Women, perhaps even more than men, appreciate the ease of handling and steering the new Ford. The little need of gear changing in traffic. The ease of parking when shopping.

Women like the new Ford's positive four-wheel brakes with stop light. The quick acceleration and speed with safety. The unsplinterable glass windscreen. The protecting steel bumpers and steel running boards.

Women, especially, like the pleasing choice of colours. The graceful low streamlines. The everlasting brightness of the rustless steel lamps, radiator shell and hub caps. They like the quality of the upholstery. The roominess and comfort of the car.

We recommend that you study the new Ford cars at your dealer's. Then, in one of the new closed or open body styles, enjoy a trial run to-day.

Prices (investigate low Ford insurance charges): Tourer £180; Tudor Saloon £195; Coupé £215; Cabriolet £225; Fordor Saloon (3-window) £225; De Luxe Fordor with sliding roof £245. All prices at Works, Manchester.

Ford Motor Company Limited, London & Manchester.

An overview of this item would be that the 1930 advertisement makes its appeal in terms of the 'pride' of owning one of the new Fords, but is most noticeable for its hand-designed illustration, its relatively 'wordy' text and its differentiated gender appeal. However, like some modern ads, it focuses keenly on technical, safety and aesthetic features.

The initial scrutiny for a written text like this would be best carried out by annotating a copy, to identify useful features and issues in the language use, as shown in Table 8.

Table 8 *Analysis of Ford advertisement*

Ford advertisement text	Analytical notes
The new fordor saloon (3-window) £225, at works, Manchester	Pun/blend – Ford/door
	Pic hand-drawn/print – implies modernity of car Town v. country? - male driving – farmer admires/envies – status? Separation from text: 50:50 text/image split
Growing pride of ownership	Slogan? Focus on 'pride'/status symbol. Minor sentence Font – quite formal, serious
Men who are owners of new Ford cars appreciate their advanced, modern design – also the unusual uses of fine steels – for strength and safety.	'Own' - anaphoric ref to 'ownership' Focus on men – semantics/connotations – strength (steels, safety). Polysyllabic – 'appreciate'

Men like the robust chassis of the new Ford car. The strong steel bodies. The practice of avoiding seasonal models. The policy of building the cars to last a long time.	Connotations of strength continued (robust). Register – continued polysyllabic phrasing – 'practice of avoiding …' Listing – parallel minor sentences – the practice of…the policy of…
Men like the new Ford's low petrol consumption, low insurance and depreciation costs.	Parallelism –'men like…' – synonymy – appreciate men – economy (semantics) – repetition – 'low' – specialist lexical field
Women, perhaps even more than men, appreciate the ease of handling and steering the new Ford. The little need of gear changing in traffic. The ease of parking when shopping.	Gender issues – pragmatics – lexical repetition – 'appreciate'. Implies gender roles: men cautious, sensible, practical, save money; women – weak ('ease of handling … little need of gear changing'), spend money (assumes not working!)
Women like the new Ford's positive four-wheel brakes with stop light. The quick acceleration and speed with safety. The unsplinterable glass windscreen. The protecting steel bumpers and steel running boards.	Tech – were 'brakes with stop light' a big deal? semantics – stress on safety – implies protectiveness. Unsplinterable/rustless – negative prefix/suffix – implies faults in other makes of car
Women, especially, like the pleasing choice of colours. The graceful low streamlines. The everlasting brightness of the rustless steel lamps, radiator shell and hub caps. They like the quality of the upholstery. The roominess and comfort of the car.	Implies women preoccupied also with appearance and domesticity (upholstery/colours). Stereotype?
We recommend that you study the new Ford cars at your dealer's. Then, in one of the new closed or open body styles, enjoy a trial run to-day.	'We' – 1st person plural – voice of Ford? Formal, sales tone in 'recommend' 'study'
Prices (investigate low Ford insurance charges): Tourer £180; Tudor Saloon £195; Coupé £215; Cabriolet £225; Fordor Saloon (3-window) £225; De Luxe Fordor with sliding roof £245. All prices at Works, Manchester.	Model names: 'Tudor' – connotations? Cf modern names

 Classroom activity 13

Use the investigation brief and sample data below to carry out the same process of overview and initial analysis as that performed above for the car advertisement.

- **Area for investigation:** Student interested in the development of his twin brothers' reading skills.
- **Focus question/hypothesis:** What does miscue analysis of 5-year-old readers reveal about the process of learning to read?
- **Key ideas/issues/contexts:** Early literacy studies and 'phonics' debate about learning to read.

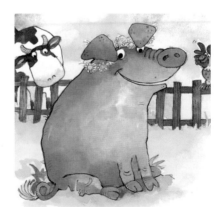

Fig. 13 *'This is Silly Pig. Everyone calls her Silly Pig because she does silly things!'*

■ **Methodology:** Brothers recorded reading aloud from the same part of a book aimed at their stage of development called *Silly Pig*. Transcription of about 1 minute of data per child. Investigation to focus on miscue analysis.

■ **Data source:** *Silly Pig* by Laura Rader (Sterling, 2005) provided by researcher. Subjects recorded at home.

Table 9 *A side-by-side comparison of transcriptions of the two readers*

Source text: *Silly Pig*	Child X's reading	Child Y's reading
This is Silly Pig. Everyone calls her Silly Pig because she does silly things!	this silly **pig** everyone calls her silly pig (3) because they (1) she doesn't silly **things**	this tha this is silly **pig** everyone calls him silly pig because he says silly **things**
'You silly pig!' said Horse. 'Pigs don't put flowers on their head!'	(2) you **silly** pig (.) said (.) **horse** (.) pigs don't put things **flowers** on their heads	(3) you silly pig said pig pigs (2) don't put flowers on their heads
One day, Silly Pig had an idea. She went to tell the other animals about her idea.	(1) one day silly pig had an **idea** (1) she went to (2) tell the other animals about her idea	(3) one day silly pig had an idea (1) she went to the (2) tell the other animals about her **idea**
'I'm going to look for treasure on the farm,' she said. 'I'm going to find lots and lots of treasure.'	(.) I am going to look for **treasure** on the farm (.) she said (.) I am going to find lots and lots of **treasure**	(2) I am going to look for things (3) **treasure** and the farm see she said (1) I am going to (2) feed (1) find lots and lots of **treasure**
'You silly pig!' said the other animals. 'You won't find treasure on the farm.'	you silly pig said (3) the other animals you won't find treasure on the **farm**	(2) you silly **pig** said the other animals you (2) won't find (1) treasure on the **farm**
Silly Pig set off to find treasure. She went out to the farmyard and up the lane.	(3) silly pig (3) tha set off to look for **treasure** (5) she went on out of the farm gate (3) and up the hill urm (2) **lane**	(4) silly pig shi set off to find (1) look for treasure she went out the farm (1) yard but (1) and up the lane
Suddenly Silly Pig stopped. She saw something sparkling in the tree.	(4) suddenly silly pig (4) **stooped** (1) she saw something (1) **sparkling** in the tree	(5) suddenly said silly pig (7) she saw something (3) spa (4) **sparkling** in the tree
'Ooh, I can see a sparkling necklace in the tree. A sparkling necklace is treasure. I shall put it around my neck.'	(2) ooh no I can see a (4) sparkling **necklace** in the tree (1) a sparkling necklace is the **treasure** (1) I will put (1) it around my neck	(1) ooh I can see a sparkling (2) **necklace** in the tree asked (5) a sparkling necklace is the **treasure** (1) I (2) shall put it round my neck
But the sparkling necklace wasn't really a necklace. It was a spider's web.	(3) but the sparkling necklace doesn't wasn't (2) really a necklace it was a spider's web	(.) but the sparkling necklace (.) wasn't (2) really a necklace it was a spiders **web**
The web was sparkling with raindrops. Spider was very cross.	(1) the web was sparkling with (1) rain drops (2) the spider was very cross	(2) the web was sparkling with (1) raindrops spider was very cross
'What a silly thing to do,' he said. 'You silly pig!' Silly Pig felt very silly. She set off up the lane.	(1) what a silly pig (1) thing to do he said you silly pig (2) silly pig (2) felt very silly she set off up the (1) lane	what a silly thing to do you silly pig silly (1) pig felt very silly she set off up the lane
Suddenly Silly Pig stopped. She saw something sparkling in the hedge.	(3) suddenly silly pig stooped (1) she saw something sparkling in the (1) don't know that word	(3) suddenly silly pig (1) sto stopped (1) she saw something **sparkling** in the bushes
'Ooh, I can see sparkling earrings in the hedge,' she said. 'Sparkling earrings are treasure. I shall put them on my ears.'	(2) ooh no I can see sparkling ears **earrings** in the hedge (1) she said (1) sparkling earrings are the treasure I (*inaudible*)	(1) ooh I can see something (1) sparkling earrings in the hed (1) she said (1) sparkling earrings are **treasure** I sha shall put them (1) on my ears

◤ Developing a structure for analysis

There are many different ways to break down your analysis into sections. Doing this will help you to tackle your analysis systematically, make your findings more easily accessible to an examiner or any other person reading your report, and also help you to be in control of the range and depth of analysis you achieve.

The nature of your investigation, hypothesis, question and data will shape the best way to tackle your analysis, but consider the following approaches, to help you settle on a good method for your own work. You might even find a combination of methods will fit your data well.

- **By text:** using the separate pieces of data as subheadings and tackling each in turn. For example: *FHM* magazine extract; *Cosmopolitan* magazine extract, etc.
- **By theme:** your hypothesis or question might have thrown up more than one area of enquiry. For example, virtuous errors in child speech, parent use of child-directed speech, etc.
- **By method:** a popular and powerful choice is to focus on one particular linguistic method at a time, for example lexis, grammar, semantics, etc. You could even take this a stage further by using specific features you have set out in your aims, for example noun modification, sentence moods, etc.
- **By chronology:** your data may have been collected over a period of time, or from different historical periods, or may be enough to warrant simply tackling it from beginning to end. Here you can use sections that describe particular parts of the data in order, for example Early Modern English letter, 1540; Late Modern English letter, 1790; contemporary English letter, 2008.

> **AQA Examiner's tip**
>
> Breaking your analysis down into different sections is very important, rather than presenting it as a continuous 1,000+ word essay.

Using a numbered system (e.g. 1.1, 1.2, etc.) of sections and sub-sections helps you to keep sight of the overall structure of your analysis – and also breaks down the task into manageable units of work which you can have the satisfaction of 'ticking off' as you go along.

Here, for example, is how one student decided to organise his analysis of his car advertisement as a hierarchy of sections and sub-sections. Within each section and sub-section he would go on to discuss all pieces of data:

Analysis structure

1 *Visual and graphological aspects*

    1.1 Text: Image ratio

    1.2 Nature and implications of image in relation to text

    1.3 Text font/size

2 *The nature of the appeal: pragmatic and discourse aspects*

    2.1 Discourse structure and organisation (inc. paragraphing)

    2.2 Implied values of car and audience – lexis/semantics/pragmatics

3 *Style and register*

    3.1 Lexical formality

    3.2 Technical lexis

    3.3 Evidence of lexical and semantic change

    3.4 Sentence type and length

■ Informing your analysis: background reading

At this stage you will need to boost your understanding and knowledge with some background reading related to the data you are studying and the issues it raises. For example, the miscue data raises questions like:

■ What are the mental and physical processes involved in reading?

■ What methods are used to teach children to read?

■ What can we learn from a 'miscue analysis' of a child's reading aloud about the reading strategies a child is learning to use when reading?

■ How are children's reading abilities measured, and what standards are they expected to achieve by the age of 7?

■ Analysis techniques

Once you have your analysis structure in place, you can concentrate on just one aspect of the data at a time. However, there is a difference between the analytical technique you might use in a routine essay, and the approach needed in a more scientific investigation.

Overall, it is important to establish a more objective and measurable way of analysing the data – which is where the use of quantitative analysis comes in. This means not settling either for subjective observations or just looking for one or two random examples to illustrate a point, but surveying the data comprehensively to establish if there really is a pattern or trend.

Quantitive and qualitative analysis

Qualitative and quantitive analysis are the two main approaches you can use when analysing the data you have collected. A sound approach is often to blend the two – setting out a statistical view of your data using quantitive methods, and then qualitatively examining individual instances that represent your figures. For example, if you are trying to define formality in a text, you could analyse the following specific features:

■ What proportion of the open-class words used are monosyllabic as opposed to polysyllabic?

■ What proportion of the lexis is from the common register and what proportion from a specialised or technical register?

■ How frequently are phrasal verbs used instead of their single-word equivalents (e.g.'go in' or 'enter')?

■ How often are contracted forms like 'we're' preferred to the full-length 'we are'?

■ How frequently are slang/idiomatic phrases used?

■ How frequently is non-standard language used?

Many of these criteria can, of course, be measured quantitively. This kind of quantitive work is not an end in itself, but can be used as a starting point for meaningful comparisons and more qualitative analysis which tries to explain and understand the findings it has revealed.

Look at the following examples of the two different kinds of analysis in use from the work of some of the linguists mentioned earlier on.

An example of quantitive analysis is Jenny Cheshire's presentation of the frequency of non-standard grammatical features by the boys and girls she was observing in her Reading study.

Table 10 *Extract from findings of Cheshire's Reading study*

Non-standard variable	Example of non-standard use	Group A girls	Group B girls
Non-standard –s	They calls me all the names under the sun.	25.84	57.27
Non-standard has	You just has to do what the teachers tell you.	36.36	35.85
Non-standard was	You was with me, wasn't you?	63.64	80.95
Negative concord	It ain't got no pedigree or nothing.	12.50	58.70
Non-standard never	I never went to school today.	45.45	41.07
Non-standard what	Are you the ones what hit my friend?	33.33	5.56
Non-standard come	I come down here yesterday.	30.77	90.63
Ain't = copula	You ain't no boss.	14.29	67.12

Adapted from *Jenny Cheshire*, Variation in an English dialect: a sociolinguistic study, 1982

Here, Cheshire has calculated percentages to show the frequency of each use of non-standard English by two groups of girls she gathered data from. Using this form of data, it is possible to identify larger patterns, **trends** and anomalies in the overall data.

Data response exercise 2

Look at Cheshire's quantitive data above. Compare the percentages given for Group A and Group B girls.

1 What patterns can you see emerging from the figures?

2 Are there any possible anomalies in the data?

The following example is from Joanna Przedlacka's work on Estuary English and shows a qualitative approach, discussing specific instances of certain vowel pronunciations based around the /u/ and /oo/ sounds. Przedlacka's data consisted of recordings of speakers from four towns outside of central London, to test how far Estuary English was being used in those places.

Key terms

Trend: patterns in data that seem to show something in particular tending to happen.

> Vowel **fronting**: The word 'blue' uttered by a speaker from Buckinghamshire, has a front realisation of the vowel, while other front realisations can be heard in 'boots', pronounced by a Kent female and 'roof' (Essex female). A **central vowel** can be heard in 'new', uttered by a male teenager from Essex. **Back realisations** of the vowel, as in 'cucumber', uttered by a Kent teenager are infrequent. The vowel in 'butter' has a back realisation in the speech of an Essex speaker, but can be realised as a front vowel, as in 'dust' or 'cousins', both uttered by teenage girls from Buckinghamshire.

www.phon.ox.ac.uk

Although this is phonological, it is the sort of analysis that would complement the sort of statistical table used in Cheshire's extract, by bringing out individual instances found in the data, for closer analysis and discussion.

Another example of the sort of qualitative analysis you might employ comes from Mark Sebba's investigation into London Jamaican, where quotations from data are brought into the analysis:

> Of particular interest are J.'s questions *im did phone you*? and *did 'im give you what you a look for*? Both are obviously intended to be Creole, as shown by the form of the subject pronoun (*him*) and the phonology. The first of these, *im did phone you*? would certainly pass for Creole in Jamaica, as it uses the same word order as the corresponding statement. The tense marker *did*, which corresponds to other Jamaican forms like *bin* and *en*, has to be treated with Jamaican Creole grammar as an invariant particle, not the past tense of an auxiliary verb *do* as in English. However, *did 'im give you what you a look for*? seems to be modelled on the English *did he give you ...* with subject-auxiliary inversion moving *did* to first position.

Mark Sebba, Contact Languages, 1997

This might be the sort of analysis that you are more used to carrying out in language analysis essays. However, the important thing to remember is that both quantitive and qualitative approaches can benefit your investigation, especially if they are blended.

You can, and should, test and explore many of your initial ideas about your data by carrying out some quantification. In general, if you find yourself writing about a feature that 'often', 'sometimes' or 'always' occurs; if you are tempted to suggest that there are 'many', 'few', 'several' or even a 'vast number' of examples; or if you use phrases such as 'a majority of' or 'mainly' – then the chances are you should be justifying your claims by providing the appropriate statistical and quantifiable evidence. You can then go on to interpret and comment on the trends revealed by your quantification. A common approach will be to set out some quantitive findings in tables, and then to bring out individual examples of quoted evidence from your data, to analyse linguistic features more deeply – helping you to achieve both range and depth.

Surveying, listing, classifying and tabulating

Another way in which an investigation differs from a traditional essay is in the use of lists and tables to survey, sift and sort through the data. For example, in the case of the Ford advertisement, you might decide to investigate the adjectival pre-modification used in the text.

A traditional essay might begin to touch on this topic like this:

> As an advertisement, the Ford text uses a range of pre-modifying adjectives both to convey factual information about the product (such as 'four-wheel brakes' and 'steel bumpers')and to persuade potential purchasers of its desirability ('quick acceleration … pleasing choice of colours').

However, an investigative approach might start by listing *all* noun phrases in the text, showing the pre-modifying adjectives/adjectival phrases used alongside the head noun they describe (determiners omitted here), as in the example in Table 11, for the Ford car advertisement.

Classroom activity 15

Identify as many interesting or significant patterns and trends in the pre-modification data as you can, quantifying any of your observations as appropriate.

Now we can go further by organising these listed examples into categories of your own, that will allow you to offer a full qualitative and quantitive analysis of the major trends and patterns of pre-modification. Table 12 (on page 157) is one possible version.

Table 12 (overleaf) certainly helps to reveal the differentiated approach to the marketing of the car to men and women. The factual pre-modification related to men focuses on economical factors, whereas those aimed at women stress either safety or aesthetic concerns. Interestingly, the word 'low' is used differently, applying to costs for the men and the 'streamline' of the car for the women. This expectation that men, not women, would be concerned with financial matters may reflect the very different ideas about gender roles in society at this time. Similarly, the more subjective, persuasive pre-modifiers (which significantly outnumber the factual ones) differentiate between the semantics of strength, toughness and modernity (targeting men) and effortlessness, attractiveness and security (aimed at women). Here again we can see reflected in the data some contemporary stereotypical assumptions about gender roles.

Table 11 *Noun phrases appearing in the Ford car advert*

Number	Pre-modification	Head noun
1	n/a	men
2	new	Ford cars
3	advanced modern	design
4	unusual	uses
5	fine	steels
6	n/a	strength
7	n/a	safety
8	n/a	men
9	robust	chassis
10	new	Ford car
11	strong steel	bodies
12	n/a	practice
13	seasonal	models
14	n/a	policy
15	n/a	cars
16	long	time
17	n/a	men
18	new	Ford
19	low	petrol consumption
20	low	insurance and depreciation costs
21	n/a	women
22	n/a	men
23	ease of	handling and steering
24	new	Ford
25	little	need

Number	Pre-modification	Head noun
26	gear	changing
27	n/a	traffic
28	ease of	parking
29	n/a	women
30	new	Ford
31	positive four-wheel	brakes
32	stop	light
33	quick	acceleration
34	unsplinterable glass	windscreen
35	protecting steel	bumpers
36	steel	running-boards
37	n/a	women
38	pleasing	choice of colours
39	graceful low	streamlines
40	everlasting	brightness
41	rustless steel	radiator shell hub caps lamps
42		quality of the upholstery
43		roominess and comfort
44	new	Ford cars
45	new	Ford cars
46	new closed or open	body styles

Table 12 *Trends and patterns of pre-modification in the Ford car advert*

Factual pre-modification		Subjective/opinionative pre-modification	
Associated with men	*Associated with women*	*Associated with men*	*Associated with women*
(not) seasonal models	four-wheel brakes	advanced, modern design	ease of handling/steering
low (?) petrol consumption	glass windscreen	unusual uses	little need of gear changing
low insurance	steel bumpers	fine (or factual?) steels	ease of parking
	steel running boards	robust chassis	positive brakes
	low streamlines		unsplinterable windscreen
	rustless (?) steel lamps		protecting bumpers
			pleasing choice of colours
			graceful streamlines
			everlasting brightness

■ Systematic analysis in practice

Looking back at the miscue analysis data, focusing on the pauses as a particular variable can lead to the following blend of quantitive and qualitative analysis, to answer specific aspects of language use:

1 How often do pauses correspond with sentence boundaries?

2 How often are pauses associated with a 'difficult' word?

3 How often are pauses associated with other miscues?

The following is an example of a write-up of each of these lines of analytical enquiry:

4 **Pauses corresponding to sentence/clause/phrase boundaries**

Child X paused at sentence boundaries on 21 out of 27 possible occasions, whereas Child Y paused on 15. Both children show some security in recognising the syntactic function of full stops, but Child X is significantly more confident, with Child Y tending to rush over these towards the end.

5 **Pauses associated with 'difficult' words**

The only individual words that really seem to cause Child X to pause are 'because', 'stopped', 'sparkling', 'farmyard' and 'raindrops'. He pauses after substituting 'farm gate' for 'farmyard', before substituting 'stooped' for 'stopped' and after suggesting 'something' for 'sparkling'. Two further pauses of 4 and 1 seconds precede the next two occurrences of 'sparkling' in the text, but the word is read without difficulty after that. Child Y also has trouble with 'sparkling', pausing before and after its first occurrence, and again after encountering the word a second time, and with stopped/stooped; he also pauses before other polysyllabic words such as 'treasure' (he pauses for 3 seconds after recognising his substitution of 'things', but deals with the word without difficulty on each subsequent encounter), 'farmyard' (a pause between the two parts of the word suggests the child may recognise each word separately but not as a compound) and 'raindrops' (another pause before a compound).

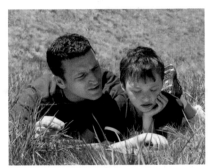

Fig. 14 *Children's early reading can make an excellent topic for a language investigation*

6 Pauses associated with other miscues

On three occasions Child X pauses between making an incorrect substitution and then making the self-correction (for example, 'up the hill urm (2) lane'), suggesting an active self-monitoring strategy. Interestingly, he pauses again before the second occurrence of 'lane', but this time avoids the substitution, clearly learning from his earlier self-correction. On at least one occasion a pause occurs after the self-correction has been made (for example, 'doesn't'– 'wasn't') and also immediately after a sentence boundary has been ignored – a trend much more noticeable in Child Y, who does this on three occasions (e.g. 'you silly pig said the other animals you (2)…') as if the failure to note the beginning of a sentence has interfered with his ability to read ahead. Child Y also pauses on 12 occasions immediately after making a substitution and prior to making a self-correction ('pig' for 'horse', 'the' for 'tell', 'things' for 'treasure', etc.). This also shows a self-monitoring process working effectively which allows him to check his reading against both sense and context. On just three occasions a pause occurs before a miscue (such as before his substitution of 'bushes' for 'hedge'). It seems that on the whole, Child Y prefers to 'have a go' and correct errors as he goes along, but is somewhat less accurate and fluent in his reading.

Classroom activity 16

Using the raw miscue analysis data, carry out a systematic analysis of each child's substitutions. Present your findings as a quantitive table, before going on to discuss and explain the results qualitatively.

Conclusion and evaluation

In this topic you will:

- learn what your conclusion section should contain

- learn how to finish off your investigation in the evaluation.

Reflecting on what you have learned

After carrying out your analysis, the conclusions section that follows allows you to provide a summary of what you have found, and reflect on how this relates to the original quesion or hypothesis you set out. You are also able to put your investigation into context and suggest what future research could be done as a result of your findings.

Conclusion

The balance between your conclusion and your analysis can be difficult to strike, as there will be things that you find could be sensibly placed in either section, if given the right treatment. However, the following guidelines may help you decide what should be in your conclusion:

- Use your hypothesis, question and aims to help structure your conclusion by commenting on your findings in relation to the points you raised at the start of your investigation.

- Don't repeat points already made in your analysis – if you find this happening, look carefully at the analysis and decide where that particular point should go.

- Be prepared to deal with anomalies thrown up by your data and put forward some suggestions as to why these appeared.

- Place your investigation in context and be realistic about what you have found only being relevant to the particular data you were able to collect. You can speculate about what your findings mean in the wider context, but show an awareness of the difference between the two.

- If your investigation has gone largely against your hypothesis, that doesn't make what you have done invalid, or even jeopardise its ability to be a strong piece of coursework. However, you must present what you found and deal with it in just as systematic and objective a way as if you had found what you expected.

Evaluation

Your evaluation gives you the opportunity to foreground your successes – and challenges – and place your work into a wider context. Although there are not as many marks on offer here as in the main body of the investigation, it is important to end your investigation strongly. If you evaluate well, you will be able to leave your reader feeling that you have understood your work and have achieved something worthwhile. Your evaluation should include:

- a reflection on the sucess of your methodology and investigation design, discussing any alterations you had to make

- observations about how your findings and work might fit in with that of other linguists and research, especially any you mentioned in your introduction

- a consideration of how your findings fit into the context of wider English language use

- suggestions for relevant further research – either improvements to your own investigation, or ideas for entirely new lines of research to develop what you have found.

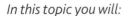

AQA Examiner's tip

Don't be afraid to edit your analysis and conclusions section at the end of your investigation, to make the most of the work you have done. 'Cutting and pasting' might help you not to repeat points, and to ensure that the relationship between your analysis and conclusions works well.

AQA Examiner's tip

Make sure that you don't waste your evaluation by stating things that are obvious and too general. Make points that are distinct to your investigation and based on specific experiences and ideas you had. In particular, avoid slipping into writing a wishlist of 'If I had more time/money/data …'.

Coursework preparation and practice

In this topic you will:

- learn how to present your investigation report

- practise using a suitably academic register

- learn how to reference your work

- apply the assessment criteria to extracts of students' work.

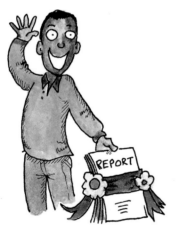

Fig. 15 *The presentation of your investigation report is very important*

Once you have gone through the stages described, it is time to put your investigation together as a whole. This is a process in which you will aim to make your work communicate its ideas as clearly as possible, proofread and edit your material and submit it correctly and on time.

How to present your investigation

The report of the investigation that you submit for assessment should be presented as professionally as possible, using the appropriate style and conventions of academic documents. Think of your audience not just as your teacher/supervisor, but the wider academic community of specialist teachers and students with expertise and interest in the topic you have been studying.

Below is a summary of what each section of your report should contain:

- **Cover page:** The title and scope of your investigation, and your name.

- **Contents:** A list of the main section headings and page numbers.

- **Acknowledgements:** Briefly acknowledge the sources of your data, thanking people who have given permission for you to use materials, and any other assistance you have received in the preparation of your investigation.

- **Introduction (guide 400 words):** Explain the background and context to your investigation, including your reasons for choosing to explore the topic you have, and the aims and focus of your investigation, including your initial questions/hypothesis.

- **Methodology (guide 250 words):** Explain how you decided on what data you needed to collect, and the methods you used to collect/ sample it. Note here also any limitations or difficulty you experienced with the collection of the data.

- **Analysis (with sub-sections, guide 1,450 words):** The bulk of your investigation. You will need to create sub-section headings according to the different levels of analysis you are carrying out. These headings may correspond to different frameworks/questions.

  Use this section to present analysis of the data in detail, identifying and presenting the evidence for patterns, then interpreting and explaining them in terms of the relevant linguistic and contextual factors. As well as full verbal analysis and explanation of the data, you may wish to use statistical and diagrammatic forms, such as tables, bar charts and any other graphic devices which seem appropriate.

  Remember, it is not enough to offer an observation with an odd example – in a scientific investigation you need to test your ideas rigorously by thorough surveys of the data. The quality of your analysis and explanation will largely determine the mark your investigation receives.

- **Conclusion and evaluation (guide 400 words):** As you started your investigation by asking some questions about your data, or by setting out to test a theory or hypothesis, your analysis should lead you towards some answers to these queries.

You should also reflect on your findings – was there anything surprising in your findings, and if so, what might explain them? Remember, a good scientist will keep an open mind about the investigation, not allowing prior assumptions to influence the conclusions you come to. It is quite likely that you will find something surprising, or even inconclusive. Don't worry. Remember, it is the quality of the process of investigation which matters. So, in drawing your conclusions:

- be open-minded: don't make the data fit your preconceptions
- be cautious: how true a sample, and how representative of all the possible material you could have collected is your data?
- be tentative: use expressions such as –
  - there is a tendency for …
  - on the whole, this seems to be …
  - we can perhaps conclude …
- be self-critical: how effective and revealing have your chosen methods of analysis been?
- explore what is next: suggest ways in which your investigation could be developed or extended given the opportunity.

■ **Bibliography:** As noted earlier, a comprehensive list of all print- and web-based sources consulted.

■ **Appendices:** Present your data, clearly labelled and with the sources clearly identified and dated. It is useful, also, to provide line numbers for ease of reference in your analysis sections. These should be clean copies free of your working annotations.

🔍 Using an academic register

AO1 requires you to 'communicate relevant knowledge using appropriate terminology and coherent, accurate written expression'. Think of your investigation report as a formal, academic document with a specialist audience – teachers, researchers and students with a strong interest in and prior knowledge of language studies. This means they will expect you to use the shared, technical language of experts in the field – so there's no need to explain or define the terms you use (though this will be a different matter when you come to write your media text). The nature of the task also presumes that you will use a reasonably formal register of Standard English, and 'coherent, accurate, written expression' implies a high level of accuracy and precision in your writing.

Let's consider two versions of an extract from an investigation arising from our sample data on the Ford text.

■ **Version A:** In my opinion, the first piece of data is very old-fashioned– no-one would accept an advert like that today. It appeals to sexist snobs who just want to look down on people who can't afford cars, and who think all their wives are good for is going shopping. But I do think it is interesting that the adverts does think of women driving at all.

The language is all very formal and nothing like the modern adverts with their witty slogans and colloquial language. There is too much text and no-one nowadays would bother to read all of that print, as they would expect just to look at a glamorous photograph.

There are many describing words in the text. These are called adjectives. When adjectives are placed with nouns we call these noun phrases.

■ **Version B:** The first piece of data seems to reflect the values and contexts of its day. Its stress on 'pride' and 'ownership' reminds us of the prestige of car-ownership at a time when this was the preserve of an affluent minority, Although the gender values it encodes strike a modern reader as sexist, as it implies that women are preoccupied with appearances, consumption and protection, not economy and practicality, it is nevertheless interesting that they are still acknowledged as potential drivers, if not owners. The register tends towards formality and verbosity, with just occasional hints of the more colloquial style that would come to dominate the more image-oriented advertisements of the future.

Classroom activity 17

Suggest which of the versions above satisfies AO1 most successfully, and state precisely why.

The criteria for achieving the upper mark bands also refer to 'suitably tentative' conclusions. The academic register is characterised by caution; beware of making sweeping generalisations, overstating and exaggerating, and claiming over-emphatically the truth of what you are saying. After all, you are carrying out your study based on a tiny fragment of data, so you really will not be able to claim many earth-shattering discoveries. You may find the following table useful as a style guide:

Table 13 *Comparison of over-assertive and tentative conclusion styles*

Over-assertive	Suitably tentative
This is …	This seems to be …
This must be because …	This may be because … is likely to be because
Most people at this time believed …	There seems to have been a common belief at this time that …
My study proves the previous research is wrong …	The findings of my study appear to contradict those of earlier researchers …
There is a vast number of examples	There are many examples … There is a clear tendency towards …
There can only be one explanation	The most probable explanation is …

Classroom activity 18

Look at the following extract from a conclusion written by a student who had investigated the language used by employees in different parts of a restaurant. Rewrite it in a more suitably academic register and comment on the reasons for your changes:

'In the restaurant, I found that just about everybody used loads of questions which there was only a couple possible answers to, whereas the ones in the kitchen were always more open. This must be because the waitresses really needed to know stuff like where their plates were etc. I also found that there was loads of slang used in both places. I guess this was to create a friendly informal atmosphere with the customers. I noticed a vast number of cases where there was lexical repetition; waiters did this a lot when taking customers' orders, obviously to check they had taken the order down right.'

■ Quoting from your data

You will need to make a good deal of reference to your data throughout your investigation – in the analysis and conclusion sections particularly. There are several conventions that you can use to make this efficient, help you to make a range of different points quickly, and to make your investigation clear to any reader. Look at the following tools that you can make use of, and think about which will be most useful in your own data handling.

■ **Line references:** If you are working with continuous spoken or written data, numbering the lines will help you to be able to refer to particular sections quickly and easily in your write-up, particularly if you want to refer to larger sections or passages of data.

■ **Short quotation and extracts:** You can use the standard essay-style method of directly quoting language from the data you have collected.

■ **Statistical:** Including quantitive analysis of your findings gives your investigation an additional dimension and allows you to use tables and graphical forms of presentation to make some strong overall points and comparisons about data.

■ **Appendices:** You should provide copies of all the data you have collected and refer to it in the appendix of your investigation, and number the pieces. In this way, you will also be able to refer to particular supporting data or information quickly by referencing the specific part of your appendices.

■ **Footnotes:** Sometimes footnotes can be used to add information and references to particular data. These are notes that support a point you are making in the main text but are placed at the bottom of a page, or at the end of a section.

As with many of these different approaches, it is often best to use several of the different forms available to tailor to the particular needs of your project.

Extension activity 8

Look for examples of these different conventions being used in your wider reading, whether in books, articles or webpages. When you have come across several different uses, apply the ones that you think will help you in your own investigation.

■ Bibliography and sources

There are various accepted methods for identifying any sources you refer to or quote from in an academic study, but the most commonly used is the Harvard referencing system.

As your research proceeds, compile your bibliography by listing sources according to author (listed alphabetically), date of publication, title (and source if referring to an article in a magazine, newspaper or journal). Don't forget also to include the details of websites you visited. It will begin to look something like this:

A. Browne, 2001, *Developing Language and Literacy* (2nd edition), Paul Chapman

D. Crystal, 1988, *Rediscover Grammar*, Longman

> M. Whitehead, 2002, *Developing Language and Literacy with Young Children*, Paul Chapman
>
> www.mantex.co.uk/ou/resource/lit-term.htm, 2004 (Checklist of literary terms)

As long as you have listed a source in your bibliography, whenever you quote or refer to it in your text all you need to do is to place the author and date of publication in brackets immediately after the reference; so if the student in the example above wanted to reference *Developing Language and Literacy with Young Children*, she would just have to put 'Whitehead (2002)'.

Applying the assessment criteria

Your work will be assessed according to how successfully it satisfies the assessment objectives set by the exam board: use Table 14 for reference at every stage of your work.

Table 14 *Assessment criteria for the investigation report, with commentary and advice*

	Assessment criteria	Commentary and advice
AO1	Select and apply a range of linguistic methods, to communicate relevant knowledge using appropriate terminology and coherent, accurate written expression (5%)	In your investigation report, write clearly, accurately and in depth about your data; go into considerable detail, using the areas of language and terminology you need to be precise and rigorous in your analysis. This should represent the best writing you are capable of at the end of two years of Advanced Level study, and show lots of evidence of the learning you have been engaged in throughout the course.
AO2	Demonstrate critical understanding of a range of concepts and issues relating to the construction and analysis of meanings in spoken and written language, using knowledge of linguistic approaches (5%)	Show in your report that you have studied and understood the main theoretical ideas about language relevant to your investigation, and applied these using suitable methods of linguistic analysis. You need to show you can analyse and discuss the most interesting aspects of language using the ideas and terminology you have learnt over the previous two years.
AO3	Analyse and evaluate the influence of contextual factors on the production and reception of spoken and written language, showing knowledge of the key constituents of language (2.5%)	Show in your report that you have understood the importance of various contextual factors in influencing how language is used in the particular situation you have investigated. You also need to demonstrate knowledge of different linguistic methods and apply these productively to your data.
AO4	Demonstrate expertise and creativity in the use of English in a range of different contexts informed by linguistic study (7.5%)	When you write your media text, adopt a suitable approach and style to make the subject of your investigation interesting and accessible for a wider non-specialist audience.

A full breakdown of the AOs and marks can be found in the Language B Specification on the AQA website, but the maximum possible marks that can be scored for each AO in your language investigation are as follows:

- Maximum total marks for AO1 – 20 marks
- Maximum total marks for AO2 – 20 marks
- Maximum total marks for AO3 – 10 marks
- Maximum total for language investigation – 50 marks

Some extracts from Clare's investigation report are set out in Table 15. She chose to explore how four texts from a child's reading scheme (The Oxford Reading Tree) systematically introduced children to an increasingly challenging range of language. The section reprinted here focuses on the increasing degree to which the lexical content of texts introduces irregular spelling patterns.

The following extracts from her investigation are matched up to an assessor's comments, making use of the criteria of the assessment objectives and showing plus (+) and minus (−) points.

Table 15 *Extracts from a student's investigation with assessor's comments*

Investigation report extracts	Assessor's comments
Section 2.2 Lexical Range: Phonemic Predictability Even though we only have 26 letters in our alphabet there are actually 44 sounds that we use in our speech. When reading, the child has to make the links between graphemes and the phonemes they represent. Some words are easily predictable because their phoneme and grapheme correspondence is very close (e.g. 'red' = /red/). Words get more difficult as this correspondence becomes less obvious, making the process of deciphering longer. We have features such as silent letters, digraphs and unusual grapheme: phoneme correspondence.	+ AO1/2: Sound intro to section: shows understanding of relevant concepts and uses relevant terminology accurately. + AO1/2: Uses relevant knowledge (phonetic spelling) effectively to analyse her data.
Text A Being the first stage we would not expect any unpredictable words so the ones that are featured can easily be 'sounded out' from their graphemic form. One word which may cause a problem, is 'Who'. The digraph 'wh' is common but is sounded differently in different words. 'Where' is an example where it represents /w/ whereas in 'who' it represents /h/. Introducing this very common word at this stage is a good idea, as all 'wh' question words are regularly found in books and so this will be the basis for their knowledge in the area.	− But could demonstrate predictability of other words by examples. + AO3: sensible comments re context (early stage of reading development).
Text B The English spelling system is not particularly phonemic and has many anomalies and irregularities so the scheme soon starts to introduce more unusual sets of phoneme: grapheme correspondences. This stage involves the words 'bought', 'statue' and 'said' which are less straightforward. The use of the four letters 'ough' is a new challenge because if you tried to spell them out separately as you came across them in the word, you would not get the correct word at all. In 'bought' this group of letters represents /-aw/. Here, it is used twice within the same text to help embed it. The word 'statue' shows that /u:/ can be represented by the two letters 'ue' though the same sound is represented differently in more common words such as 'moon' and 'do'. By including 'statue' alongside words like 'balloon', 'new' and 'blew', the child is exposed to different ways of spelling the same sound idea. 'Said' = /sed/ is also another common word in books and so this is the best time to expose a child to it, as it isn't the easiest word to know how to spell and recognise as 'ai' does not often express the sound /e/.	+ AO1: sub-sections show highly systematic approach to analysis – effective. Expression is coherent and accurate.
Text C The amount of words with a close relationship between spelling and sound is still high but the proportion of more 'difficult' words has risen now at stage 5. Six words are less conventional for children: 'Read', 'laughed', 'laugh', 'photographs', 'believe' and 'watched'. Once again the author has picked up on a certain sound /f/ and is repeating it in different digraph forms 'gh', 'ph' to allow the child to become familiar with it.	+ AO3/2: Insight into how context (i.e. the position of the text in a graded reader scheme) has affected selection of lexis and phonemic patterns. Good understanding of relevant concepts. + AO1: some attempt to quantify data here – systematic.
Text D This text is now able to use words from a large vocabulary list because the child will have built up an adequate dictionary in their minds. There are a number of phonemically unpredictable words whose graphemic state and phonemic sound are quite distant: machine engine right knocked captain However due to the steady way in which the *Tree* introduces these types of words the child has the set basis to make knowledgeable guesses about their sound.	− But what is the proportion, exactly? + AO2: Perceptively observes patterns which illuminate data. + AO1: fair observations on data. − AO1: but not analysed here. Could note −ine pattern, for example.

■ **Further reading**

General

Articles at www.emagazine.org.uk

Bragg, M. *The Adventure of English*, Hodder and Stoughton, 2003

Crystal, D. *Encyclopedia of Language*, CUP, 1997

Crystal, D. *Encyclopedia of the English Language*, CUP, 2003

Crystal, D. *How Language Works: How Babies Babble, Words Change Meaning and Languages Live or Die*, Penguin, 2007

Fromkin, V. and Rodman, R. *An Introduction to Language* (7th edition), Thomson, 2002

Jackson, H. and Stockwell, P. *The Nature and Functions of Language*, Stanley Thornes, 1996

The Oxford English Dictionary (www.oed.com)

Thorn, S. *Mastering Advanced English Language*, Palgrave, 2008

Language investigation

British National Corpus (www.natcorp.ox.ac.uk)

Carter, R. *et al. Working with Texts: A Core Book for Language Analysis*, Routledge, 2008

Collect Britain (www.collectbritain.co.uk)

Engelmann, S. *Teach your Child to Read in 100 Easy Lessons*, Simon and Schuster, 1986

Freeborn, D. *From Old English to Standard English*, Macmillan, 2006

Garfield, A. *Teach Your Child to Read: A Phonic Reading Guide for Parents and Teachers*, Vermilion, 2007

Goddard, A. *Researching Language*, Heinemann, 2000

Jager Adams, M. *Beginning to Read*, MIT, 1994

Keith, G. and Shuttleworth, J. *Living Language*, Hodder and Stoughton, 1997

Langford, D. *Analysing Talk: Investigating Interaction in English*, Macmillan, 1994

Leith, D. *A Social History of English*, Routledge, 1997

McDonald, C. *English Language Project Work*, Macmillan 1992

Sealey, A. *Researching English Language: A Resource Book for Students*, Routledge 2008

B Media text

Introduction

In this section you will:

- consider the range of media texts open to you to write

- understand the different assessment criteria for the media text.

You have already been researching widely in your chosen language topic, and have been producing an academic report for a specialist audience of fellow language experts. The second text you are required to produce (of 750 to 1,000 words) must also be on the linguistic topic of your choice, but written in a more popular medium and for a less specialist audience.

This means it could be:

- an article for a newspaper or magazine
- a pamphlet for general information and distribution
- a script for an audio medium, such as radio or podcast
- a script and handouts/slides for a 'live' presentation.

Although you do not simply have to represent and rewrite the material of your language investigation report, it is likely that you will wish to make use of the research and reading you have done to produce a text that presents the topic you have been studying for people with little prior specialist knowledge.

Think of the media text task as a lively and accessible spin-off in which you find an interesting angle on your chosen topic, which will have a wide appeal. If the investigation report draws on many of the concepts and skills developed through Units 1 and 3, to satisfy the assessment objectives for the media text you will be developing many of the skills you practised in Unit 2:

AO4: Demonstrate expertise and creativity in the use of English in a range of different contexts informed by linguistic study (7.5%).

What this means is that when you write your media text, you should adopt a suitable approach and style to make the subject of your investigation interesting and accessible for a wider non-specialist audience. As with the texts you produced for Unit 2, this means you have to:

- select, organise and present material appropriately
- research and study suitable style models
- adopt the relevant genre conventions for your text
- write in a style that is lively and engaging as well as informative
- produce a text that is genuinely 'original' and creative
- produce a coherent text with very high standards of expression and accuracy
- present your work as professionally as possible.

The nature of the media text you will write will clearly be quite different from the document you produce as your language investigation report. It is in a different **genre** (which you will decide), will be published in a different **medium**, will have a different kind of **audience**, and will have a different **purpose**, as it needs not only to inform but also to engage the interest of and perhaps even advise or entertain its readers.

Preparing to write

In this topic you will:

- consider how to adapt a language topic for a media text

- study an example of a style model

- practise editorial skills of writing and presentation

- prepare to write your own media text.

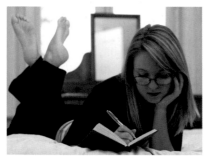

Fig. 1 *Reworking and drafting your writing will help produce something you're happy with*

When you tackle your media text in earnest, there are a few things that might help you to keep the right sort of approach in mind. Whether you find it difficult to start writing a language production piece, or you find it difficult to make it sufficiently linguistic, or you don't find it comfortable producing 'creative' writing, the following points should help you.

- **Value originality**: Go with your own ideas and try to keep what you write lively and varied. Once you've typed it out, it is easy to rework it, get second opinions and generally shape what you've got – so make what you've got raw and experimental, and then hone it. If you start off with cautious writing, there won't be so much you can do with it.

- **Remember that drafting is your friend**: Don't agonise over 'first sentences' or 'the right word' to the point that you come to a complete standstill. Try to get writing and sustain it. The way you will create a really strong piece is through honest and thoughtful drafting of your material.

- **Think 'process' not 'perfect'**: This sums up both of the previous two. Embrace your media text as a writing process and don't get hung up on it being perfect in the first couple of drafts.

💡 Finding an angle

To produce a successful text that really engages a more general audience you will need to find an angle on your topic of study that raises thought-provoking issues and connects with interests your audience already has. Let's take the two investigations we were working with in Unit 4, Section A (car advertisements and child reading miscues) as examples:

1 If you had been working on the changing language and style of car adverts in the 20th century, you might write an article for a magazine about the changing styles of adverts, possibly for readers with an interest in cars but no prior specialist knowledge of language.

2 If you had been studying the development of reading skills in twin brothers, you could produce an article for a parenting magazine, or a pamphlet to be given away by nurseries, or even the script for a presentation to be given to the parents of 3 to 4-year-olds, about the importance of shared reading experiences for the development of children's reading. Alternatively, you could write a newspaper article contributing to the debate about the merits of phonics-based teaching methods.

Some more suggestions that might arise from some of the investigations suggested earlier are offered in Table 1.

Table 1 *Some suggestions for media texts*

Topic area	Language investigation	Possible angles for media texts
Language varieties	Studies of broadcast and/or print-based news media.	Article for newspaper/magazine about contrasting styles (and bias?) of the news. Is it being 'dumbed down'? Is it truly neutral?
	Studies of persuasion in spoken/written texts.	Advisory article for fellow students about how to make their writing (and speeches) effective.
	Studies of teacher talk and/or classroom discourse.	Article about teaching styles and the language of the classroom, possibly for your own school or college magazine. Could be lively and amusing but also ask questions about teaching and learning.
	Studies of the language of humour, for example *The Office* or *Extras*.	Script for a broadcast or podcast discussing issues along the lines of language and comedy.
Language and gender	Studies of male and female language use.	Newspaper feature (perhaps for the weekend magazine section) about the myths and reality of language and gender. Are men really from Mars and women from Venus, or do they just *talk* like they're from different planets?
Language and power	Studies of pragmatics, status and power in conversational discourse and/or written texts.	An article about the hidden meanings, codes and power games that exist beneath the surface of everyday conversations – perhaps for your fellow students.
Language and technology	Studies of the evolution of language conventions in new technologies.	A script for a talk or presentation you might give to parents and teachers who are worried about the apparently harmful influence of new technologies on standards of literacy.
Language acquisition	Studies in the development of literacy.	A newspaper article that contributes to the current debate about approaches to the teaching of reading.
Language change	Studies in the change reflected in 20th- and 21st-century spoken and written sources.	A weekend newspaper or magazine article reflecting nostalgically on changing times and our changing language.
Topics arising from individual interests	Studies in individuals' language use at work.	An article about the language of the workplace – perhaps in the form of a light-hearted piece on 'How to talk the talk' at work, aimed at students about to take up a part-time job.

Classroom activity 1

For each of the following investigations, suggest an angle for a possible media text that might arise:

1. A study of the language used in a reality TV show.

2. A study of how males and females describe themselves and their ideal partner in an online dating site.

3. A study of the differences between the styles of radio and television sports commentaries.

4. A study of the language development of a child between 2 and $2\frac{1}{2}$ years.

🔍 Looking at style models

Not only is your media text going to be significantly shorter than your investigation report, it will, in many other respects, provide a new kind of writing challenge. It will differ in terms of:

■ layout and presentation
■ degree of linguistic detail
■ tone and style
■ use of specialist terminology.

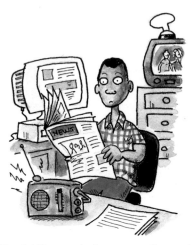

Fig. 2 *When producing your media text, it is useful to observe how the professionals do it*

An excellent way to approach creating your own original media text is to look carefully at the way professional writers manipulate language in their published and broadcast pieces. If you find some texts that appeal to you, you can use them as a style model to learn the conventions of that particular genre, and get some ideas for generating subtle effects like humour or creating a debate.

The following extracts showcase this kind of lively, original way of presenting a linguistic topic to a non-specialist audience. Remember that you have the opportunity to produce a text of a spoken or written mode in your media piece, and these extracts will provide you with an example of each.

Mind your language

I was relaxing in an Old Compton Street café when the waiter jogged my elbow, sending a hot stream of cappuccino up my nose. As I gave him a piece of my mind, he announced to the floor, 'God, she is soooo butch!' and whisked away, chortling. I was irked by this poisonous retort, but my gay friend was reassuring.

'He doesn't mean you're dykey. Butch is Polari for upfront, strong,' he said. 'It's the lingo, innit? Like "vada the bona casa". Or "get a load of her lallies."'

He could have donned a bowler hat and spoken in Droog for all I understood, but Polari did strike me as something novel and, well, fantabulosa (a useful Polari adjective). Paul Baker, a research associate at Lancaster University who is writing a PhD on Polari, has noticed something of a revival of interest in Polari in certain circles, as well as increasing interest in gay linguistics among academics …

Peter Gilliver, associate editor of the Oxford English Dictionary, tells me that Polari is actually more than 200 years old, and that the roots of some words are older still. Reference to the verb 'troll' (to take a walk) is to be found in a 14th-century text (although Polari gave us the derived noun 'trollette'). The ubiquitous 'bona' (good, attractive) was absorbed into English as long ago as Shakespeare's Henry IV Part II, where it appears as 'bona roba' (a wench, apparently, one wearing a lovely dress).

An extract from 'Mind your language', **Beverley D'Silva**, The Observer, *10 December 2000*

D'Silva's piece provides some excellent examples of how it is possible to blend original writing with linguistic content. It is based on the language variety of Polari, used by homosexual men in the mid-20th century, and the research carried out by Dr Paul Baker. The commentary in Table 2 picks out some of the main techniques and features that achieve this combination of flair and linguistic depth.

Table 2 *Commentary on main techniques and features used in 'Mind your language'*

Technique/feature	Commentary on effect
1. Dropping in examples of language use related to your chosen subject. Examples: 'soooo butch', 'vada the bona casa', 'lallies', 'fantabulosa', 'the derived noun "trollette"', 'bona roba'.	With an area that offers as much inventive vocabulary as Polari, D'Silva uses words from its lexicon like 'vada de bona casa' (probably 'look at the lovely house' in this context) and 'lallies' (legs) to set an informal, lively tone, but also to interest a non-specialist audience with words that are unfamiliar and exotic. This also shows a depth of knowledge of the subject.
2. Using original wider references for effects or depth. Examples: *Oxford English Dictionary*, 'could have donned a bowler hat and spoken in Droog', Shakespeare's *Henry IV Part II*.	By referencing such bastions of the English language as the *OED* and Shakespeare, D'Silva lends a weight of credibility to her article. However, she also makes a subtle and less well-known **allusion** to Anthony Burgess's novel *A Clockwork Orange*. This works particularly well as it has much in common with Polari as they both occurred largely in London; use their own invented vocabulary; and are about **anti-language** and **subculture.**
3. Employing varied, articulate and distinctive vocabulary. Examples: jogged, cappuccino, announced, whisked, chortling, irked, poisonous retort, donned, novel, fantabulosa, revival, ubiquitous, absorbed.	D'Silva creates a number of effects with her vocabulary choices. They range from an informal, entertaining register ('jogged', 'chortling') through to a formal, academic one ('donned', 'ubiquitous') which helps the piece gain credibility in each of these purposes. She also makes use of Polari-specific vocabulary herself, not just to exhibit it, but also incorporating it in her own style, as in the use of 'fantabulosa'. There are also some clever references: 'cappuccino' is Italian-derived, like much of Polari, and 'donned' perhaps alludes to the world of universities and PhDs that appear in the paragraph it is in. All of these make the piece work well, but also show a depth of linguistic awareness behind the writing.
4. Showing depth of knowledge in your chosen area of language study. Examples: Polari, Paul Baker, Lancaster University, gay linguistics, Peter Gilliver.	D'Silva makes it clear to her audience that Polari is a subject that has undergone recent academic study by using a term like 'gay linguistics' and name-dropping Paul Baker. She also adds range with Peter Gilliver, by placing Polari into the wider context of the English language.

The following text is an extract from the script for an episode of BBC Radio 4's *Word of Mouth* programme, presented by Michael Rosen and contributed to by Ian Peacock:

The problem with prepositions

Michael Rosen: And now WITHOUT any further ado, we arrive AT the contentious issue OF English prepositions UPON which Ian Peacock has disturbingly strident views which are somewhat OFF the wall, OVER the top, and BEYOND the realms of sanity. Frankly, Ian's opinions drive me UP the wall and ROUND the bend. In fact I suspect he may be OUT OF his depth and OUT OF his tree. And possibly OFF his face and OFF his rocker ...

Ian Peacock: That is the sort of introduction up with which I will not put. To what do you think you're up? You've no idea through what I've been. Anyway: welcome to ... aboard ... into this feature on ... about ... regarding prepositions and issues around them, by means of and as a consequence of which you may feel a little confused.

Under ... in the circumstances ... I went out-and-about and to-and-fro and hither-and-thither, over-and-above the call of duty and set off erelong, in a good mood and a taxi, sitting abaft, athwart the back-seat, betwixt Scylla and Charybdis, pondering prepositions we no longer use.

[...]

Key terms

Allusion: a subtle reference to a story or factual aspect outside of the text.

Anti-language: language that is used by a particular group to prevent others from understanding them.

Subculture: a cultural pursuit engaged in that happens outside of the mainstream, accepted values of society.

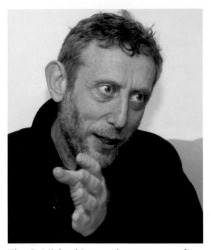

Fig. 3 *Michael Rosen, the presenter of BBC Radio Four's* Word of Mouth

Gosh. It's almost time to quickly wrap up ... up with which quickly to wrap ... which brings me to TIME prepositions. Just for the record ... the clock does not stand still at ten BEFORE three, nor ten AFTER three. Nor is it logically possible to arrive at 6.30 FOR 7. I refuse to work Monday THROUGH Friday or to do anything ACROSS the weekend. I suspect we got these expressions off of the Americans. They're certainly completely different than ... from ... to ... the grammar up with which I was brought.

Michael Rosen and Ian Peacock, Word of Mouth, BBC Radio 4, 2007

In discussing the use of prepositions in the English language, this piece also makes use of original phrasing and specific linguistic content, and it is interesting to compare how a more explicitly spoken mode piece goes about this in comparison to D'Silva's largely written mode text. The commentary in Table 3 looks at the way Rosen and Peacock make use of the same four strategies:

Table 3 *Commentary on main techniques and features used in **Word of Mouth***

Technique/feature	Commentary on effect
1. Dropping in examples of language use related to your chosen subject. Examples: 'WITHOUT' and other prepositions used, 'abaft' and other **archaic** prepositions.	Rosen makes repeated, even exaggerated, use of a range of prepositions, like 'without' in his introduction to the topic, which is entertaining, as well as showing good knowledge of the range of use of the word class. This is given depth by putting the prepositions used in common idioms, and by Peacock later distinguishing archaic prepositions like 'abaft'.
2. Using original wider references for effects or depth. Examples: 'in a good mood and a taxi', Scylla and Charybdis.	Peacock sets a certain scene with his phrase 'in a good mood and a taxi', painting a kind of **word picture** of his surroundings and continuing a lively, informal narrative style. He also uses a **classical allusion** to the mythical monsters of Scylla and Charybdis, which works subtly as it refers to being stuck between two difficult problems that require you to find a balance between them – much like the problem of preposition use being defined.
3. Employing varied, articulate and distinctive vocabulary. Examples: ado, contentious, disturbingly strident, sanity, off his rocker, to-and-fro, athwart, pondering prepositions.	Because this is a broadcast piece, rather than in print, the sound of the words can be used to even greater effect. Rosen and Peacock's text therefore strikes a balance between an informal/formal register with contrasting phrases like 'off his rocker' and 'disturbingly strident'. Preposition phrases are also used to good effect to double up the entertainment and linguistic purposes of the script. An example of the sound of words being foregrounded comes in Peacock's use of alliteration in 'pondering prepositions'.
4. Showing depth of knowledge in your chosen area of language study. Examples: Ian Peacock, 'To what do you think you're up?', 'ten BEFORE three', 'the Americans. They're certainly completely different than ... from ... to ... the grammar up'.	Both Rosen and Peacock make wide use of prepositions and related phrases, but Peacock takes this a step further by including some non-standard phrases like 'ten before three' to illustrate his knowledge of the potential prescriptivist debate over such use. Peacock himself is included as a contributor as he has done some specialist work in the field, and he develops his point further by linking preposition use to the wider debate about **Americanisms** and their influence on British English usage.

Editorial skills

Once you have a clear idea for your media text and have found some style models to work with, the writing process will involve exercising a range of editorial skills. You will be aiming to make your media text achieve many different things: address a non-specialist audience, provide a convincing and subtle focus on a linguistic topic, and create an original style, written with flair.

Genre conventions

In addition to these, it will be important to produce an authentic version of the particular genre of text you are writing. Different genres can be identified by the conventions and features they use, which can involve graphological elements, particular textual segments, as well as the style of language and content. Look at Table 4 for a guide to the conventions for some of the media texts you might write.

Table 4 *Conventions and features of various genres*

Media genre	Conventions and segments	Style and content
Newspaper article	Bold, large font in main title Use of bold or italics for emphasis Images with captions Text layout in columns Title, subtitles and main text	Objective approach Use of factual information Summary and interpretation of main concepts Integration of short quotation
Editorial	Bold, large font in main title Photo of writer Images or supporting graphics Email address or website for readers to send comment to	Lively, discursive style Generation of debate Contains opinion and subjective material Use of wordplay, humour and figurative devices
Webpage	Use of colour and font style variation Images and graphical elements Website menu Website banner Advertisement boxes and panels	Style can vary widely depending on nature of text Quotations and statistics from reader contributions Hyperlinks to related subjects, previous pages, video and audio

Key terms

Archaic: a word from an earlier period of English usage that is rarely used in the modern contemporary language.

Word picture: a feature of radio broadcasting where a presenter will put forward a visual scene using verbal narrative description.

Classical allusion: a reference to a character or event in classic Greek or Roman mythology.

Americanisms: examples of language use distinct to American English speakers.

Effective writing and rhetorical techniques

Never lose sight of the fact that writing effectively and inventively is at the heart of your media text production piece. Outside of the use of style models and preparing good linguistic content, you might remind yourself of some basic techniques that can go a long way to helping you write an original text. Here are some tips:

■ Keep in mind the importance of variety. This should be evident in your punctuation, paragraph and sentence structures and vocabulary.

■ Make use of specific rhetorical devices and effects, for example: alliteration, assonance, metaphor, simile, anaphora, litotes, synecdoche, tripling, and others you have encountered.

■ Experiment with register by using a range of spoken and written mode features, varying manner elements like formality for effect.

■ Think of the impact of your text across the frameworks. This means trying to make sure that you show originality in terms of your choice of lexis, semantic and phonological effects, grammatical structures and layout and graphology.

Extension activity 2

Revise your knowledge of the language devices you can make use of, like those mentioned above and others you can unearth.

Coursework preparation and practice

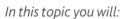

In this topic you will:

■ learn how to present your media text

■ learn how to reference your work

■ apply the assessment criteria to examples of students' work.

Now that you have explored a range of techniques for putting your media text together, this topic will provide a few tips on how to complete and submit your media text coursework piece, as well as presenting you with the assessment criteria that your piece will be judged against, with a worked example of a final piece being assessed.

How to present your media text

The media text is a relatively simple piece to put together and submit. Here is a checklist for you to use as you enter the final stages:

■ Is the topic link to your investigation clear?

■ What is the word count – is it between 750 and 1,000 words?

■ Have you typed up your piece and formatted the text?

■ Do you have a record of the style models and source texts you used?

■ Are you sure you have 'transformed' the language of the style models and source texts and avoided any risk of plagiarism?

Bibliography and sources

Just as you did in your investigation, you will need to give a record of the sources that you used to help you with your media text. It may well be that some are 'doubled up' from your investigation, but you should provide a brief bibliography either immediately after your text, or on a separate, titled sheet, detailing any books, articles or webpages you used, either as a style model, or as a source for the information in your piece.

Applying the assessment criteria

Only one assessment objective (AO4) is used in assessing your media text, and it is worth 30 marks in total. Although it is only a single AO, it covers several threads in your piece, including:

■ showing expertise in your writing, by controlling your accuracy and expression

■ recreating a particular genre of text convincingly

■ exhibiting creativity and originality in the stylistic choices that you make

■ maintaining a focus on a relevant language topic.

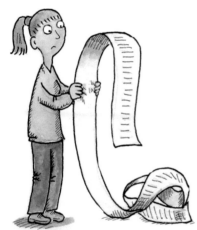

Fig. 4 *Make sure you've checked off everything you need to do before submitting your media text*

Table 5 *Assessment criteria and breakdown of marks for the media text*

Mark	AO4: Demonstrate expertise and creativity in the use of English in a range of different contexts informed by linguistic study.
28–30	Originality in the deployment of the structures and conventions associated with media texts.
	Sensitive and convincing manipulation of register to meet demands of audience and purpose.
	Successful, effective and convincing new text; demonstrates ingenuity and finesse in the use of original materials and ideas.
26–27	Confident, controlled deployment of the structures and genre conventions.
	Appropriate control of register, demonstrating sophisticated awareness of the demands of audience and purpose.
	Effective and sustained adaptation of original materials; sources manipulated and integrated into entirely new text.
22–24	Sustained deployment of appropriate structures and genre conventions; strong clarity and control of writing.
	Coherent register, secure writing style – effective for audience and purpose.
	Effective adaptation of original materials for new audience and purpose.
19–21	Competent deployment of structures and genre conventions – good clarity and control of writing.
	Growing sophistication in control of register – article likely to be effective for audience and purpose.
	Largely effective adaptation of original materials for new audience and purpose.
16–18	Demonstrates control of genre requirements; good clarity and control in writing.
	Effective register, demonstrating the ability to adapt writing to engage and interest audience.
	Source original materials shaped to suit new audience/purpose – some lack of control at times.
13–15	Language choices generally effective and appropriate, demonstrating increasing control; some awareness of structures and genre conventions.
	Register mainly appropriate; some ability to adapt writing to engage and interest audience.
	Partly effective transformation; attempts to shape original materials for new audience/purpose.
10–12	Some ability to control genre requirements for audience and purpose – likely to be inconsistent.
	Mainly appropriate register – possibly oversimplified at times or overly complex.
	Some transformation – demonstrates awareness of the need to shape original materials for new audience/purpose.
7–9	Knowledge of genre, and purpose demonstrated; oversimplified audience awareness.
	Beginnings of appropriate register – likely to be inconsistent across writing.
	Some transformation for new audience/purpose, likely to shadow original materials.
4–6	Some limited understanding of audience, purpose and genre.
	Some limited control over writing – attempts to develop appropriate register.
	Some limited attempt to transform original materials, though not very successfully; very dependent on original sources.
1–3	Little understanding of writing activity – inappropriate content; limited awareness of genre, audience and purpose.
	Ineffective register; imprecise language choices, little control over writing.
	Little transformation of original materials leading to inappropriate content for task.
0	Nothing written/totally inappropriate for tasks.

It is a sensible idea to familiarise yourself with the contents of Table 5 in order to get an accurate impression of the quality of text expected to achieve good marks. The example in Table 6 of an extract from a media text shows the way that the assessment criteria might be applied to a coursework piece, and what particular marks 'look like' in practice.

This piece is based on the car advertisement investigation idea explored in Unit 4, Section A of this book. It is an article discussing the power and influence of slogans in advertising that would appear in a newspaper supplement magazine or similar.

Table 6 *Extracts from a student's media text with AO4 criteria comments*

Media text extracts	AO4 criteria comments
Probably the best slogan in the world? Joe Bloggs on how advertising's catchy phrases conquered the globe.	+ Use of headline and sub-headed introduction provides clear opening. (22–24 band for 'appropriate structures')
Slogans appear to be an inescapable part of the backdrop to the modern world. Towns and cities have become galleries for the corporate masterpieces of the advertising era, with constantly changing exhibitions of the latest works from the easel of Sony or Nike or Volkswagen. And, as we walk around the aisles and take it all in, our radios, televisions – even our friends – provide a running commentary of the latest adspeak. From 'Every Little Helps' (Tesco) to 'Where do you want to go today?' (Microsoft) the reassuring voices of advertising are everywhere – but just how do these mantras, bon-mots and one-liners make such a lasting impression on us, and why do we keep coming back for more?	+ Articulate tone set up with variation in vocabulary: 'inescapable', 'backdrop'. (19–21 band for 'good clarity and control of writing') + Use of metaphor to describe advertisements as 'exhibitions' in 'galleries' shows sophistication. (28–30 band for 'use of original ... ideas') + Use of question to address audience develops reader relationship. (22–24 band for 'effective for audience and purpose')
Apparently, the word slogan is derived from a couple of ancient Gaelic words for host 'sluagh' and cry 'gairm' that realised they were made for each other and gradually sidled up closer to become the word we know and love today. In the original Gaelic setting, 'slaugh-gairm' was a full-throated battle cry – a far cry now, perhaps, from the subtler, if no-less-powerful stealth of the world's marketing departments. And so, we now live in the world of 'The World's Online Market Place' (eBay), where 'Life's Good' (LG) and 'The Future's Bright, The Future's ---' (Orange, right?).	+ Etymological detail of the word 'slogan' provides depth and linguistic weight. (28–30 band for 'convincing new text') + Including quoted slogans shows evidence of research and knowledge in chosen field. (22–24 band for 'adaptation of original materials') – Over-exaggerated style and attempt at humour at end perhaps does not fit with tone. (19–21 band for just 'largely effective adaptation')

This is only an extract of what would be the opening 25–30% of an entire media text, and it is important to note that the overall mark out of 30 is awarded by balancing the quality of the entire piece, rather than 'counting up' particularly successful sections. Even so, the comments column above should give you a feel for the fact that this piece is meeting the criteria for the top few bands consistently, and would be likely to continue to become a piece worth in the region of 24–30 marks overall.

 Classroom activity 3

The following piece is an extract from a media text arising out of the other investigation idea from the first section, on the language use of young children. It is the first part of a leaflet (again approximately 25–30% of the overall piece) to promote the value of shared reading between parents and young children. It would be aimed at the parents and would appear in public places like local libraries, nurseries and schools.

Read it carefully and use the assessment criteria from Table 5 on page 176 to 'mark' the piece. Make notes of particular things it achieves and the band you think each is described by, and also any problems you can see.

Reading together

How to share books with your child

Reading with your children is one of the most important and enjoyable things you can do with them. As your child grows older, being able to read well will help them a great deal in their schooling and life – as well as being good fun! Sharing books is worth doing at any age, even with very young babies, and this leaflet will give you a few tips on how to do it well, and why it is so valuable.

The value of reading

Reading is great for growing children for many reasons:

- It introduces young babies to the sounds of words and language.
- Stories give lively young minds lots to think about and enjoy.
- Sitting together reading is a lovely time to bond with your child.
- Reading from an early age helps develop your child's literacy skills.

Some tips for shared reading

Sitting and reading with your child will probably come very naturally. Here are some tips to help you both get the most from it:

- Let your child choose books he or she would like to read.
- Visit the library or the bookshop together every week or so.
- Reading can happen at any time, but try to build in a regular slot each day.
- Encourage your child to talk about books and stories and ask questions.

Further reading

General

Articles at www.emagazine.org.uk

Bragg, M. *The Adventure of English*, Hodder and Stoughton, 2003

Crystal, D. *Encyclopedia of Language*, CUP, 1997

Crystal, D. *Encyclopedia of the English Language*, CUP, 2003

Crystal, D. *How Language Works: How Babies Babble, Words Change Meaning and Languages Live or Die*, Penguin, 2007

Fromkin, V. and Rodman, R. *An Introduction to Language (7th Edition)*, Thomson, 2002

Jackson, H. and Stockwell, P. *The Nature and Functions of Language*, Stanley Thornes, 1996

The Oxford English Dictionary (www.oed.com)

Thorn, S. *Mastering Advanced English Language*, Palgrave, 2008

Media text

Clark, U. *Introducing Stylistics,* Stanley Thornes, 1996

Cook, G. *The Discourse of Advertising*, Routledge, 2001

Freeborn, D., Langford, D. and French, P. *Varieties of English*, Macmillan, 1993

Goddard, A. *The Language of Advertising*, Routledge, 2002

Morkane, S. *Original Writing*, Routledge, 2004

Russell, S. *Grammar, Structure and Style*, OUP, 2001

Feedback on the activities

Unit 3, Section A Language acquisition

Developing speech

Classroom activity 1

Stage	Lexis/semantics	Phonology	Grammar	Pragmatics/ discourse
Pre-verbal		Vocal skills are vital to producing phonemes. Combining sounds to produce recognisable words is practised.		By practising pitch, intonation and volume, children prepare themselves for conversation and rehearse ways to make meanings clear in their speech acts.
Holophrastic/ one-word	At the proto-word and holophrastic stages, the lexical process is under way.	With only one word, phonology is still important to conveying meaning.		
Two-word	Successfully joining words and phrases involves understanding the meanings of words (semantics).		Once two words can be combined, then syntactical and grammatical advances can be made.	Discourse skills such as turn-taking develop as conversations become possible and politeness skills encouraged by parents may appear.
Telegraphic	More words are needed to combine together, so vocabulary is likely to be developing rapidly.		Grammatical ability will become more important at this stage to combine words together in the correct order.	Discourse and pragmatic awareness become more sophisticated as children learn to interpret other people's speech and meanings.
Post-telegraphic			More complex utterances are created accurately. Skills being refined and practised.	

Classroom activity 2

Plosives form most of the first sounds produced by 24 months, but the sounds produced are mainly those created by using the tongue and teeth (n, m) and the lips (p, b). These sounds mostly fall into the 'stop' consonants and voiced categories, with their voiceless counterparts (f, s) produced later. Fricatives appear later because physical control of speech organs is needed, especially a more delicate control of the tongue and the lips; children often replace fricatives with stop consonants in early sounds. Understanding the order in which children acquire consonant sounds, and the ways the sounds are produced, helps in interpreting the typical phonological 'errors' they make.

Classroom activity 3

Some ways in which you may have grouped the words:

Proper nouns: 'Jasper', 'Daddy', 'Laa-Laa', 'Nana', etc.

Food/drink words: 'juice', 'jam', 'biscuits', 'cup', etc.

Social words: 'bye-bye', 'hello', 'hiya'

Politeness words: 'ta', 'please'

Requests: 'cuddle', 'wassat', 'more'

Animals: 'duck', 'quack', 'woof', 'cat'

Interestingly, you were probably able to group them quite easily, which shows that there are patterns to first words. These may be influenced by social interaction and the contexts (situations) of children's development. Notice amongst the first 50 words here are 'Laa-Laa' (from the television programme Teletubbies) and 'book', displaying Rachel's early cultural experiences.

Classroom activity 4

Example	Meaning relation
More cat	Recurrence
Daddy sit	Agent + action
No dolly	Negation
Brush hair	Action + affected
Mummy key	Possessor + possession
Ball big	Entity + attribute
There Jack	Nomination
Biscuit floor	Entity + location
Sit buggy	Action + location
Drop juice	Agent + affected

Classroom activity 5

This data does not support Skinner's views about imitation. Here, the child wants to say 'another spoon', but expresses this request using two determiners ('other one'). The message is unclear to the father, who tries to correct the child's speech by breaking the phrase into separate words. Despite the correction the child continues uttering the same noun phrase ('other one spoon'), which seems to support Piaget's view that thought influences language development and that this child has not grasped the concepts surrounding the varieties of determiners that can suggest quantity, etc. But, for Chomsky, this child has engaged with a key syntactical rule, i.e. that determiners are used before nouns in order to make a more precise message, even if they have not fully mastered this yet.

Coursework activity 6

There are no right or wrong answers to some of the utterances because you don't have the full context and can't see or hear the children. Here are some conclusions you may have made.

Utterance	Context	Halliday's function	Dore's function
Look at me, I superman	Child playing	Imaginative	Requesting
Mummy	Mummy returns home from work	Representational	Labelling or greeting
Want juice	Child is thirsty	Instrumental	Requesting
Put down	Father is holding child	Regulatory	Requesting or protesting
Me like that	Child looks at toy in a shop	Personal	Answering or labelling
Why?	Child asks why she has to get her shoes on	Heuristic	Requesting action (i.e. response to question)
Night night daddy, love you	Being put to bed	Interactional	Answering or repeating
No	Child wants to stay at the park	Personal	Protesting

Classroom activity 7

The girls' role-play is based around idealised female stereotypes of a 'princess' and a 'fairy' and feminine roles ('mother'), starting with the use of the fairy outfits as props. The storyline acted out is connected to their understanding of bedtime routines; Anya, as 'mummy', cajoles Keri's 'baby' character to sleep with a story and a kiss. The roles are negotiated straightaway in the declarative adjacency pairs:

Anya: I can be the mother (.) right

Keri: I can be a princess

Although neither agrees directly to the other's role-taking, agreement is implicit in Keri's statement after Anya's tag question ('right'). The modal verb ('can') also offers politeness strategies, suggesting the possibility of refusal from the other player.

By using directives ('lie in you bed now princess' and 'your had to kiss me') they control each other's behaviour, and add to their view of the required elements of the role-play. Anya's commanding behaviour fits her motherly role as she attempts to get baby to sleep ('go to sleep now', 'go back to sleep now'). She also adopts features of parental behaviour with the soothing sounds ('shh') and her choice of vocatives ('fairy', baby') mimics a mother's lexical address to her child; this behaviour will be covered later when evaluating the role of carers (see page 28).

You might also have noticed, when applying your knowledge of gender studies, that the modifiers used ('lovely') conform to Robin Lakoff's list of typical features of women's language.

Classroom activity 8

In Text A the mother repeats utterances ('what a noise', 'it is a long time') and uses lexical repetition ('dear'). She uses the present tense ('is it a long time', 'let's go') and her utterances are simple sentences ('are you hungry') with simple verbs such as the copula ('is') and other verbs ('get', 'let' 'are', etc.). Yes/no interrogatives ('are you hungry', 'you're all right aren't you') simulate imagined responses from the baby, modelling discourse structure in adjacency pairs – despite his inability to apply this at this early developmental stage. The mother treats the baby's sounds as responses to her utterances, teaching Michael that communication is two-way (dyadic). Surprisingly, she doesn't use the baby's name and uses few concrete nouns, perhaps because the baby is young and she is responding to sounds that represent his basic food and comfort needs.

The mother's linguistic choices in Text B support the view that CDS adapts as the child develops. She constructs more sophisticated interrogatives ('how many chickens are there') requiring a more developed response. Her discussion of chickens expands the conversation, asking Tom to count how many, and recalls their earlier experience of seeing chickens and his actions of stroking the chicken. Here the mother uses lexical repetition more consistently ('Pascale', 'chicken', 'stroke') than Michael's mother to help Tom learn new labels and terms to describe his actions.

Developing reading

Classroom activity 9

First books do not resemble adult books. They are often made of soft material, thick card or even plastic, and exploit the tactile and physical nature of children's early experiences. Interactivity is important in children's books because reading is usually shared with adults. Children actively engage with reading books by pointing to objects in the text, lifting a flap to reveal the words and images underneath, or guessing rhymes.

Sound effects, and other phonological/poetic devices, are common features. Children delight in the sounds of words and the effects of rhythm and rhyme. Books also offer explicit learning, both of language itself, and of the world around them; they can be used by carers to support – or to use Bruner's term 'scaffold' – development of the spoken word by giving young children new lexical terms for objects around them and to describe their feelings and experiences.

These books also assist children's social and pragmatic development, modelling the handling of real-life situations. Books also encourage children's imagination and their use of play to represent their understanding of the surrounding world.

Classroom activity 10

Some of the advantages and disadvantages that you might have discussed:

Method	Advantages	Disadvantages
Whole-word	Children learn visual methods to read words. Good for beginners, mirroring the ways children learn their name.	Children don't have strategies for working out new words. Not all children have good visual memories.
Phonics	Children: ■ become good spellers ■ tackle new words effectively by breaking them down into smaller units ■ can self-teach by applying rules they have been taught.	Not all English words fit patterns neatly.
Analytic phonics	Children: ■ learn the patterns and rules of English spelling and sound/grapheme correspondence, applying these to unseen words ■ can use the rhymes of words to read and spell unfamiliar words, comparing their knowledge of similar word patterns ■ develop an excellent sight vocabulary for both reading and spelling ■ benefit from having phonics combined with other teaching methods and exposure to reading books.	It takes time to learn all the sounds/letters and combinations of vowels and consonants. Not all children have good rhyming skills. Not effective if children can't apply their knowledge to unfamiliar words and words that are not accompanied by a picture.
Synthetic phonics	Children: ■ benefit from the speed at which they learn all phonemes, encouraging reading and spelling skills immediately ■ can apply knowledge to unseen words quickly as the blending of sounds is taught early on.	Existing research has not found any disadvantages.

Classroom activity 11

The book has a traditional narrative structure with the setting clearly stated in the first sentence, providing a recognisable context for a school-age child. However, unlike story books there is little descriptive language, and plot development relies on the use of direct speech. Recapping the storyline is a key, as characters repeat sentences and lexical features ('race') as a way of foregrounding both the stages of the story and the new vocabulary being introduced; this means that there are fewer deictic references than would appear in naturally occurring speech. Although simple reporting clauses ('asked', 'said') are usually used, here the speech tags suggest the prosody of speech ('shouted'). Inverting reporting clauses only occur when a noun is used (as in 'shouted Mr March').

The lexical choices are context-dependent, forming a sports-day related semantic field. Colloquial lexis is included ('dad') and contractions ('it's') add to the informality. Nouns and verbs are repeated as they are new words introduced in this book ('race', 'gym' and 'train'). Pronouns ('he') are used anaphorically once a proper noun ('Ben', 'dad') has been introduced; this makes the text cohesive and helps the child to connect the noun and pronoun. Simple and compound sentences are used, and the repetition of sentences reinforces new vocabulary and creates predictable patterns. Graphologically, the sentences are laid out mainly on one line, running on only after a conjunction ('and', 'but'); children already recognise that these function as linking words. Pictures visually represent the words and allow children to 'cue'.

Developing writing

Classroom activity 12

The written text summarises the story viewed on television into a compound sentence using adverbials ('one day', 'on a trip', 'in the Tardis'). He has captured the main plot elements and uses words lexically relevant to Dr Who. He has not elaborated on the story descriptively, using pictures to show the stages of the story and help the reader visualise the events. Cameron's graphological choice of a storyboard is interesting. It is unlikely he has been taught this; perhaps he has used his cultural experiences of watching or reading comic-strips and cartoons. This supports researchers' links between cultural experience and literacy. Cameron shows awareness that different representations of the same information are possible by using other symbol systems; the text is still multimodal and the images support the text's meanings, adding cohesion.

Understanding of writing processes is demonstrated in his use of a title ('Doctor Who Story') and claiming authorship at the bottom of the text. Cameron understands lineation and directionality. His writing is fairly neat and letter formation is generally secure, including some understanding of both upper- and lower-case letters. Some mirroring of letters ('d'/'b') is evident. Typically of an early learning stage, his separation of letters and words is inconsistent, possibly reflecting his mental re-composition of the story. For an audience, he has not presented his message clearly enough and the transliteration is required for it to make sense to someone who was not present when he wrote this.

His spelling shows phonetic awareness, indicating that he knows some strategies for guessing unfamiliar words. He has to spell 'Shakespeare' because it is polysyllabic and has many separate sounds that cannot be replicated phonetically. This will require further knowledge of English spelling rules to produce accurately. Importantly, he has created a complete text but has yet to progress in writing an extended piece of discourse with cohesive links.

Classroom activity 13

The first text 'Our trip to Chatsworth Farm' is a 4-year-old's recount of a school trip to a farm. Because of the child's age, the orientation is typed at the top by the teacher. The child structures their recount into simple sentences, following a subject, verb, object pattern. It has a list-like layout, with each sentence beginning with the first person pronoun ('I') on a new line. You might question whether it meets Rothery's definition of a recount as chronological, as it is difficult to conclude whether this is the order of the child's experiences or everything that they recalled about their trip. You might perceive that the child's use of the adjective ('favourite') is an evaluation of their experience.

This choice of adjective along with other descriptive lexis suggests that 'My favourite place' is an observation/comment genre. Although it could have evolved into a report-type task, this was obviously intended to allow the child to explore and evaluate their experiences, suggested by the extensive use of modifiers ('warm', 'lovely', 'delicious', 'most wonderful').

'Hedgehogs' fulfils some of the genre criteria for a report, being factual and not sequencing the events chronologically. The dynamic verbs ('eat', 'wander', 'curl') describe the hedgehog's actions, demonstrating the child's understanding that these, rather than any descriptive lexical choices, are more relevant for the task. The 8-year-old's graphological choices show awareness of the appropriate layout for a report, seemingly into bullet points and separate paragraphs. She has edited her writing, crossing out her statement ('because I like them') which reveals that she knows that you don't need this evaluative comment in a report.

Classroom activity 14

Child's spelling	Actual spelling	Type of spelling error (s)
suddnly	suddenly	Omission of salient sounds
peculier/ perculiar	peculiar	Phonetic
cloke	cloak	Phonetic
kitchin	kitchen	Phonetic
discusting	disgusting	Phonetic
(golf) corse	course	Omission/phonetic
shale (shall)	shall	Overgeneralising/ phonetic
exspensis	expensive	Phonetic/salient sounds
twincling	twinkling	Substitution/phonetic
butifull	beautiful	Omission/ overgeneralising
kitins	kittens	Phonetic
fraindly	friendly	Phonetic/transposition
becuase	because	Transposition
correg (meaning bravery)	courage	Phonetic/over- generalising
bissnis	business	Phonetic/over- and undergeneralising
chearful	cheerful	Overgeneralising
intelgent	intelligent	Salient sounds

Your findings indicate that children make a range of errors based on their phonetic, grammatical and visual memories. There is usually a logical reason for these errors, making them 'virtuous' rather than random.

■ Unit 3, Section B Language change

Changes in context, lexis and semantics

■ Classroom activity 1

Word	Origin	Word	Origin
poncho, hammock, mosquitoes, guitar, tortilla	Spain, or South America	marmalade	Portugal
anorak, parka, igloo, kayak	Arctic Region/Inuit	shish kebab, sherbert	Turkey
dungarees, pyjamas	India	sushi, kamikaze	Japan
ski	Norway	tea	China
chocolate	France	moussaka	Greece
knapsack, cruise	Holland	safari, trekked	Africa
tobogganing	Canada	barbecue, cannibal	Caribbean
anonymous	Greece	tattooed	Polynesia
pow-wow	North America	assassin	Egypt
zero, coffee	Arabic origin		

From this you can see just how wide-ranging English borrowing has been, as this passage only represents a few. Some clues lie in the consonant combinations used more commonly in other languages ('kk'). The words seem to fall into semantic fields: clothes ('poncho', 'anorak') and food ('tortilla', 'coffee') being the main ones. These would indicate the influence of travel and different cultural experiences, which English did not have existing words to describe.

Some have been borrowed because of colonisation and empire-building, such as the Indian words 'dungarees', 'pyjamas'. Mainly we use their native, non-anglicised form as loan words using the relevant orthography ('ski', 'kamikaze'), but sometimes we anglicise them in both spelling and pronunciation ('chocolate' instead of 'chocolat').

This exercise has introduced the importance of etymology, the study of the origins and history of words and their meanings. This helps us understand how speakers and writers have used English over time and is vital when analysing historic texts in a detailed and informed manner.

■ Classroom activity 2

Blend	Blended words	Blend	Blended words
motel	motor + hotel	skort	skirt + short
brunch	breakfast + lunch	Oxbridge	Oxford + Cambridge
Wikipedia	Wiki + encyclopedia	labradoodle	labrador + poodle
docusoap	documentary + soap	boxercise	box + exercise
guesstimate	guess + estimate	netiquette	internet + etiquette
Chunnel	Channel + tunnel	confuzzle	confuse + puzzle

Blends are based on the idea of merging objects together ('labradoodle', 'skort', 'Oxbridge'). Another technique is to use the first letter from one word with the majority of another ('motel', 'brunch'). Sometimes whole words are blended with parts of others ('guesstimate', 'boxercise').

Classroom activity 3

Word	Semantic change	Word	Semantic change
doctor	**Narrowing** The word once referring to teachers, now mainly used for the medical profession and academics	web	**Metaphor** Now most commonly used to refer to the internet, metaphorically suggesting ideas of thin, invisible, interlinked webs. Still has its existing meaning, so arguably has also broadened
gay	**Pejoration** Originally meaning 'happy', it ameliorated, and used metaphorically, in reference to homosexuality. In current slang it now refers to something defective or unfashionable, e.g. 'that's gay'	mouse	**Broadening/Metaphor** As well as the small animal, the meaning now includes the object used to interface with the computer
virus	**Metaphor/broadening** Once only associated with an illness transmitted from people, but now also refers to the infecting of computers by bugs	a domestic	**Euphemism/narrowing** Now used euphemistically to refer to arguments between spouses, probably a shortening of a longer phrase such as 'a domestic incident'
guts	**Amelioration** Once referred to animal/human entrails and now is more positively associated with courage	friendly fire	**Euphemism** A phrase used to refer to killing allies accidentally in a war context
punk	**Broadening/semantic shift** Used to mean a prostitute. In US slang it now means a petty criminal or thug, as well as a coward. In UK use it is now associated with a music sub-culture	hoodie	**Metaphor/broadening/pejoration** Refers to an item of clothing, the colloquial term for a hooded top. However, it is now associated with the type of person wearing it and the associated anti-social behaviour
vulgar	**Pejoration** Used to mean popular and now means in rather bad taste	starve	**Narrowing** Once meant to die, and now refers to death by not eating

Classroom activity 4

	1747	1852	1998
neologisms			nutrition, calories, protein, carbohydrate
borrowings/ loan words	currey		wan kai thai-style curry, soy sauce, mangetout
compound	tea spoonful, sauce-pan, stew-pan	table-spoonfuls, piled-up	supermarkets, non-stick
archaism	enough	broth, fat pot	
narrowing	fowls, shovel	liquor	
broadening	scum		'in'
conversion		salt	

Changes in written style

Classroom activity 5

The earliest texts shows surprisingly few differences from modern spelling, with the only unusual orthographical representation being the letter 's'. The short 's' appears at the ends of words ('companies', 'delicious') and the long in the initial or medial position ('ʃlave', 'taʃk').

Dorothy Wordsworth's journal shows more variation, perhaps because it was originally handwritten rather than printed. Use of the –e at the end of words is different from modern usage (it is used in 'sate' but not in 'headach'). Both spellings are used consistently but don't follow yet the rule for long and short vowel sounds.

The 2004 message shows many features of non-standard spelling: phonetic ('foreva', 'iz'); vowel deletions ('wy', 'thnk'); substitutions ('faze', 'dis'). These give the message a more informal and conversational tone, but are still based on certain evolving conventions of text usage despite their non-conformity to Standard English.

Classroom activity 6

Punctuation

When reporting direct speech, Stedman uses speech marks on every line on the left of the page only, as well as to open and close the speech tag ('said he'). Other noticeable differences are that the semicolons mark subordinate clauses (into this hospital; 'where I beheld'…) and before the translation ('dogo tay Tamara; The sun is just going to sleep'). Punctuation is inconsistent in these cases as the determiner ('The') is capitalised in the second example. The first sentence is much longer than would be typical now, using semicolons, colons and dashes to add further clauses in the first paragraph.

All sentences begin with the same adverb ('here'), arguably because this is a 'real' account, rather than a literary, fictional representation and so stylistic variety is not important.

Mary Kingsley's travel writing from the late 19th century suggests that the use of semicolons and colons had declined. However, many commas still separate clauses, often being used to convey her opinions ('I should say', 'however much I may deplore') and the majority of sentences are complex. Both texts show that capitalisation had been standardised to proper nouns only. Punctuation in the 2008 travel blog has become more non-standard with missing apostrophes ('cant', 'its'), use of the slash ('on/off') and the use of brackets adds the humorous tone and afterthoughts for the audience, a feature Mary Kingsley also employs. Commas divide clause elements but are used less frequently in the text and there are more simple and elliptical sentences ('Time to go I thought').

Graphology

The use of italics for place names and other languages is an interesting graphological feature; in the 2008 blog capital letters are used for a speech-like emphasis ('WRONG') rather than to signal important information. The placing of one word on the last line ('morrow') is typical of the time and the word would be repeated on the next page to provide cohesion for the reader.

Orthography/spelling

The long 's' is still evident in 1796 and has clearly died out by the 1897 piece. Number and letter homophones ('U' '4') in 2008 reveal the influence of text/online chat styles.

Classroom activity 7

He told me in our journey… She was small of her age	Prepositions
She say you to the day? She doubted not…	Auxiliary verbs
It is a nothing of a part… To be taken into the account…	Articles
Fanny shrunk back and much was ate…	Irregular verbs
I am so glad we are got acquainted. So you are come at last!	Tense usage
The properest manner… The richest of the two…	Comparative/ superlative adjectives
Will not it be a good plan? It would quite shock you…would not it?	Contractions
I stood for a moment, felling dreadfully. It is really very well for a novel.	Adverbs

Classroom activity 8

All three extracts have a female audience, but use pronouns to create different relationships.

'Summer Preview' adopts an instructional tone, offering the writer's expert opinion to her audience through the use of the first person. ('I think we can all manage', 'I have'). The instructional and informative advice is given in imperatives using direct address ('give you', 'help you'), although some inclusive pronouns ('let's') present a more equal relationship. Patronising as it seems to us, it appears that access to fashionable clothes couldn't be taken for granted in this post-war period.

'Beauty is where Beauty is' is written from the reader's perspective. The contractions ('let's', 'don't'), the speech-like interjections ('oh') and the dashes suggesting the writer's personal asides ('– well, my chat –') are in an informal register. Other interactive features are the rhetorical interrogatives, often introduced as non-standard sentences beginning with conjunctions ('And how about pretty chocolate boxes for stockings and hankies?'). Although written in the first person ('I'), direct address ('you') is used; this is intended in a matey style to highlight the writer's shared experiences with the reader. Indeed some language choices hint at an existing relationship between the writer and reader ('like I always do'). The pronoun choices support the pragmatics, as in the inclusive pronouns ('we all use hair rollers' and 'let's face it'); here the shared knowledge centres on the awfulness of 'hair rollers' to 1960s girls. Some lexical choices, like the compound ('hair rollers'), seem dated today, as do some of the ideas offered – again showing how attitudes and language change. Apart from the pronouns, adjectival repetition ('pretty') reinforces the writer's engagement with the audience.

The problem page letter is different; it doesn't just entertain, but advises not only the individual addressee but, pragmatically, the wider readership, who have similar problems. 1970s' attitudes to girls' work and educational opportunities seem old-fashioned to us and the writers' pronoun choices appear patronising ('we sympathise, but we think that you should look at it from your parents' point of view', 'we hope you appreciate it'). The direct address ('you') is repeated, emphasising the advice offered, and the plural pronoun ('we') is not used inclusively, but to show the writers' joint perspective.

 ## Classroom activity 9

Font	Connotations
Graphology is important	Comic Sans creates a playful and informal font
Graphology is important	Fonts such as Times New Roman and Arial can be used to connote a more academic and traditional style
Graphology is important	The bold perhaps creates a sense of the text's importance, but the style contradicts this and suggests a light-hearted message
Graphology is important	The handwritten effect connotes a friendly font and would suit a more personal message

Changes in speech style

Classroom activity 10

The convict's language shows his dialect and social class, with lexical choices suggesting his accent. Instead of 'victuals' (an archaism for food), the convict offers an alternative word ('wittles'); Dickens presents this using eye dialect for his audience's interpretation. This could also suggest assimilation in the sounds typical of his accent or his lack of knowledge. The use of elision ('em') also reinforces his mode of speech. The verb choice is also interesting ('lookee'), possibly elision of 'look' and 'thee', suggesting the archaic pronoun used in some dialectal forms. Dickens chooses to make the distinction between the speech of the boy and the convict, showing the divergence between them. Note the boy's polite reply, using the pragmatics of polite speech with the conditional ('if'), modal auxiliaries ('would') and an adverb to suggest possibility ('perhaps'). This hesitancy shows the boy's fear but also marks him as more educated.

Why does language change?

 ## Classroom activity 11

Swift uses very emotive lexis to describe his fears ('corruptions', 'abuses', 'absurdities'). His worries centre in this extract on young male university graduates, who presumably enjoyed high social status at the time, who wanted to use the popular and fashionable colloquial language of the day not only in their speech but also in their writing, in order to be seen as both funny and clever. Although his criticisms are specific, his negative view of youth sociolect and slang seem very familiar!

Johnson, on the other hand, realised that he couldn't fix meanings in a prescriptive way – by stopping them changing – and could only reflect current ones (a more descriptive approach to how words were being used at that time). This still resonates with us now as dictionaries are continually updated.

Classroom activity 12

Non-standard English	Standard English	Feedback
I didn't do nothing wrong	I didn't do anything wrong	Standard English views a double negative as forming a positive
Who are you going out with?	With whom are you going out?	Ending a sentence with a preposition is deemed ungrammatical
Can you borrow me this pen?	Can you lend me this pen?	Lexical confusion with the words 'borrow' and 'lend'
You was right, wasn't you?	You were right, weren't you?	In Standard English the second person agreement would be the plural form
That was sick.	That was very good.	The slang use of the word 'sick' is not recognised in Standard English
r u goin 2 james house l8er	Are you going to James' house later?	Words in the non-standard form are spelt phonetically or use number/letter homophones
Den im goin 2 da cinemas	Then I'm going to the cinema	Youth sociolect and instant messaging/text language choices are not recognised in Standard English

Some of these could be thought of as dialectal, as in the multiple negation and number agreement, and are probably left over from regional or historic usage. Other examples show how slang and youth sociolect have an impact on language use and the effect of text messaging and instant messaging chat on the phonetic spellings of words, the lack of punctuation and the use of number/letter homophones.

Classroom activity 13

Humphrys' language is highly rhetorical, with exaggerated comparisons between texters and the medieval Mongol warlord, Genghis Khan, well known for his violence towards his enemies. This semantic field of violence is reinforced in the tripartite ('pillaging', 'savaging', 'raping') and the military choices make the discourse more cohesive ('quiver', 'arrow'). It is also humorously self-effacing in the way he pokes fun at his own attitudes through the imagined direct speech of a texter ('granddad', 'quill pen'), appealing to the readers who agree with him by explaining the initialism ('SMS Short Messaging Service') and using the archaic pronoun ('one') to give a mock RP air. Humphrys use a conversion ('texters'), which perhaps shows his more modern use of lexis; he also uses the root word as an adjective to qualify the type of message ('text')!

Humphrys' lexical choices are interesting too for semantic change, as with the noun ('vandals') which once referred to an invading Germanic tribe and now means someone who destroys something, usually property. This example of an eponym has been used metaphorically and, perhaps, narrowed in meaning as the tribe no longer exists. The blend 'emoticon' (from emotion + icon) indicates Humphrys' knowledge of the new terms used in text language; and the 'smiley', although annoying to him, is evidence of a graphological (and typographical) style possible because of technology. Both emoticons and smileys are ways that graphology provides visual presentations of paralinguistic features in text messages.

The two orthographical choices ('answerphone', 'ansafone') visually portray the influence of text spelling choices based on phonetics and the desire to use fewer letters; both are unhyphenated compounds, showing how the words entered the language separately but have combined to describe a recent invention. Later in the article, Humphrys acknowledges that some people will say that 'language changes', but worries about the lasting effect on written language caused by text and netspeak.

Unit 4, Section A Language investigation

Focusing your investigation

Classroom activity 1

The focus in each of these investigations should be limited to just one or two stories.

1 An effective advertising investigation will usually focus on a single product – cars, cosmetics, chocolate or whatever – and if gender is the issue, then the adverts should be broadly aimed at people of a similar age and socio-economic group. So you could look at car/cosmetic/chocolate adverts in magazines with a primarily young male/young female readership (perhaps *Cosmopolitan* and *FHM*?). However, modern adverts in print media tend to have minimal text content so you may need to collect quite a few.

2 If you enjoy sport, this could be an attractive option: take the same game or event, pick out one or two specific incidents, and record and transcribe the commentary on radio and television. As the variable here is medium, try to avoid any other variations. Other commentary-related possibilities include comparing commentary styles of different commentators (same game, same medium) or even comparing professionals and amateurs – tape the 'fan zone' amateur commentaries which are a feature of some Sky TV broadcasts and compare with the professional version of the same match. Yet another alternative approach is to vary the sport and investigate the differences between the commentary on a darts match with one on a horse race, for example.

3 Magazine-based studies need to limit the scope and range of the data; if you are looking at the 'age' variable, you might stick to a single gender and magazine feature, perhaps comparing the advice page, true-life story, horoscopes or fashion tips found in publications aimed at boys (or girls) of different ages – say, *Sugar, J17* and *Elle*.

4 This kind of investigation is likely to appeal as the data is close to hand, but you will need to be clear about the focus of the study. You could take a single teacher who teaches the same subject to several different age groups, and record a similar *kind* of lesson, perhaps concentrating on the opening few minutes, or on a class discussion. An alternative might be to keep the age range constant, and focus on how a variation in the subject affects language choice – how, for example, a chemistry lesson differs from an English lesson.

Classroom activity 2

Three examples of the data required to tackle a question from the list are:

■ **How true is it that males use less phatic talk than females?** This would require working with spoken and then transcribed data from both male and female speakers. The data would need to be drawn from interactions, and it would be necessary to try to gather data that is as realistic as possible, and that involves a similar audience, purpose and context. It would also be important to decide if the investigation was going to focus on mixed or single-sex interaction, or include a comparison of the two. Ideally, data from at least three different speakers in each sex would be needed to provide some basis for comparison.

■ **How does the language of legal texts convey power and authority?** At first glance this seems to be about written texts, although the investigation could compare or make use of spoken legal texts as well. In the case of written texts, a small corpus of texts would be useful, either ranging across legal genres, or narrowing the focus of the investigation to look at one particular kind of text.

■ **Are texting and email more like speech or writing?** A range of authentic text messages and emails would need to be sourced, preferably ones that had been written without the investigation itself in mind. A decent amount would be needed to set up the sort of quantitive analysis that would work well in this kind of approach, so a minimum of four of each text type would be necessary – and more would be beneficial.

Classroom activity 3

- **Child speech development**: Any study of early reading materials is likely to be informed by the current debate about teaching methods and the influence of phonics-based approaches in particular. Sampling three or four texts from different stages of the Oxford Reading Tree would be one approach, or you could include a couple of examples of early 'readers' from the 1950s and 1960s for a potentially rewarding language change element in such a study. Working directly with children and asking them to read a short passage aloud is likely to produce a more interesting study; a miscue analysis – transcribing and analysing the results – can be one of the most productive of all studies in this area (see page 149–150 for an example).

- **Child literacy studies**: Children's writing can be sampled and analysed in various ways – across the primary age range, for example, taking a couple of similar pieces from an 'average' child in each year, or sampling the ability range within a single class to gauge the variation in writing skills at a given age. There may even be interesting gender issues to explore here.

- **Language change**: The best approach to a study of changing report styles is to take a single type of report – a sports report, or crime, or major disaster – and find two or three examples from the same publication at perhaps 20-year intervals. (You can track down examples of historic newspapers online, or using the local archive – usually a department attached to the central library in major towns and cities – which usually has local and national newspapers stretching back to the 19th century). The archive may also be able to help you turn up examples of other genres, such as children's literature. Other sources would also include online archives, such as that of the British Library, Project Gutenburg and the British Museum. Comparing television or film texts can work well, with good access to high-quality archive material available on DVD, or by acquiring second-hand VHS tapes. The only disadvantage can be the often time-consuming process of transcribing from a video source, although the advantage to this is that you can tailor the transcription to precisely the features that you would like to record on paper for analysis. In addition, scripts are widely available either published in books, or through internet sources, for example the Internet Movie Script Database, along with other enthusiast sites.

Data response exercise 1

Non-standard features that you might have identified in the Scouse transcript are:

- h-dropping in the word 'ow' and 'im'
- slang contraction in the words 'gonna' and 'ain't'
- possible dialect words in 'friggin'' and 'youse'
- g-dropping in 'friggin''
- non-standard verb form (3rd person instead of 1st person) used in 'knows'
- t-dropping or possible glottalling on 'wha''
- multiple negative construction in 'ain't never'
- ellipsis of auxilliary verb 'had' in 'you better'.

Classroom activity 4

1. Agard's poem could be compared with Standard English poets from a similar time, with an investigation into their distinctive styles.

2. Agard's poem could be compared with spoken data from speakers using Jamaican creole to see how far his poem has accurately reproduced it, or to provide evidence of how Jamaican creole has changed since the poem was written.

3. Agard's poem could be used alongside other black English forms to research attitudes towards these varieties and particular features.

4. Agard's poem could be compared with Sebba's data on London Jamaican and the concept of code-switching.

Classroom activity 5

Some of the many possibilities for Mark would include:

Details about Mark's life	Potential investigation ideas
Part-time job: Helps out on his dad's market stall on Saturdays.	The family market stall would be an interesting place to base an investigation into the interaction between stall holders and customers (in so-called 'service encounters') and the use of occupationally-specific sales talk.
Interests and hobbies: Football – plays for local team in Sunday league and supports Manchester City. Cars – has recently passed test. Music – plays guitar in a band with friends.	There are also many possibilities within the world of football: the banter between his fellow players in the dressing room before and after a match (how does winning, or losing, affect this?), or the manager's half-time team talk, for example. Then there's the colourful language of the terraces, or the contrast between fanzine language and that of the official programme. Mark may even be able to access match programmes from the distant past and make these the subject of a language change study. The online supporters' forum may also provide rich material for a study of e-discourse.
Media habits: Enjoys a variety of music; reads car magazines; contributes to online Manchester City supporters' forum. Favourite programmes: enjoys reality TV shows such as *I'm a Celebrity …* and *Big Brother*.	Mark could compare the language associated with various kinds of music media – the speech of DJs live or on radio, the reviews of new music or gigs, or the contrasting styles and language of publications catering for specialist tastes, to suggest but a few. Mark's preferred television programmes do offer some interesting possibilities: reality TV allows us unproblematic access to an abundance of spontaneous speech, and can often yield rich material in terms of discourse and pragmatics.

Classroom activity 6

1 Here, the hypothesis provides a specific and well-informed point of departure for the investigation, as it refers to a well-documented trend in the style of reporting and defines three specific linguistic elements for the investigation.

2 This is a suitably 'open' question which would lead to a wide-ranging investigation, though the 'member' of the 'family' and the 'different contexts' would need to be specified, as would the aspects of 'talk' to be studied (Turn-taking? Dialectal/idiomatic/slang usage? Politeness features and observance of Grice's Maxims?)

3 The question here is too limiting: 'what do they have in common?' invites a simplistic response and seems to exclude discussion of a range of similarities and differences. A better question might be 'To what extent does Blair's oratory use similar rhetorical techniques to Churchill's, and to what extent does he depart from these?'

Classroom activity 7

The following table sums up the range of each proposal put forward by Maxine, with discussion below of the advice she would need.

Investigation criteria	Proposal 2	Proposal 3
1. Your link to, or interest in the investigation area.	Favourite topic from AS.	Originally from Birmingham.
2. The sort of data you plan to collect – if you can provide a sample, even better.	Male and female descriptions of pictures.	Spoken language from three generations of family.
3. Where and how you plan to gather your data.	Show males and females a series of colourful pictures and ask them to describe what they see.	From immediate family.
4. The main linguistic frameworks and features you aim to work with.	Semantics in detail and also lexis.	Phonology in depth but also some other areas.
5. The question or hypothesis at the heart of your idea.	Testing out Lakoff's theory.	Comparing accents in the family against original Brummie accent to see how much it has changed.
6. Details of any related linguistic research or theories.	Robin Lakoff and women's use of language to describe colours.	Estuary English awareness.

Advice for proposal 2:

This sort of idea has worked well before, Maxine, and male and female data is fine and would be good to compare.

- Bear in mind that exactly what sort of data you would collect needs to be defined more clearly. It could be spoken or written, for example.
- The stimulus pictures would need to be carefully chosen to fairly test both male and female interests and knowledge.
- Your link to Lakoff's theory is purposeful, although focusing on only the colour terms part might be too narrow to provide a full analysis.
- Begin thinking about more specific language features that you would like to focus on from the frameworks that you mention, and think if it would be possible to extend the aims a bit to include some deeper grammatical data and analysis.

Advice for proposal 3:

This is a lively topic, Maxine, and there is a good research base you could make use of.

- Remember that you should not analyse your own language – perhaps your sister could take your place as the data for the youngest generation.
- You have good ideas about Estuary English, especially being based in London – look into Paul Kerswill's research as your investigation could look for evidence of Estuary English in each speaker.
- Using spoken data would work well – although you need to think about how to obtain it reliably through recording and transcribing, so it might be time-consuming.
- Phonology will be an important framework – it would be possible and useful to open the investigation out to include some analysis of non-standard lexis or grammar use. Start to think about the particular linguistic variables you would need to test.

Classroom activity 8

- **Commentary**: Jespersen's status as a 'respected linguist' is somewhat offset by the lack of empirical evidence, and the date of the source (1922). Even if his observations were true then, much has changed in society in general and in gender roles in particular. Nevertheless, there are echoes of his ideas in more recent research-based discussions of language and gender, and the issues of taboo/vulgar and tentative expression remain interesting aspects of language study.

Methodology: collecting your data

Classroom activity 9

1. This really is out of the question. Even if all the volunteers were over 18, it might still appear that the experiment was encouraging them to drink to excess to their possible harm or, at best, embarrassment or humiliation. Think again, Alice!

2. There are some problems with this potentially interesting investigation, mainly regarding the workplace-based conversations. Gabrielle needs to establish the ground rules for the home recordings, and then talk to her father about what kinds of conversations it may be admissible for him to record – with all the participants' permission.

3. In principle this sounds like potentially a very interesting idea, but just because the authors of the letters are dead doesn't rule out some possible sensitivities – especially if they contain very personal material. He needs to get full permission from his family, and promise to render the material anonymous.

Classroom activity 10

1. This method can only work if the situation you are aiming to capture recurs regularly at the same location with the same subjects during the week. Even if your volunteers do grant you this kind of 'open permission', you must check after your recording that they are still happy for you to use the material.

2. This method may eliminate some of the more inauthentic and self-conscious aspects of the data – but is, of course, no good to you if the very thing you are interested in is how conversations/discussions actually get started!

Classroom activity 11

1. Working with the text of both the film and book would be essential here, so a kind of corpus analysis would be the most obvious candidate. If the film script could be found online and an ebook of the novel acquired, then some quite sophisticated searching of particular lexical patterns would form the structure of the investigation and help identify the most important parts of each text for more qualitative analysis.

2. This could be set up in several possible ways. Some sort of experiment could be devised where a group of people agree to respond to text messages from the researcher and their replies are then used as data. Alternatively, people could volunteer existing messages from the 'sent' box of their mobile phone and these could even be processed to form a kind of mini-corpus for analysis. A survey or interview would also be possible, although maybe these would be more appropriate as supporting methods to the first two, as they would be less likely to yield raw text message data for analysis.

Classroom activity 12

The matches, with commentary, are:

- **1 and C**: Well-chosen visual stimuli – such as those featuring colourful items of clothing, or members of the opposite sex of varying degrees of attractiveness, can be effective in provoking responses which test received ideas about language and gender. Make the stimulus a series of controversial/outrageous statements like 'the death penalty should be re-introduced for paedophiles' and you may elicit a useful corpus of data related to the expression of opinion.

- **2 and B**: Games are useful for any age group, providing they require plenty of verbal communication. One student recorded a group of friends during a game of Monopoly to investigate the balance between game-focused and social talk, and to see whether the dynamics and style of the usual group 'banter' changed once clear 'winners' and 'losers' started to emerge. With younger children, engaging them in some kind of productive activity is a good way of overcoming their self-consciousness.

- **3 and A**: Whether confining your study to children, or investigating storytelling more generally, you need to settle on a specific task or stimulus. Inviting older people to reminisce about specific experiences can yield fascinating data, whether your focus is narrative skills or the use of regional dialect. Just don't tell them you're interested in their language – you could present your investigation as being about local history, for example.

Analysis: exploring your data

Classroom activity 13

Overview: Both children successfully negotiate the text provided without any prompting, demonstrating a number of competencies in terms of reading skills. This is interesting as the text uses a mixture of narrative and dialogue, and the young readers need to recognise the function of speech marks. However, there are many examples of hesitations and other miscues in their reading, and some interesting differences between these which indicate that the twins are using different reading strategies.

Initial scrutiny:

Child X	Analytical notes
this silly **pig** everyone calls her silly pig (3) because they (1) she doesn't silly **things**	Omits verb 'to be' and doesn't observe punctuation – micropauses for thought, not at punctuation marks – takes 3 secs to recognise visual shape of 'because'. Substitutes 'she' for 'they' after everyone – but self-corrects. Then negates – 'doesn't' for 'does'. Reading for sense?
(2) you **silly** pig (.) said (.) **horse** (.) pigs don't put things **flowers** on their heads	Micropauses possibly reflect recognition of speech marks? Substitutes 'things' for 'flowers' – makes syntactic/semantic sense – predictive reading, influenced by an echo from previous line?
(1) one day silly pig had an **idea** (1) she went to (2) tell the other animals about her idea	Recognises sentence boundary at 'idea' – pause + stress. Pause before 'tell' – reading ahead?
(.) I am going to look for **treasure** on the farm (.) she said (1.) I am going to find lots and lots of **treasure**	Confident recognition of 'treasure' – stress shows understanding. Again, micropauses recognise speech marks? Again – 'treasure' stressed – but sentence boundary not recognised here.
you silly pig said (3) the other animals you won't find treasure on the **farm**	Longer pause – reading ahead?
(3) silly pig (3) tha set off to look for **treasure** (5) she went on out of the farm gate (3) and up the hill urm (2) **lane**	Longer pause followed by miscue – that? Then? Predictive reading but self-corrects. Longest pause so far – sentence boundary – followed by three miscues – suggests reading ahead and spotting 'obstacles'. Substitutes 'on' for 'out', 'of' for 'to' and 'farm gate' for 'farm yard'. Gate/yard – semantically OK – visually similar (four letters, initial letter with descender, second letter 'a'). Filled pause marks self-correction of substitution – predicts semantically possible 'hill' (from collocation 'up the hill').
(4) suddenly silly pig (4) **stooped** (1) she saw something (1) **sparkling** in the tree	Longer pause (4) prior to miscue – substitution of 'stooped' for 'stopped'. Semantically/syntactically possible – visual confusion of 'stopped' and 'stooped'. Pauses before 'sparkling' on three occasions.
(2) ooh no I can see a (4) sparkling **necklace** in the tree (1) a sparkling necklace is the **treasure** (1) I will put (1) it around my neck	Longest of three 'sparkling' pauses before 'sparkling necklace' – word recognition. Insertion of 'the' – predicts syntax. Substitutes 'will' for 'shall' – more commonly used.
(3) but the sparkling necklace doesn't wasn't (2) really a necklace it was a spider's web	Self-corrects wasn't/doesn't – realises syntactic impossibility of 'the necklace doesn't really a necklace'?
(1) the web was sparkling with (1) rain drops (2) the spider was very cross	Insertion of 'the' – syntactically/semantically reasonable.
(1) what a silly pig (1) thing to do he said you silly pig (2) silly pig (2) felt very silly she set off up the (1) lane	Pauses/self-corrects after substitution, influenced by repeated collocation of 'silly pig'.
(3) suddenly silly pig stooped (1) she saw something sparkling in the (1) don't know that word	Longer pause correctly observes sentence boundary punctuation. Avoids earlier 'hill'/'lane' substitution. Repeats previous 'stopped'/'stooped' confusion – not really semantically OK here. Sense? Which word? Hedge? Or earrings? More likely – reading ahead.
(2) ooh no I can see sparkling ears **earrings** in the hedge (1) she said (1) sparkling earrings are the treasure I [*inaudible*]	False start – takes cue form beginning of word – self-corrects (semantically impossible).

Child Y	Analytical notes
this tha this is silly **pig** everyone calls him silly pig because he says silly **things**	Initial hesitation – then fails to observe punctuation at sentence boundary. Substitutes male for female pronouns. Substitutes 'says' for 'does' – both semantically/syntactically OK.
(3) you silly pig said pig pigs (2) don't put flowers on their heads	Substitutes 'pig' for 'horse'. Inserts plural suffix on 'heads' – logical concord with subject 'pigs'.
(3) one day silly pig had an idea (1) she went to the (2) tell the other animals about her **idea**	Gender pronoun OK now! Seems to jump ahead to 'the other animals' – self-corrects with 'tell' – suggests reading ahead. Secure recognition of sentence boundary by stress.
(2) I am going to look for things (3) **treasure** and the farm see she said (1) I am going to (2) feed (1) find lots and lots of **treasure**	Substitutes 'things' for 'treasure' – semantically possible – longer word, initial letter – but self-corrects. Substitutes 'and' for 'on' – sense? Phonetic confusion of 'she' and 'see' next to 'said' – tongue twist effect. Substitutes 'feed' for 'find' – triggered by initial letter recognition and semantic context (animals, farm).
(2) you silly **pig** said the other animals you (2) won't find (1) treasure on the **farm**	Slight hesitation on polysyllabic 'treasure'.
(4) silly pig shi set off to find (1) look for treasure she went out the farm (1) yard but (1) and up the lane	Hesitates – 'shi'/ 'set' – tempted to substitute subject pronoun. Inserts 'look for' alongside 'find'. Substitutes/self-corrects conjunction 'but' for 'and'.
(5) suddenly said silly pig (7) she saw something (3) spa (4) **sparkling** in the tree	Substitutes entire phrase 'said silly Pig' for 'Silly Pig stopped'. False start and pause before 'sparkling' – word recognition.
(1) Ooh I can see a sparkling (2) **necklace** in the tree asked (5) a sparkling necklace is the **treasure** (1) I (2) shall put it round my neck	Insertion of 'asked' (nb. check word class) followed by long pause – insertion of 'the'. Deletion of initial vowel of 'around'.
(.) but the sparkling necklace (.) wasn't (2) really a necklace it was a spiders **web**	Occasional micropauses but mainly observes sense and sentence boundaries.
(2) the web was sparkling with (1) raindrops spider was very cross	Pause before 'raindrops' (recognition?).
what a silly thing to do you silly pig silly (1) pig felt very silly she set off up the lane	Sentence boundary/punctuation not observed. Deletion of phrase 'he said'.
(3) suddenly silly pig (1) sto stopped (1) she saw something **sparkling** in the bushes	Correctly observes sentence boundary. Slight hesitation on 'stopped'. Substitutes 'bushes' for 'hedge' – semantic prediction.
(1) ooh I can see something (1) sparkling earrings in the hed (1) she said (1) sparkling earrings are **treasure** I sha shall put them (1) on my ears	Substitutes 'something' for 'sparkling' – influenced by previous sentence – self-corrects. This time correctly reads as 'hedge', though with deletion of final consonant. Slight hesitation on (unfamiliar?) 'shall'.

Classroom activity 14

There is, of course, no single 'correct' way of organising the analysis, but the versions suggested here would certainly provide a robust structure for a comprehensive investigation.

Sample: Children reading

1 Pauses in reading
  1.1 Correct recognition of sentence boundaries and other phrase/clauses
  1.2 Pausing associated with 'challenging' words
  1.3 Pausing associated with miscues
2 Substitutions
  2.1 Resulting from visual miscue
  2.2 Resulting from semantic prediction
3 Analysis and explanation of omissions/deletions
4 Analysis and explanation of self-corrections
5 Analysis and explanation of false starts, hesitation (non-fluency)
6 Analysis and explanation of evidence from prosodic features (stress and intonation pattern of understanding)
7 Overall conclusions

Data response exercise 2

1 In general, the Group B girls show a trend of using non-standard language more frequently, with significantly higher percentages in the use of the non-standard '–s', 'was', negative concord, 'come' and 'ain't' features.

2 The most striking anomaly is in the Group B girls' frequency of use for the non-standard 'what' feature. This seems a very low frequency of use compared with the more general trend of the Group B girls to use a higher frequency of non-standard forms.

Classroom activity 15

Of the examples listed, the overwhelming majority of nouns (37/48) are pre-modified in some way; there are five cases of double pre-modification ('design', 'bodies', 'windscreen', 'bodies', 'streamlines'), three of which are concentrated in the description of features thought to appeal to women. Where this occurs, the pair of adjectives are semantically related, as with 'steel' and 'protecting' when applied to the 'bumpers'. We will explore the different kinds of pre-modification next; it's worth noting here that every time the word 'Ford' or phrase 'Ford car' appears, it is preceded by 'new' – six times in all, with a seventh when it describes the 'open or closed body styles': this repeats the association of the brand name with the modernity, supporting the theme of the image used.

Classroom activity 16

Text	Child X	Self-corrects?	Cause of substitution?	Text	Child Y	Self-corrects?	Cause?
she	they	yes	Assumes 'everyone' is plural subject of sentence.	this	tha	yes	Visual miscue of 'this'/'that'?
does	doesn't	no	Adds negation – cause unclear.	she	he	no	Imposes expectation of gender.
flowers	things	yes	Semantic prediction.	does	says	no	Semantic prediction.
set off	tha	yes	They? Then?	horse	pig	no	Repeats previous word.
out to the farmyard	on out of the farm gate	no	Unfamiliar with 'farmyard'. Assumes journey begins by going 'out of'.	head	heads	no	Logical – assumes plural subject 'pigs' has plural object 'heads'.
lane	hill	yes	Semantic prediction.	treasure	things	yes	Semantic prediction.
stopped	stooped	no	Visual confusion of similar verbs.	she	se	yes	Phonic slip?
shall	will	no	Replaces less familiar with more commonly used modal verb.	find	feed	yes	Semantic prediction compatible with farm context.
wasn't	doesn't	yes	Visual miscue?	set off	she	yes	Predicts subject of sentence.
thing	pig	yes	Collocation? 'Silly pig' already used several times.	and	but	yes	Grammatical/lexical prediction of conjunction.
stopped	stooped	no	As above.	silly pig stopped	said silly pig	no	Discourse prediction.
earrings	ears	yes	Recognises first part of word.	hedge	bushes	no	Semantic synonym.
				sparkling	something	yes	Partial visual miscue (–ing)?

From the table we can see that both children make a similar number of substitutions, and both immediately self-correct about 50 per cent of the time. It is also clear that both children use a number of different strategies when reading, including making several creative but semantically sound predictions. Neither child seems to be 'sounding out' words in a phonics-influenced way, but some of the substitutions do suggest a reliance on visual recognition and 'reading for meaning'.

Coursework preparation and practice

Classroom activity 17

Version B is clearly much better as an academic text, for many reasons. Although there is no prohibition on the use of 1st person in your investigation report, there is nothing to be gained by using phrases like 'in my opinion' (Version A) and as a 'scientist', you should aim for a more impersonal style. The tone of condemnation and criticism in phrases like 'rather old-fashioned' and 'no-one would … today' is inappropriate; your task is not to judge, but to analyse and explain. The attack on 'sexist snobs' is also completely out of place – note how Version B deals with the issue of values and attitudes but in a much less emotional way. The comments in Version A about the register and style of the text are far too sweeping and simplistic ('all very formal'), and once again adopts an inappropriately condemnatory tone ('too much text'), as well as including lapses of style (no-one would bother to …). When using technical language, the writer explains unnecessarily the meaning of terms like 'adjective' and 'noun phrase' which can be taken for granted at this level.

Version B, on the other hand, uses an appropriate register – not particularly technical here, but with words like 'affluent', 'prestige', 'consumption' and even 'verbosity'. The discussion of language recognises that it is not all black and white, and suggests an alertness to subtlety and detail totally lacking from Version A.

Classroom activity 18

Original version	Suggested version	Commentary
In the restaurant, I found that just about everybody used loads of questions which there was only a couple possible answers to, whereas the ones in the kitchen were always more open. This must be because the waitresses really needed to know stuff like where their plates were etc. I also found that there was loads of slang used in both places. I guess this was to create a friendly informal atmosphere with the customers. I noticed a vast number of cases where there was lexical repetition; waiters did this a lot when taking customers' orders, obviously to check they had taken the order down right.	In the restaurant a large majority of staff tended to use closed questions, whereas those in the kitchen were generally open questions, quite probably because these expressed a genuine need for practical information on the part of the waitresses. There was significant use of slang, quite possibly to help create a friendly atmosphere with customers. The tendency towards significant amounts of lexical repetition noted was presumably due to the waiters' need to confirm the accuracy of the customers' orders.	No need for 'I'. 'A large majority' better than 'just about everybody'. Closed questions – use the terminology. No need to explain. 'Quite probably because' – more tentative than 'this must be'. Get rid of vague, casual expression – 'know stuff'. 'Significant use of' much better than 'loads of'. 'I guess' too personal/casual. 'Tendency towards' – much more tentative than 'vast number'. 'Presumably' more tentative than 'obviously'.

Unit 4, Section B Media text

Preparing to write

Classroom activity 1

1 One obvious option would be an article for a television listings magazine or television review page of a newspaper; it could focus on what the participants reveal about themselves through their language and conversational behaviour.

2 This topic would lend itself to a light-hearted look at the subject of gender differences in language for a school or college magazine.

3 An article aimed at sports fans, or even the script for a podcast from a newspaper or radio station like Radio 5 Live would be possibilities here.

4 The subject of early child language will be of interest to any parent or carer, and you could consider any genre that would reach this audience, such as an article for an appropriate magazine, an informative pamphlet available in clinics and surgeries, or the script for a possible talk/presentation to first-time parents.

Classroom activity 2

■ **Layout and presentation**: This will depend entirely on the genre/medium you choose. As with your work for Unit 2, you should study a suitable style model carefully and aim to emulate its distinctive presentational features.

■ **Degree of linguistic detail**: There will obviously be a lot less technical detail in your text, though you will still need to use suitable illustrations and quotations to enliven and illustrate your piece.

■ **Tone and style**: For a non-specialist audience, the tone needs to be less intensely serious; a lively, journalistic touch is needed, with the occasional light-hearted observation or anecdote.

■ **Use of specialist terminology**: As for terminology, you can no longer assume your readers will understand the more technical linguistic vocabulary; you may need to introduce a few useful terms, but it would be a mistake to bombard your readers with jargon.

Coursework preparation and practice

Classroom activity 3

Overall, the piece seems to work well, with clear communication. Some specific achievements and problems are noted below, with reference to the sort of criteria that might be most relevant to them. Although the piece feels very competent, it could lack the flair and originality to get it into the top few bands, so an overall mark of between 18 and 22 would be appropriate if it continued in a similar vein.

Achievements:

■ Very clear sections to the text, using headings and bullet points. (19–21 band, 'deployment of structures and genre conventions')

■ Convincing style and tone reads clearly and well. (19–21 band, 'article likely to be effective for audience and purpose')

■ Some overview of the value of reading to child language development given. (19–21 band, 'largely effective adaptation of original materials')

Some problems:

■ Some confusion of using pronouns to refer to the 'child' – on one occasion the plural 'their' is used. (16–18 band, 'some lack of control at times')

■ The subject and genre might limit the opportunities to show 'top band' flair in the language.

Glossary

A

accent: the distinctive pronunciation patterns used by a particular group of people 132

allusion: a subtle reference to a story or factual aspect outside of the text 175

Americanisms: examples of language use distinct to American English speakers 177

anomalies: strange, one-off or unexpected results in your data 149

anti-language: language that is used by a particular group to prevent others from understanding them 175

archaic: a word from an earlier period of English usage that is rarely used in the modern contemporary language 177

archaism: an old word or phrase no longer in general spoken or written use 85

ascender: the typographical feature where a portion of the letter goes above the usual height for letters in any font 49

assimilation: the influence exercised by one sound upon the articulation of another, so that the sounds become more alike 103

B

backing: moving the place in which a vowel is pronounced towards the back of the mouth 157

behaviourists: those who believe that language is acquired through imitation and reinforcement 11

bound morpheme: one that cannot stand alone as an independent word, but must be attached to another morpheme/word (affixes, such as the plural '–s', are always bound, as is the comparative adjective inflection '–er') 20

C

care giver: the term used to refer to the main adult who looks after a child 132

central vowel: a vowel pronounced roughly in the 'middle' of the mouth cavity 157

child directed speech: a distinctive form of language use employed by adults when interacting with young children 132

classical allusion: a reference to a character or event in classic Greek or Roman mythology 177

Cockney: a distinctive accent spoken in London 132

code-switching: a language skill that enables the user to change between different languages and language varieties while speaking 134

cognitive theorists: those who believe that language acquisition is part of a wider development of understanding 21

cohesion: the way in which a text appears logical and well constructed 38

consonant: a speech sound that is produced when the vocal tract is either blocked or so restricted that there is audible friction 6

content word: a type of word that has an independent 'dictionary' meaning, also called a lexical word 11

convergence: a process of linguistic change in which people adjust their dialect, accent or speech style to those of others, often occurring to express solidarity and understanding 47

copula verb: verb used to join or 'couple' a subject to complement 17

corpus: a large, text-based collection of data, usually stored electronically so that it can be quickly analysed and searched 128

corpus analysis: conclusions and findings drawn from running tests against a fairly large body of language material, often stored and assessed electronically 145

covert prestige: refers to the status speakers who choose not to adopt a standard dialect get from a particular group within society 75

creole: a language variety created by contact between one or more language forms and becoming established over several generations of users 133

cueing: the strategies used to help decode written texts successfully 42

cursive handwriting: handwriting in which the characters are joined in rounded and flowing strokes 47

D

data: examples of any kind of language in use collected, sourced, or presented for analysis 126

deixis: lexical items that 'point' towards something and place words in context 19

derivational morphology: the creation of new words by adding prefixes and suffixes 15

descender: where part of a letter goes below the baseline of a font 49

descriptivism: an attitude to language use that seeks to describe it without making value judgements 113

diachronic change: refers to the study of historical laguage change occuring over a span of time 70

dialect: the lexical, semantic and grammatical patterns of language use distinctive to a particular group of people 132

digraph: a graphic unit in which two symbols combine, or any sequence of two letters produced as a single sound, e.g. 'sh' 57

diphthong: a vowel in which there is a perceptible change in quality during a syllable 6

discourse: a stretch of communication 3

divergence: when a person's speech patterns become more individualised and less like those of the other person in a conversation 104

drift: a process of linguistic change over a period of time 81

dummy auxiliary: the verb 'do' which is used to form questions and negatives or to add emphasis in a statement 94

dynamic verb: a type of verb that expresses activities and changes of state, allowing such forms as the progressive 22

E

egocentric speech: the running discourse style of speech used by children where no listener is directly addressed and the talk is focused on the child's activities 24

emergent writing: children's early scribble writing, a stage of their literacy development 49

emoticons: the online means of showing facial expressions and gestures 100

empirical: work that comes from observation and experience, rather than pure theory 126

Estuary English: a variety of English with its roots in the Thames estuary area, but seen to be spreading to many other parts of the UK 133

ethically sound: this refers to the methods of gathering data and conducting an investigation that make sure it won't mislead or offend anyone 128

ethnographic study: a research method involving observing the 'real life' behaviour of the people being studied 145

euphemism: inoffensive word or phrase used to suggest something **less pleasant** 82

expansion: the development of a child's utterance into a longer, more meaningful form 29

experiment: an artificial and controlled situation or activity designed to test a specific idea or hypothesis 145

extrapolate: to draw conclusions based on a sample of data which might apply more widely 144

eye dialect: a way of spelling words that suggests a regional or social way of talking 105

F

fascicle: one of the divisions of a book published in parts 111

free morpheme: one that can stand alone as an independent word, e.g. apple 20

fronting: moving the place in which a vowel is pronounced towards the front of the mouth 157

function word: a word whose role is largely or wholly to express a grammatical relationship 11

G

grapheme: a written symbol, letter or combination of letters that is used to represent a phoneme 38

H

holophrase: a single word expressing a whole idea 10

homophone: a lexical item that has the same pronunciation as another 57

hypernym: a superordinate, i.e. a word that is more generic or general and can have more specific words under it 13

hyponym: a more specific word within a category or under a hypernym 13

hyponymy: the hierarchical structure that exists between lexical items 13

hypothesis: a statement of theory to be tested by research and data analysis 126

I

idiolect: an individual's own 'linguistic fingerprint' 2

idiom: a speech form or an expression of a given language that is peculiar to itself grammatically or cannot be understood from

the individual meanings of its elements 82

inflectional morphology: the alteration of words to make new grammatical forms 15

influential power: power used to influence or persuade others 102

informalisation: the way in which language is becoming increasingly informal in all areas of society 103

instrumental power: power used to maintain and enforce authority 102

interview: an interaction between two or more people for a specific purpose 144

L

Language Acquisition Device (LAD): the human brain's inbuilt capacity to acquire language 5

Language Acquisition Support System (LASS): this refers to the child's interaction with the adults around them and how this interaction supports language development. 29

lexicon: the vocabulary of a language 72

lexis: the vocabulary of a language 3

linguistic variables: specific linguistic features identified as markers for possible variation in an investigation 129

London Jamaican: a distinctive variety of language blending Cockney, Jamaican creole and Standard English forms 134

longitudinal study: a data-gathering exercise for investigation that takes place over a significant period of time, for example recording the same child's language use over several weeks or months 132

M

mean length utterance (MLU): a measure of children's ability to produce stretches of language; the number of morphemes is divided by the total number of utterances to find the average length. A higher MLU is taken to indicate a higher level of language proficiency 15

methodology: the design of an investigation and the stages it goes through 127

micropause: a pause of about half a second or less 148

miscue: errors made by children when reading 44

mixed-mode: features of printed text combined with features expected in conversation 70

morphology: the area of language study that deals with the formation of words from smaller units called morphemes 3

multimodal texts: texts that combine word, image and sound to produce meaning 1

N

nativists: those who believe that humans have an inbuilt capacity to acquire language 32

negative reinforcement: when an undesirable behaviour is unrewarded with the intention that it will not be repeated 11

non-standard: language use of any kind that differs from standard grammatical, lexical, semantic, phonological or graphological uses 132

O

object permanence: the awareness that objects continue to exist even when they are no longer visible 30

objective: an unbiased, factual view of a subject 126

observer's paradox: the difficulty of gaining examples of real language data, when the presence of an observer or a contrived situation might change the way people would normally use language 143

obsolete: no longer having any use 80

omission: the leaving out of a phoneme in a group of phonemes clustered together 103

orthography: the study of the use of letters and the rules of spelling in a language 48

overextension: a feature of a child's language where the word used to label something is 'stretched' to include things that aren't normally part of that word's meaning 12

overgeneralisation: a learner's extension of a word meaning or grammatical rule beyond its normal use 21

overt prestige: refers to the status speakers get from using the most official and standard form of a language. Received Pronunciation and Standard English are accepted as the most prestigious English accent and dialect 75

P

paralinguistics: aspects of speech in addition to the actual words and word-sounds said 148

phoneme: the smallest contrastive unit in the sound system of a language 3

phonemic contraction: the variety of sounds is reduced to the sounds of the main language used 5

phonemic expansion: the variety of sounds produced increases 5

phonetic spelling: a way of writing down speech to show the way it was pronounced by using letters and symbols to represent single sounds 148

phonetics: the study of the sounds used in speech, including how they are produced 3

phonics: a system of teaching reading and spelling that stresses basic symbol–sound relationships and their use in decoding words; a system used especially in the early stages of reading 40

phonology: the study of the sound systems of language and how they communicate meaning 3

political correctness: words or phrases used to replace those that are deemed offensive 74

positive reinforcement: when a behaviour is rewarded, including verbal praise to encourage this behviour to be repeated 11

pragmatics: the factors that influence the choices that speakers make in their use of language – why we choose to say one thing rather than another 3

prescriptivism: an attitude to language use that makes judgements about what is right and wrong and holds language up to an ideal standard that should be maintained 108

primary data: spoken or written data collected by a researcher 128

proto-word: an invented word that has a consistent meaning 9

Q

Qualitative: data analysis that focuses on individual instances of language use and analyses them closely and in context 127

Quantitive: data analysis that summarises findings in larger sets of data and presents statistical findings 127

R

recast: the commenting on, extending and rephrasing of a child's utterance 29

received pronunciation (RP): the prestige form of English pronunciation, sometimes considered as the 'accent' of Standard English 103

register: a variety of language appropriate to a particular purpose and context 2

reliable: used to refer to data that is an accurate reflection of real language use 126

S

scaffolding: the process of transferring a skill from adult to child and then withdrawing support once the skill has been mastered 31

Scouse: a distinctive accent spoken in Merseyside 132

secondary data: data that has already been collected by another researcher, that is made use of in a new investigation 130

semantics: the study of meaning 3

social interactionists: those who believe that child language develops through interaction with carers 11

social variables: the ways in which the context of data differs by social factors like age, gender, ethnicity and social class 129

sociolect: a defined use of language as a result of membership of a social group 47, 132

standardisation: making all variations of language conform to the standard language 70

stative verb: verb that describes a state; stative verbs are not usually used in the progresive aspect, which is used for incomplete actions in progress 22

subculture: a cultural pursuit engaged in that happens outside of the mainstream, accepted values of society 175

subjective: a view of a subject that includes personal opinion 126

survey: gathering data on attitudes or knowledge by asking many people to respond to questions and information through a questionnaire or some other method 144

synchronic change: refers to an approach that studies language at the theoretical point in time without considering the historical context 70

synonyms: words with very similar semantic value 39

synoptic: bringing together a full range of skills and viewpoints 125

syntax: the way words are arranged to make sentences 3

T

trend: patterns in data that seem to show something in particular tending to happen 156

typography: the study of the graphic features of the printed page 40

U

underextension: a feature of a child's language where the word used to label is 'reduced' to include only part of its normal meaning 12

universal grammar: the explanation that all world languages share the principles of grammar despite surface differences in lexis and phonology. Sometimes called linguistic universals 5

V

virtuous error: syntactic errors made by young children in which the non-standard utterance reveals some understanding, though incomplete, of standard syntax 21

vocative: a form (especially a noun) used to address a person 11

vowel: a sound made without closure or audible friction 6

W

word picture: a feature of radio broadcasting where a presenter will put forward a visual scene using verbal narrative description 177